Acute Liver Failure

Editor

NIKOLAOS T. PYRSOPOULOS

CLINICS IN
LIVER DISEASE

www.liver.theclinics.com

Consulting Editor
NORMAN GITLIN

May 2018 • Volume 22 • Number 2

ELSEVIER

1600 John F. Kennedy Boulevard • Suite 1800 • Philadelphia, Pennsylvania, 19103-2899

http://www.theclinics.com

CLINICS IN LIVER DISEASE Volume 22, Number 2
May 2018 ISSN 1089-3261, ISBN-13: 978-0-323-58360-2

Editor: Kerry Holland
Developmental Editor: Meredith Madeira

Clinics in Liver Disease (ISSN 1089-3261) is published quarterly by Elsevier Inc., 360 Park Avenue South, New York, NY 10010-1710. Months of issue are February, May, August, and November. Business and Editorial Offices: 1600 John F. Kennedy Blvd., Ste. 1800, Philadelphia, PA 19103-2899. Customer Service Office: 3251 Riverport Lane, Maryland Heights, MO 63043. Periodicals postage paid at New York, NY and additional mailing offices. Subscription prices are $292.00 per year (U.S. individuals), $100.00 per year (U.S. student/resident), $509.00 per year (U.S. institutions), $403.00 per year (international individuals), $200.00 per year (international student/resident), $631.00 per year (international instituitions), $338.00 per year (Canadian individuals), $200.00 per year (Canadian student/resident), and $631.00 per year (Canadian institutions). Foreign air speed delivery is included in all Clinics subscription prices. All prices are subject to change without notice. **POSTMASTER:** Send address changes to Clinics in Liver Disease, Elsevier Health Sciences Division, Subscription Customer Service, 3251 Riverport Lane, Maryland Heights, MO 63043. **Customer Service: Telephone: 1-800-654-2452 (U.S. and Canada); 314-447-8871 (outside U.S. and Canada). Fax: 314-447-8029. E-mail: journalscustomer service-usa@elsevier.com (for print support); journalsonlinesupport-usa@elsevier.com (for online support).**

Reprints. For copies of 100 or more of articles in this publication, please contact the Commercial Reprints Department, Elsevier Inc., 360 Park Avenue South, New York, NY 10010-1710. Tel.: 212-633-3874; Fax: 212-633-3820; E-mail: reprints@elsevier.com.

Clinics in Liver Disease is covered in MEDLINE/PubMed (Index Medicus), Science Citation Index Expanded, Journal Citation Reports/Science Edition, and Current Contents/Clinical Medicine.

Contributors

CONSULTING EDITOR

NORMAN GITLIN, MD, FRCP (LONDON), FRCPE (EDINBURGH), FAASLD, FACP, FACG
Formerly, Professor, Department of Medicine, Chief of Hepatology, Emory University, Currently, Consultant, Atlanta Gastroenterology Associates, Atlanta, Georgia, USA

EDITOR

NIKOLAOS T. PYRSOPOULOS, MD, PhD, MBA, FACP, AGAF, FAASLD, FRCP (Edin)
Professor of Medicine, Chief, Division of Gastroenterology and Hepatology, Medical Director, Liver Transplantation, Rutgers New Jersey Medical School, University Hospital, Newark, New Jersey, USA

AUTHORS

ROBERT S. BROWN Jr, MD, MPH
Gladys and Roland Harriman Professor of Medicine, Clinical Chief, Division of Gastroenterology and Hepatology, Weill Cornell Medical College, New York, New York, USA

CHALERMRAT BUNCHORNTAVAKUL, MD
Division of Gastroenterology and Hepatology, Department of Medicine, University of Pennsylvania, Philadelphia, Pennsylvania, USA; Assistant Professor, Division of Gastroenterology and Hepatology, Department of Medicine, Rajavithi Hospital, College of Medicine, Rangsit University, Ratchathewi, Bangkok, Thailand

ANDRES F. CARRION, MD
Director of Hepatology, Assistant Professor of Medicine, Texas Tech University Health Sciences Center El Paso, El Paso, Texas, USA

MELROY D'SOUZA, MD
Department of Internal Medicine, Rutgers Robert Wood Johnson Medical School, New Brunswick, New Jersey, USA

BILLIE FYFE, MD
Professor, Department of Pathology, Rutgers Robert Wood Johnson Medical School, New Brunswick, New Jersey, USA

JAMES V. GUARRERA, MD, FACS
Professor of Surgery, Chief, Division of Liver Transplant and Hepatobiliary Surgery, Program Director Liver Transplantation, Rutgers New Jersey Medical School, Newark, New Jersey, USA

ELIZABETH JOHN, MD
Department of Internal Medicine, Rutgers Robert Wood Johnson Medical School, New Brunswick, New Jersey, USA

SCOTT KIZY, MD
Department of Surgery, University of Minnesota Medical School, Minneapolis, Minnesota, USA

STEVEN KRAWITZ, MD
Assistant Professor, Department of Medicine, Division of Gastroenterology and Hepatology, Rutgers New Jersey Medical School, Newark, New Jersey, USA

JAMES H. LEWIS, MD, FACP, FACG, AGAF, FAASLD
Professor of Medicine, Director of Hepatology, Division of Gastroenterology, MedStar Georgetown University Hospital, Washington, DC, USA

VIVEK LINGIAH, MD
Assistant Professor, Department of Medicine, Division of Gastroenterology and Hepatology, Rutgers New Jersey Medical School, Newark, New Jersey, USA

CHEN LIU, MD, PhD
Professor, Department of Pathology, Rutgers Robert Wood Johnson Medical School, New Brunswick, New Jersey, USA

SARAH ZAHRA MAHER, MD
Resident, Internal Medicine, Penn State Health Milton S. Hershey Medical Center, Hershey, Pennsylvania, USA

PAUL MARTIN, MD, FRCP, FRCPI
Chief, Gastroenterology and Hepatology, Professor of Medicine, University of Miami Miller School of Medicine, Miami, Florida, USA

AVANTIKA MISHRA, MD
Division of Gastroenterology and Hepatology, Rutgers Robert Wood Johnson University Hospital, New Brunswick, New Jersey, USA

NNEOMA OKORONKWO, MD
Gastroenterology Fellow, Division of Gastroenterology and Hepatology, Rutgers New Jersey Medical School, Newark, New Jersey, USA

RAQUEL OLIVO, MD
Assistant Professor, Division of Gastroenterology and Hepatology, Rutgers New Jersey Medical School, Newark, New Jersey, USA

PAVAN PATEL, MD
Gastroenterology Fellow, Division of Gastroenterology and Hepatology, Rutgers New Jersey Medical School, Newark, New Jersey, USA

DANIEL PIEVSKY, DO
Division of Gastroenterology and Hepatology, Rutgers New Jersey Medical School, University Hospital, Newark, New Jersey, USA

NIKOLAOS T. PYRSOPOULOS, MD, PhD, MBA, FACP, AGAF, FAASLD, FRCP (Edin)
Professor of Medicine, Chief, Division of Gastroenterology and Hepatology, Medical Director, Liver Transplantation, Rutgers New Jersey Medical School, University Hospital, Newark, New Jersey, USA

PRIYANKA RAJARAM, MD
Department of Medicine, Emory University School of Medicine, Atlanta, Georgia, USA

K. RAJENDER REDDY, MD
Professor, Division of Gastroenterology and Hepatology, Department of Medicine, University of Pennsylvania, Hospital of the University of Pennsylvania, Philadelphia, Pennsylvania, USA

RUSSELL ROSENBLATT, MD
Fellow, Division of Gastroenterology and Hepatology, Weill Cornell Medical College, New York, New York, USA

NEIL RUSTGI, BA
Eastern Virginia Medical School, Norfolk, Virginia, USA

VINOD RUSTGI, MD, MBA
Division of Gastroenterology and Hepatology, Rutgers Robert Wood Johnson Medical School, New Brunswick, New Jersey, USA

IAN ROY SCHREIBMAN, MD, FACG, FAGA
Associate Professor of Medicine, Division of Gastroenterology and Hepatology, Penn State Health Milton S. Hershey Medical Center, Hershey, Pennsylvania, USA

DANIEL SEDHOM, MD
Department of Internal Medicine, Rutgers Robert Wood Johnson Medical School, New Brunswick, New Jersey, USA

CLIFFORD J. STEER, MD
Departments of Medicine and Genetics, Cell Biology and Development, University of Minnesota Medical School, Minneapolis, Minnesota, USA

RAM SUBRAMANIAN, MD
Department of Medicine, Emory University School of Medicine, Atlanta, Georgia, USA

ARUL M. THOMAS, MD
MedStar Georgetown Transplant Institute, MedStar Georgetown University Hospital, Washington, DC, USA

KEITH M. WIRTH, MD
Department of Surgery, University of Minnesota Medical School, Minneapolis, Minnesota, USA

FRANCISCO ZALDANA, DO
Resident, Department of Pathology, Rutgers Robert Wood Johnson Medical School, New Brunswick, New Jersey, USA

Contents

Preface: Acute Liver Failure   xiii

Nikolaos T. Pyrsopoulos

Classification and Epidemiologic Aspects of Acute Liver Failure   229

Daniel Pievsky, Neil Rustgi, and Nikolaos T. Pyrsopoulos

> Acute liver failure is a rare condition with high short-term morbidity and
> mortality. The most widely accepted definition is an abnormality in coagu-
> lation with any degree of encephalopathy in a patient without cirrhosis and
> an illness duration of less than 26 weeks. Multiple classification systems
> are currently in use to help categorize the condition. This article reviews
> the most commonly used systems. The epidemiologic aspects of the dis-
> ease are also reviewed, including incidence, prevalence, demographics,
> geographic distribution, and racial and cultural factors, and are discussed
> for the various subtypes of acute liver failure.

Acute Liver Failure: Mechanisms of Disease and Multisystemic Involvement   243

Steven Krawitz, Vivek Lingiah, and Nikolaos T. Pyrsopoulos

> Acute liver failure is accompanied by a pathologic syndrome common to
> numerous different causes of liver injury. This acute liver failure syndrome
> leads to potentially widespread devastating end-organ consequences.
> Systemic dysregulation and dysfunction is likely propagated via inflamma-
> tion as well as the underlying hepatic failure itself. Decoding the mecha-
> nisms of the disease process and multisystemic involvement of acute
> liver failure offers potential for targeted treatment opportunities and
> improved clinical outcomes in this sick population.

The Pathology of Acute Liver Failure   257

Billie Fyfe, Francisco Zaldana, and Chen Liu

> Varied injuries may manifest clinically as acute liver failure. The pathologic
> features include variable amounts of necrosis and regeneration. This
> article reviews pathologic classification of patterns of necrosis and asso-
> ciated inflammatory and regenerative responses in specimens from pa-
> tients with acute liver failure. Detailed pathologic examination of these
> specimens with clinical pathologic correlation can give the multidisci-
> plinary team vital information regarding the cause and timing, as well as
> the extent of injury and regenerative response. Pathologists are a vital
> component of the health care team for patients with acute liver failure.

Liver Regeneration in the Acute Liver Failure Patient   269

Keith M. Wirth, Scott Kizy, and Clifford J. Steer

> Liver regeneration after simple resection represents a unique process in
> which the organ returns to its original size and histologic structure. Over
> the past 30 years, there has been significant progress in elucidating the

mechanisms associated with regeneration after loss of hepatic mass. Liver regeneration after acute liver failure shares several of these classical pathways. It differs, however, in key processes, including the role of both differentiated and stemlike cells. This article outlines these differences in addition to new molecular mechanisms, including immunomodulation, microRNAs, and the gut-liver axis. In addition, applications to the patient population, including prognostication and stem cell therapies, are explored.

Viral Hepatitis and Acute Liver Failure: Still a Problem   289

Daniel Sedhom, Melroy D'Souza, Elizabeth John, and Vinod Rustgi

Although the overall prevalence of viral hepatitis is on the decline, the condition still plays a major role in the development of acute liver failure (ALF) worldwide. Hepatitis A, B, D, and E contribute to most fulminant viral courses. These viruses have not gained much attention in recent years yet remain relevant from a clinical perspective, as the incidence in certain populations is on the increase. Other viral therapies and immunotherapies are currently being examined as treatments for hepatitis D and hepatitis E. Clinicians should still maintain a high index of suspicion for viral causes in approaching patients with ALF.

Nonacetaminophen Drug-Induced Acute Liver Failure   301

Arul M. Thomas and James H. Lewis

Acute liver failure of all causes is diagnosed in between 2000 and 2500 patients annually in the United States. Drug-induced acute liver failure is the leading cause of acute liver failure, accounting for more than 50% of cases. Nonacetaminophen drug injury represents 11% of all cases in the latest registry from the US Acute Liver Failure Study Group. Although acute liver failure is rare, it is clinically dramatic when it occurs and requires a multidisciplinary approach to management. In contrast with acetaminophen-induced acute liver failure, non–acetaminophen-induced acute liver failure has a more ominous prognosis with a lower liver transplant-free survival.

Acetaminophen (APAP or *N*-Acetyl-*p*-Aminophenol) and Acute Liver Failure   325

Chalermrat Bunchorntavakul and K. Rajender Reddy

Acetaminophen (APAP) is the leading cause of acute liver failure (ALF), although the worldwide frequency is variable. APAP hepatotoxicity develops either following intentional overdose or unintentional ingestion (therapeutic misadventure) in the background of several factors, such as concomitant use of alcohol and certain medications that facilitate the formation of reactive and toxic metabolites. Spontaneous survival is more common in APAP-induced ALF compared with non-APAP causes. *N*-acetylcysteine is recommended for all patients with APAP-induced ALF, and it reduces mortality. Liver transplant should be offered early to those who are unlikely to survive based on described prognostic criteria.

Nonviral or Drug-Induced Etiologies of Acute Liver Failure   347

Russell Rosenblatt and Robert S. Brown Jr

Acute liver failure (ALF) is a rare but highly fatal condition. The most common causes include drug-induced and viral hepatitis, but other less common causes, especially autoimmune hepatitis, Budd-Chiari syndrome, and Wilson disease, need to be considered. Because diagnosis is frequently tied to potential for reversibility of ALF and prognosis, early identification in a timely manner is crucial. Other causes of ALF are more easily recognizable based on specific circumstances, such as ALF in pregnancy or ischemic hepatitis. Ultimately, maintaining a wide differential diagnosis in patients with ALF is essential to identifying the proper treatment and prognosis.

The Clinical Spectrum and Manifestations of Acute Liver Failure   361

Sarah Zahra Maher and Ian Roy Schreibman

Acute liver failure (ALF) is a rare life-threatening condition characterized by rapid progression and death. Causes vary according to geographic region, with acetaminophen and drug-induced ALF being the most common causes in the United States. Determining the cause aids in predicting the prognosis and the presentation of manifestations and guides providers to perform cause-specific management. At initial presentation, nonspecific symptoms are present but may progress to complications, including cerebral edema, infection, coagulopathy, renal failure, cardiopulmonary failure, and acid-base and/or metabolic disturbances. Although some cases of ALF resolve with conservative measures, liver transplant is the ultimate treatment in many cases.

Prognostic Models in Acute Liver Failure   375

Avantika Mishra and Vinod Rustgi

There is a strong imperative to develop valid and accurate prognostic modeling for acute liver failure (ALF). Despite the numerous clinical models that have been proposed thus far and the use of some such models, that is, King's College Criteria and Model for End-Stage Liver Disease, in clinical practice to aid decision making, there is a significant need for improvement for determining patients' clinical course, survival, and requirement for liver transplant. Future prognostic models shall need a stronger statistical foundation and accountability for time and variability in the clinical course of ALF and be applied for pretransplant and post-transplant outcomes.

Non–Intensive Care Unit Management of Acute Liver Failure   389

Andres F. Carrion and Paul Martin

Acute liver failure (ALF) is an uncommon syndrome with a highly variable and unpredictable clinical course. The initial diagnostic evaluation is typically performed in a non–intensive care unit (ICU) setting, such as the emergency department or general hospital ward. Prompt restoration of intravascular volume with intravenous fluids and correction of electrolyte, metabolic, and acid-base disturbances are important initial interventions in the management of ALF and can be safely accomplished in non-ICU settings in many patients. Similarly, therapies such as administration of N-acetylcysteine for acetaminophen-induced ALF and other cause-specific interventions can also be administered in non-ICU settings, thus minimizing delay.

Management of Acute Liver Failure in the Intensive Care Unit Setting   403

Priyanka Rajaram and Ram Subramanian

This article discusses the intensive care unit management of patients with acute liver failure. It focuses on the clinical presentation, identification, and management of the myriad of complications seen in patients with acute liver failure.

Liver Transplantation for Acute Liver Failure   409

Raquel Olivo, James V. Guarrera, and Nikolaos T. Pyrsopoulos

With the advent of liver transplant for acute liver failure (ALF), survival rate has improved drastically. Liver transplant for ALF accounts for 8% of all transplant cases. The 1-year survival rates are 79% in Europe and 84% in the United States. Some patients with ALF may recover spontaneously, and approximately half will undergo liver transplant. It is imperative to identify patients with ALF as soon as possible to transfer them to a liver transplant center for a thorough evaluation. Emergent liver transplant in a patient with ALF may place the patient at risk for severe complications in the postoperative period.

Future Approaches and Therapeutic Modalities for Acute Liver Failure   419

Pavan Patel, Nneoma Okoronkwo, and Nikolaos T. Pyrsopoulos

The current gold standard for the management of acute liver failure is liver transplant. However, because of organ shortages, other modalities of therapy are necessary as a possible bridge. This article discusses the current modalities as well as the future management of acute liver failure. Liver assist devices, hepatocyte transplant, stem cell transplant, organogenesis, and repopulation of decellularized organs are discussed.

CLINICS IN LIVER DISEASE

FORTHCOMING ISSUES

August 2018
Primary Biliary Cholangitis
Cynthia Levy and Elizabeth J. Carey,
Editors

November 2018
Pediatric Liver Disease
Philip Rosenthal, *Editor*

February 2019
Alcoholic Liver Disease
Norman L. Sussman and Michael R. Lucey,
Editors

RECENT ISSUES

February 2018
NASH and NAFLD
David E. Bernstein, *Editor*

November 2017
Consultations in Liver Disease
Steven L. Flamm, *Editor*

August 2017
**Hepatitis C Infection as a Systemic Disease:
Extra-Hepatic Manifestation of Hepatitis C**
Zobair M. Younossi, *Editor*

ISSUE OF RELATED INTEREST

Infectious Disease Clinics of North America, June 2018 (Vol. 32, Issue 2)
Overcoming Barriers to Eliminate Hepatitis C
Camilla S. Graham and Stacey B. Trooskin, *Editors*
Available at: http://www.id.theclinics.com/

THE CLINICS ARE AVAILABLE ONLINE!
Access your subscription at:
www.theclinics.com

Preface

Acute Liver Failure

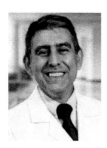

Nikolaos T. Pyrsopoulos, MD, PhD, MBA,
FACP, AGAF, FAASLD, FRCP (Edin)
Editor

Acute liver failure (ALF), formerly known as fulminant hepatic failure, is an uncommon condition with potentially devastating consequences, including an increased rate of short-term morbidity and mortality.

It has been estimated that the incidence of ALF is less than five cases per million population per year in the developed world, with approximately 2000 cases per year in the United States. It is noted that the incidence of ALF is poorly defined, which could lend itself to lower number of cases reported annually.

The clinical presentation can vary; some cases have shown a very rapid deterioration. It is imperative for the clinician to be aware of this entity, to seek expert opinion with potential transfer to centers that have experts in liver disease on staff and can offer liver transplantation as a backup.

It is noteworthy to mention that the cause of ALF varies worldwide; for example, in the United States and Europe, patients present with drug-induced liver injury, predominantly due to acetaminophen toxicity, while in other parts of the world, viral hepatitis is the main cause.

Due to increased immigration and travel worldwide, when a patient presents with ALF, clinicians must be vigilant in ascertaining the cause of ALF. They must delve not just into the patients' medical history but also into their recent travel history, as a rare disease could be the cause of ALF.

Tremendous strides have been made in successfully treating various liver diseases; however, our therapeutic momentum in treating patients with ALF has been suboptimal. Several attempts have been made in formulating prognostication formulas, especially in the pretransplant evaluation setting.

In this issue of *Clinics and Liver Disease*, expert clinicians and researchers collaborated to provide a multispectrum view of this topic.

Topics reviewed and detailed in this issue include the mechanism of the disease and its epidemiologic aspects, along with clinical manifestation, prognostic models, and

Clin Liver Dis 22 (2018) xiii–xiv
https://doi.org/10.1016/j.cld.2018.02.001
1089-3261/18/© 2018 Published by Elsevier Inc.

liver.theclinics.com

various causes. Therapeutic modalities, including liver transplantation and potential future approaches, have been comprehensively overviewed.

I am honored to be a part of this issue, and I would like to express my gratitude to the distinguished authors of these articles, who shared their experiences and expertise on this significant topic in an outstanding manner. Finally, I would like to express my appreciation to Dr Norman Gitlin for allowing me this opportunity and to Ms Kerry Holland and Ms Meredith Madeira for their tremendous assistance.

Nikolaos T. Pyrsopoulos, MD, PhD, MBA, FACP, AGAF, FAASLD, FRCP (Edin)
Division of Gastroenterology and Hepatology
Liver Transplantation
Rutgers New Jersey Medical School
University Hospital
185 South Orange Avenue
MSB H Room 536
Newark, NJ 07101-1709, USA

E-mail address:
pyrsopni@njms.rutgers.edu

Classification and Epidemiologic Aspects of Acute Liver Failure

Daniel Pievsky, DO[a], Neil Rustgi, BA[b],
Nikolaos T. Pyrsopoulos, MD, PhD, MBA, FACP, AGAF, FAASLD, FRCP (Edin)[a],*

KEYWORDS

- Acute liver failure • Fulminant liver failure • Classification • Epidemiology • Race

KEY POINTS

- Acute liver failure is a life-threatening condition that requires early recognition and transfer to specialized centers to achieve good outcomes.
- It is not a single disease, but a whole group of varied etiologies, many of which are difficult to diagnose and lack specific treatment modalities.
- Understanding the epidemiologic aspects of the various conditions that lead to acute liver failure and their subtype classifications can help clinicians better identify and manage this condition.

INTRODUCTION

Acute liver failure (ALF) is a devastating condition with a high rate of short-term morbidity and mortality.[1] The disease has been labeled by multiple names, including fulminant hepatic failure, acute hepatic necrosis, fulminant hepatitis, and fulminant necrosis, but the preferred term is ALF.[2] It is a rare condition with a reported incidence of less than 5 cases per million population per year in the developed world and an estimated 2000 cases per year in the United States.[2,3] It should be noted, however, that accurate estimates of both the incidence and the morbidity of ALF are difficult to obtain, because many patients expire before transfer to a referral center and are thus not accounted for by estimated models.[4]

ALF, originally named fulminant hepatic failure, was defined in 1970 by Charles Trey and Charles Davidson as "a potentially reversible condition, the consequence of severe liver injury, with the onset of encephalopathy within 8 weeks of the appearance of the first symptoms and in the absence of pre-existing liver disease."[5]

[a] Division of Gastroenterology and Hepatology, Rutgers New Jersey Medical School, University Hospital, 185 South Orange Avenue, Newark, NJ 07101-1709, USA; [b] Eastern Virginia Medical School, 825 Fairfax Avenue, Norfolk, VA 23507, USA
* Corresponding author.
E-mail address: pyrsopni@njms.rutgers.edu

Clin Liver Dis 22 (2018) 229–241
https://doi.org/10.1016/j.cld.2018.01.001
1089-3261/18/© 2018 Elsevier Inc. All rights reserved.

Aspects of this original definition are still in use today, although the condition has gone through multiple names and diagnostic criteria over the past 47 years. The most widely accepted definition of ALF is an abnormality in coagulation (practically an International Normalized Ratio of >1.5) with any degree of encephalopathy in a patient without cirrhosis and an illness duration of less than 26 weeks.[6] This review addresses the classification of ALF and the epidemiologic aspects of the disease, with a focus on the underlying etiology and its relationship to incidence and outcomes.

CLASSIFICATION

Since the initial definition by Trey and Davidson, there have been more than 40 different criteria that have attempted to define and subclassify ALF.[7] Of all of these definitions and classification systems, there are 4 that warrant special mention (**Table 1**). The Bernuau system, published in 1986, was the first to classify ALF into 2 subgroups: fulminant, in which less than 2 weeks pass between the onset of jaundice and symptoms of liver failure, and subfulminant, in which liver failure symptoms develop between 2 and 12 weeks after the onset of jaundice.[8]

In 1993, John O'Grady and colleagues[9] published the first classification system that accounted for the etiology, complications, and prognosis of ALF. The O'Grady system, still widely used today, subdivides ALF into hyperacute, acute, and subacute groups. Hyperacute liver failure is defined by hepatic encephalopathy (HE) developing within 1 week of the appearance of jaundice, patients in the acute group develop HE between 1 and 4 weeks, and patients with subacute liver failure develop HE between 4 and 12 weeks.

In an attempt to standardize the nomenclature and classification of ALF, the International Association for the Study of the Liver formed a subcommittee for the nomenclature of ALF and subacute liver failure. This International Association for the Study of the Liver subcommittee published their findings in 1999 and divided ALF and subacute liver failure into 2 distinct entities, rather than as subdivisions of an overarching condition.[10] ALF was defined as HE within 4 weeks of symptom onset, and subacute liver failure was defined as HE or ascites that develop between 5 weeks and 6 months of symptom onset. Because ALF was considered a separate condition from subacute liver failure by the International Association for the Study of the Liver, it was further subdivided into a hyperacute form, with the development of HE within 10 days of symptoms, and a fulminant form, with HE developing between 10 and 30 days from the first onset of symptoms.[10]

Historically, the definition and classification of ALF in Japan was different from that of Europe and the United States.[11] In an attempt to align their definitions, the Intractable Hepato-Biliary Diseases Study Group in Japan established a task force that published its revised definition and classification in 2011.[12] The Japanese defined ALF as an International Normalized Ratio of 1.5 or greater or a prothrombin time of 40% or less of the standardized value within 8 weeks of the onset of symptoms in a patient without prior liver disease. The presence of HE was not required to meet the definition of ALF; thus, ALF was subdivided into ALF with hepatic coma (grade 2 HE or higher) and ALF without hepatic coma (no HE or grade 1 HE). Those patients who had ALF with hepatic coma were further subdivided into an acute type, with HE developing within 10 days of symptoms, and a subacute type, with HE developing between 11 and 56 days after symptom onset. Patients who meet the criteria for ALF with hepatic coma but develop symptoms between 8 weeks (56 days) and 24 weeks are categorized as having late-onset hepatic failure.

Table 1
Classification systems of acute liver failure

	Bernuau System	O'Grady System	IASL System	Japanese System
Definition of ALF	≥50% decrease in factor II or V with HE	Severe liver injury with HE without prior liver disease	Severe liver Disfunction with HE within 4 wk without prior liver disease	INR ≥ 1.5 or PT ≤ 40% within 8 wk of symptoms without prior liver disease
Requirement for HE	Yes	Yes	Yes	No
Subclasses	Fulminant Subfulminant	Hyperacute Acute Subacute	Hyperacute Fulminant	With hepatic coma (Acute Subacute) Without hepatic coma
Duration between symptoms and HE	<2 wk 2–12 wk	<1 wk 1–4 wk 4–12 wk	<10 d 10–30 d	<10 d 10–56 d NA

Abbreviations: ALF, acute liver failure; HE, hepatic encephalopathy; IASL, International Association for the Study of the Liver; INR, International Normalized Ratio; NA, not applicable; PT, prothrombin time.
Data from Refs.[8–10,12]

The debate about the most appropriate definition and classification system is far from over, and all 4 of these classifications are still being used today. The O'Grady system is the most popular in the United States and Europe, whereas the Japanese system is used in Japan. Current issues of contention include a lack of consensus as to the specific cutoff in terms of coagulation parameters and the degree of alteration in consciousness required to transition from severe acute liver injury to ALF.[13] There has also been debate about whether International Normalized Ratio is the best measure of coagulation dysfunction or if it would be better to use prolongation of the prothrombin time in relation to the normal value for that particular laboratory test.[14]

Despite a lack of consensus as to the exact degree of HE required to diagnose ALF, the time frame from the onset of symptoms, usually jaundice, to encephalopathy is the basis for each of the classifications and disease phenotypes mentioned. The reason that HE plays such a central role in the classification of ALF is that the onset of HE is a marker of severe liver damage and is closely tied to increases in arterial ammonia, which itself is associated with an increased risk of intracranial hypertension and possible herniation.[15] Although the prevalence of both intracranial hypertension and cerebral edema has been decreasing, they remain deadly complications of ALF.[16,17]

Currently, there are no specific differences in the management of ALF based on the subclassification of the disease into hyperacute, acute, subacute, fulminant, or subfulminant classes. Although the most recent guidelines from the American Association for the Study of Liver Diseases state that these subclassifications are not helpful, the recently released guidelines from the European Association for the Study of the Liver state that the separation of hyperacute and ALF from subacute liver failure for prognosis and management should be considered in future guidelines.[2,14]

Hyperacute liver failure, as defined by the O'Grady system, is the development of HE within 7 days of symptom onset.[9] This is mostly commonly due to acetaminophen overdose, hepatitis A virus (HAV) infection, or hepatitis E virus (HEV) infection. Overall, the prognosis for hyperacute liver failure is good, but is highly variable based on individual etiology. Given the rapid progression of hyperacute liver failure, high grades of HE are associated with a worse prognosis.[18] The ALF presentation occurs between 1 and 4 weeks and is most commonly the result of hepatitis B virus (HBV) infection. Subacute liver failure occurs between 4 and 12 weeks and is most commonly associated with idiosyncratic nonacetaminophen drug-induced liver injury (DILI) or indeterminate causes. Unlike the hyperacute presentation, the prognosis is poor with subacute liver failure, even in the setting of minimal grades of HE.[18] It is usually the subacute liver failure cases that benefit most from emergency liver transplantation, rather than the hyperacute cases.[13]

EPIDEMIOLOGY

ALF is a condition that has undergone a great deal of change since it was formally defined in 1970, including changes to the definition, causes of the illness, treatment, and prognosis. Before the advent of liver transplantation, the death rate for ALF was greater than 80%.[19] Overall survival is now approximately 70%, and 2-year survival rates are up to 92.4% for those who undergo liver transplantation.[16,20] Not only has there been a dramatic improvement in the management and prognosis of ALF, but there has also been a major shift in the etiology of the disease. Worldwide, viral hepatitis remains as the most common cause of ALF, but its incidence has decreases tremendously over the past several decades in the developed world. Drug-induced liver failure, most commonly from acetaminophen, is now the most common cause of ALF in the United States and Europe.[18,21] Significant variation remains in the etiology of ALF worldwide, but with the large amount of travel and immigration, clinicians must be on the lookout for even the rarest causes. This factor underscores the importance of a thorough workup to identify the underlying cause, because each etiology has a distinct pattern of presentation, prognosis, and, in some cases, specific treatment (**Table 2**).

Acetaminophen

Acetaminophen, also known as paracetamol or APAP in non-US territories, is the most common cause of ALF in the United States, accounting for 42% to 46% of cases.[22,23] It is even more prevalent in the UK, where rates as high 73% were reported in the early 1990s.[24] Incidence rates of acetaminophen-induced ALF in the UK have decreased dramatically since then, largely owing to legislation passed in 1998 that restricted the sale of the drug.[25] It remains, however, as the most common cause of ALF in the UK and some parts of Europe.[26] Interestingly, in a retrospective analysis from Spain from 1992 to 2000, acetaminophen only accounted for 2% of ALF cases.[3] It has been hypothesized that this rate is so much lower than those of many other European nations because acetaminophen is not available for sale over the counter in Spain.[27] In addition, the typical reason for overdose differs between the United States and the UK. Accidental ingestion-induced ALF is seen more frequently in the United States, whereas intentional overdose is more common in the UK.[22,28]

As mentioned, acetaminophen-induced ALF tends to result in a hyperacute presentation and is characterized by large elevations of aminotransferases (>10,000 IU/L) in the setting of normal or slightly elevated bilirubin levels.[14] It is one of only a few causes of ALF that has a known treatment, and if acetaminophen overdose is suspected, N-acetylcysteine should be administered immediately, even in the setting of negative acetaminophen blood levels.[2] Acetaminophen undergoes breakdown by the CYP2E1 pathway, yielding a toxic metabolite called N-acetyl-p-benzoquinoneimine that can lead to hepatic necrosis.[29] Glutathione converts acetaminophen into mercapturic acid, a nontoxic and readily excreted byproduct, rather than N-acetyl-p-benzoquinoneimine.[30] N-Acetylcysteine replenishes the glutathione stores of the liver, which helps to prevent further hepatic toxicity.[31]

Despite severe metabolic derangement and hyperacute presentation, the prognosis in acetaminophen-induced ALF is good, with spontaneous nontransplant survival of greater than 70%, and transplant survival of greater than 80% at 1 UK site.[16] The Acute Liver Failure Study Group (ALFSG) is an ongoing observational registry of

Table 2
Etiology of acute liver failure in selected countries[a]

United States	United Kingdom	Japan	Sudan	India	Spain
Acetaminophen	Acetaminophen	Unknown	Unknown	HEV	Unknown
Unknown	Unknown	HBV	HBV	Unknown	HBV
DILI[b]	DILI[b]	DILI[b]	P. falciparum Malaria/AIH	HBV	DILI[b]
HBV	Other	Other	HEV	Other	AIH
AIH	HBV	HAV	DILI[b]	HAV	Other

Abbreviations: AIH, autoimmune hepatitis; DILI, drug-induced liver injury; HAV, hepatitis A virus; HBV, hepatitis B virus; HEV, hepatitis E virus.
[a] In descending order of incidence.
[b] Nonacetaminophen.
Data from Refs.[3,11,26,32,45,65]

ALF patients in the United States.[32] Comprehensive data are collected up to 3 weeks after enrollment, and prospective outcomes are also collected at 1 and 2 years. The 2-year survival rates were 89.5% for those with spontaneous recovery from acetaminophen-induced ALF who survived past the initial 3-week period.[20] Similarly, the 2-year survival rate for patients with acetaminophen-induced ALF who underwent liver transplantation was 88%.

In terms of demographics, the majority of patients with acetaminophen-induced ALF in the ALFSG cohort were white, and there were no differences in mortality among whites, blacks, and Asians.[33] Women were more likely to have acetaminophen-induced ALF than men within each of the 3 racial groups. Within the group of whites, Hispanics were less likely than non-Hispanic whites to develop acetaminophen-induced ALF.[33] Similar results were seen at 2 years among those who spontaneously recovered from acetaminophen-induced ALF. Spontaneous survivors tended to be younger, female, white, and non-Hispanic.[20] It was also found that spontaneous survivors were more likely to have active psychiatric and substance abuse issues at study enrollment, and there were more unintentional overdoses than intentional ones (52% vs 38%, respectively).[20]

Viral Hepatitis

ALF owing to viral hepatitis usually refers to infection with HAV, HBV, and HEV. Acute hepatitis C has been reported as a cause of ALF in Asian countries like Taiwan and Japan, but is exceedingly rare in Western countries.[34–36] Hepatitis D has also been reported to contribute to ALF in those with HBV by acting as a coinfection or as a superinfection.[37] Overall, viral hepatitis remains the most common cause of ALF worldwide, with much of the burden owing to HAV and HEV infection in the developing world.[18] Although the incidence in Europe and the United States is lower, it is not insignificant. Viral hepatitis accounts for 19% of liver transplants performed for ALF in Europe and for 12% of all cases of ALF in the United States.[32,38]

ALF from HAV typically leads to a hyperacute presentation and has a better prognosis than ALF from HBV.[23] Overall, less than 1% of those infected with HAV develop ALF, although it is more common among the elderly, for whom the outcomes are worse.[39,40] Currently, HAV accounts for about 4% of ALF cases in the United States, similar to the rates observed in Spain, Germany, Australia, Sweden, India, and the UK.[26] A higher incidence of 7% to 8% has been reported in Japan and Pakistan.[11,41] There was a significant decrease in liver transplants for HAV-induced ALF, as well as in overall cases of HAV in the United States between 1988 and 2005.[40] It has been proposed that the initiation of routine childhood vaccination for HAV has been the main driver of the decrease in HAV-induced ALF in the United States.[42]

Unlike ALF from HAV or HEV, ALF from HBV typically has an acute presentation.[13] ALF from HBV has a worse prognosis than both HAV and HEV, with 4% of acute HBV infections progressing to ALF.[43] Overall, the prognosis is worse for the elderly and those with multiple comorbidities. HBV infection can potentially cause ALF in 2 distinct ways: acute infection or reactivation of prior infection, either from spontaneous reactivation or immunosuppression owing to chemotherapy or other immunosuppressive medications.[28] Similar to HAV, the incidence of HBV-induced ALF has decreased dramatically in the United States from 23% between 1987 and 1991 to the current level of 8%.[32,44] This decrease has also been attributed to vaccination, because it mirrors the overall decrease in HBV infection in the United States.[42] Similar trends have been observed in countries throughout Europe.[26] HBV remains a leading cause of ALF in Japan, sub-Saharan Africa, Hong Kong, and Australia.[11,45,46] Of interest, Asian

Americans are more likely have ALF from viral hepatitis, in particular HBV, than are white or black Americans.[33]

ALF as a result of HEV infection, like that associated with HAV, presents as hyperacute liver failure with a good overall prognosis and low mortality.[14] Although most cases in the United States and Europe are the result of travel to endemic countries like Russia, Pakistan, China, Mexico, and India, spontaneous cases of HEV have been reported.[47,48] ALF from HEV is very rare in the United States. A recent analysis from the ALFSG demonstrated that only 0.4% of patients with ALF had an acute HEV infection.[49] Evidence of a prior HEV infection was seen in 43.4% of patients with ALF from other causes, however, which is a much higher percentage of prior HEV infection than the 21% that is seen in the general US population. A possible explanation suggested by the authors is that patients may have acquired the HEV immunoglobulin G antibody via passive transfer from blood or plasma products, which they received before being enrolled in the study.[49] Elderly patients and those with chronic liver disease tend to have worse outcomes.[50] HEV has been known to have a predilection for pregnant women, especially in the third trimester, and the classic teaching has been that pregnancy is associated with worse outcomes. Recent studies have questioned this association and demonstrated that the prognosis for pregnant women with HEV-induced ALF is the same as that of nonpregnant women or men with HEV-induced ALF.[51]

Nonacetaminophen Drug-Induced Liver Injury

ALF owing to nonacetaminophen drug intake is difficult to diagnose and treat. The condition tends to appear as a subacute presentation, which can make identifying the causative agent difficult. Overall, ALF from nonacetaminophen DILI, also called idiosyncratic DILI, accounts for 11% of ALF cases in the United States and is the second leading cause of ALF behind acetaminophen.[32] Although the incidence is a little lower in Europe, with less than 10% of DILI patients progressing to ALF, the morbidity and mortality associated with this condition are tremendous: up to 80% of these patient die or require emergency liver transplant.[52]

From a demographics standpoint, ALF from DILI is one of the few types of ALF that has a higher incidence among the elderly, those older than 60 years, than among young patients.[26] A study from the ALFSG in the United States found ALF from DILI occurs more often in women, a result that was also observed in Spain.[52,53] Racial differences in prevalence and etiology have also been noted. Asians were much more likely to develop ALF from an herbal supplement than were blacks or whites (16.0% vs 3.4% vs 3.8%, respectively), and both blacks and Asians were more likely than whites to develop ALF from DILI (24.4% vs 24.0% vs 14.9%, respectively).[33] Similarly, when the white patients were subdivided by ethnicity into Hispanic or non-Hispanic white, the Hispanic group was more likely to have DILI-induced ALF than the non-Hispanic whites (29% vs 13.4%). It should be noted that the Hispanic group was also more likely to be on tuberculosis medications at the time of ALF presentation, which may account for the increased rates of ALF from DILI.

Overall, the most common classes of medications that result in ALF from DILI in the United States are antibiotics, antituberculosis medications, and antiepileptic agents.[53] The causative agents vary greatly from region to region, with drugs like flutamide, cyproterone acetate, and nimesulide more common in Latin America and phenprocoumon as a major cause of DILI-induced ALF in Germany.[54,55] A partial list of commonly encountered prescription and illicit drugs that can induce ALF is listed in **Box 1**.

Box 1
Common medications and drugs known to cause acute liver failure
Allopurinol
Amiodarone
Carbamazepine
Ciprofloxacin
Cocaine
Efavirenz
Herbalife
Hydroxycut
Isoniazid
Kava Kava
Ketoconazole
Labetalol
Ma Juang
MDMA
Phenytoin
Pyrazinamide
Statins
Valproic acid
Abbreviation: MDMA, 3,4-methylenedioxy-*N*-methylamphetamine.

The use of herbs and supplements is increasing quickly, and currently more than 50% of the US population is taking some kind of herb or supplement.[56] Subsequently, ALF from herbs and supplements has been increasing over the past 10 years and now accounts for 20% of ALF owing to DILI, up from 12%.[57] Recent data from Hillman and colleagues[58] show that ALF owing to supplements and herbs has worse outcomes, lower transplant-free survival, and higher rates of transplant than ALF owing to prescription medications. This finding underscores the importance of a thorough history, with specific questions regarding supplement and herbal use from both the patient, if possible, and the family. In 2012, the National Institute of Diabetes and Digestive and Kidney Diseases and the National Library of Medicine created a website called Liver-Tox (www.livertox.nih.gov), which provides a free and comprehensive assessment of medications and herbal products and their potential to induce DILI.[59] It is an invaluable clinical tool that should be consulted when the diagnosis of DILI, and especially DILI-induced ALF, is suspected.

Other Etiologies

The incidence of ALF owing to other etiologies ranges from 11% to 23%, depending on the definition of "other," which varies from study to study.[28] Some of the more common conditions that fall into this category include autoimmune hepatitis (AIH), Budd-Chiari syndrome, Wilson disease, ischemic hepatitis, malignant liver infiltration, pregnancy complications, mushroom poisoning, and other viruses including herpes simplex virus, cytomegalovirus, Epstein-Barr virus, and varicella.

AIH is one of the more common causes of ALF among this group of diseases. It accounts for 5% of cases in the United States and usually has a poor spontaneous recovery rate.[32] Although AIH is technically a chronic liver disease and would normally be excluded as a possible cause of ALF, acute cases of previously unrecognized and undiagnosed AIH are considered an exception to this rule.[2,14] It is often difficult to differentiate DILI-induced ALF from AIH-induced ALF owing to their similar appearance on laboratory tests and subacute presentations.[60] A liver biopsy may be helpful to diagnosis AIH, especially when autoantibodies are negative.[2] From a demographic standpoint, patients with ALF from AIH tend to be female, Caucasian, young, and overweight or obese.[61]

Ischemic hepatitis, also called hypoxic hepatitis or shock liver, is another relatively common condition that is frequently grouped in this category. Ischemic hepatitis is considered to be a secondary form of ALF; thus, transplant is not warranted and treatment centers on correcting the underlying cause.[14] It is more common in elderly patients, especially those with comorbidities like cardiovascular disease, severe heart failure, or severe sepsis.[62] Illicit drug use with cocaine or 3,4-methylendedioxymethamphetamine have also been reported to induce ALF owing to ischemic hepatitis.[18] The ALFSG has documented that ischemic hepatitis accounts of 4% of ALF cases in the United States, although other sources have reported rates of 6%.[32,63] It should be noted that a documented episode of hypoxia is not required to make the diagnosis. Like other causes of hyperacute liver failure, ALF from ischemic hepatitis has a good prognosis with a spontaneous recovery rate of 58% to 64%.[23]

Wilson disease is a rare cause of ALF, accounting for 2% to 3% of cases of ALF in the United States.[2] Like AIH, Wilson disease is considered to be an exception to the rule that ALF cases must not have an underlying chronic liver disease. These patients tend to be young, usually less than 20 years old, with a high bilirubin to alkaline phosphatase ratio on laboratory workup.[14] ALF from Wilson disease is universally fatal without a liver transplant, so prompt recognition is of the utmost importance.[64]

SUMMARY

ALF is a life-threatening condition that requires early recognition and transfer to specialized centers to achieve good outcomes. It is not a single disease, but rather a whole group of varied etiologies, many of which are difficult to diagnose and lack specific treatment modalities. Understanding the epidemiologic aspects of the various conditions that lead to ALF, along with their subtype classifications, can help clinicians to better identify and manage this devastating condition. Further evaluation and study from groups like the ALFSG are of tremendous importance to continue to advance our understanding of ALF, with the goal of improving not only short-term survival, but also the long-term morbidity associated with this condition.

REFERENCES

1. Stravitz RT, Kramer AH, Davern T, et al. Intensive care of patients with acute liver failure: recommendations of the U.S. Acute Liver Failure Study Group. Crit Care Med 2007;35(11):2498–508.
2. Lee WM, Larson AM, Stravitz RT. AASLD position paper: the management of acute liver failure: update 2011. AASLD Sept. 2011. Available at: http://www.academia.edu/download/37105836/The_Management_of_Acute_Liver.pdf. Accessed September 26, 2017.

3. Escorsell A, Mas A, de la Mata M, Spanish Group for the Study of Acute Liver Failure. Acute liver failure in Spain: analysis of 267 cases. Liver Transpl 2007;13(10): 1389-95.

4. Craig DGN, Bates CM, Davidson JS, et al. Overdose pattern and outcome in paracetamol-induced acute severe hepatotoxicity. Br J Clin Pharmacol 2011; 71(2):273-82.

5. Trey C, Davidson CS. The management of fulminant hepatic failure. Prog Liver Dis 1970;3:282-98.

6. Polson J, Lee WM, American Association for the Study of Liver Disease. AASLD position paper: the management of acute liver failure. Hepatology 2005;41(5): 1179-97.

7. Wlodzimirow KA, Eslami S, Abu-Hanna A, et al. Systematic review: acute liver failure - one disease, more than 40 definitions. Aliment Pharmacol Ther 2012;35(11): 1245-56.

8. Bernuau J, Rueff B, Benhamou JP. Fulminant and subfulminant liver failure: definitions and causes. Semin Liver Dis 1986;6(2):97-106.

9. O'Grady JG, Schalm SW, Williams R. Acute liver failure: redefining the syndromes. Lancet 1993;342(8866):273-5.

10. Tandon BN, Bernauau J, O'Grady J, et al. Recommendations of the International Association for the Study of the Liver Subcommittee on nomenclature of acute and subacute liver failure. J Gastroenterol Hepatol 1999;14(5):403-4.

11. Sugawara K, Nakayama N, Mochida S. Acute liver failure in Japan: definition, classification, and prediction of the outcome. J Gastroenterol 2012;47(8): 849-61.

12. Mochida S, Takikawa Y, Nakayama N, et al. Diagnostic criteria of acute liver failure: a report by the intractable hepato-biliary diseases study group of Japan. Hepatol Res 2011;41(9):805-12.

13. Bernal W. Acute liver failure: review and update. Int Anesthesiol Clin 2017;55(2): 92-106.

14. European Association for the Study of the Liver. Electronic address: easloffice@easloffice.eu, Clinical practice guidelines panel, Wendon J, Panel members, Cordoba J, et al. EASL clinical practical guidelines on the management of acute (fulminant) liver failure. J Hepatol 2017;66(5):1047-81.

15. Bernal W, Hall C, Karvellas CJ, et al. Arterial ammonia and clinical risk factors for encephalopathy and intracranial hypertension in acute liver failure. Hepatology 2007;46(6):1844-52.

16. Bernal W, Hyyrylainen A, Gera A, et al. Lessons from look-back in acute liver failure? A single centre experience of 3300 patients. J Hepatol 2013;59(1): 74-80.

17. Oketani M, Ido A, Nakayama N, et al. Etiology and prognosis of fulminant hepatitis and late-onset hepatic failure in Japan: summary of the annual nationwide survey between 2004 and 2009. Hepatol Res 2013;43(2):97-105.

18. Bernal W, Wendon J. Acute liver failure. N Engl J Med 2014;370(12):1170-1.

19. Hoofnagle JH, Carithers RL, Shapiro C, et al. Fulminant hepatic failure: summary of a workshop. Hepatology 1995;21(1):240-52.

20. Fontana RJ, Ellerbe C, Durkalski VE, et al. 2-year outcomes in initial survivors with acute liver failure: results from a prospective, multicenter study. Liver Int 2015; 35(2):370-80.

21. Adams D, Fullerton K, Jajosky R, et al. Summary of notifiable infectious diseases and conditions - United States, 2013. MMWR Morb Mortal Wkly Rep 2015;62(53): 1-122.

22. Larson AM, Polson J, Fontana RJ, et al. Acetaminophen-induced acute liver failure: results of a United States multicenter, prospective study. Hepatology 2005; 42(6):1364-72.
23. Lee WM, Squires RH, Nyberg SL, et al. Acute liver failure: summary of a workshop. Hepatology 2008;47(4):1401-15.
24. Williams R. Classification, etiology, and considerations of outcome in acute liver failure. Semin Liver Dis 1996;16(4):343-8.
25. Hawton K, Bergen H, Simkin S, et al. Long term effect of reduced pack sizes of paracetamol on poisoning deaths and liver transplant activity in England and Wales: interrupted time series analyses. BMJ 2013;346:f403.
26. Bernal W, Auzinger G, Dhawan A, et al. Acute liver failure. Lancet 2010; 376(9736):190-201.
27. Polson J, Lee WM. Etiologies of acute liver failure: location, location, location! Liver Transpl 2007;13(10):1362-3.
28. Ichai P, Samuel D. Etiology and prognosis of fulminant hepatitis in adults. Liver Transpl 2008;14(Suppl 2):S67-79.
29. Jollow DJ, Mitchell JR, Potter WZ, et al. Acetaminophen-induced hepatic necrosis. II. Role of covalent binding in vivo. J Pharmacol Exp Ther 1973;187(1): 195-202.
30. Mitchell JR, Jollow DJ, Potter WZ, et al. Acetaminophen-induced hepatic necrosis. IV. Protective role of glutathione. J Pharmacol Exp Ther 1973;187(1):211-7.
31. Burgunder JM, Varriale A, Lauterburg BH. Effect of N-acetylcysteine on plasma cysteine and glutathione following paracetamol administration. Eur J Clin Pharmacol 1989;36(2):127-31.
32. Ostapowicz G, Fontana RJ, Schiødt FV, et al. Results of a prospective study of acute liver failure at 17 tertiary care centers in the United States. Ann Intern Med 2002;137(12):947-54.
33. Forde KA, Reddy KR, Troxel AB, et al, Acute Liver Failure Study Group. Racial and ethnic differences in presentation, etiology, and outcomes of acute liver failure in the United States. Clin Gastroenterol Hepatol 2009;7(10):1121-6.
34. Chu CM, Sheen IS, Liaw YF. The role of hepatitis C virus in fulminant viral hepatitis in an area with endemic hepatitis A and B. Gastroenterology 1994;107(1):189-95.
35. Yoshiba M, Dehara K, Inoue K, et al. Contribution of hepatitis C virus to non-A, non-B fulminant hepatitis in Japan. Hepatology 1994;19(4):829-35.
36. Farci P, Alter HJ, Shimoda A, et al. Hepatitis C virus-associated fulminant hepatic failure. N Engl J Med 1996;335(9):631-4.
37. Govindarajan S, Chin KP, Redeker AG, et al. Fulminant B viral hepatitis: role of delta agent. Gastroenterology 1984;86(6):1417-20.
38. Germani G, Theocharidou E, Adam R, et al. Liver transplantation for acute liver failure in Europe: outcomes over 20 years from the ELTR database. J Hepatol 2012;57(2):288-96.
39. Ajmera V, Xia G, Vaughan G, et al. What factors determine the severity of hepatitis A-related acute liver failure? J Viral Hepat 2011;18(7):e167-74.
40. Taylor RM, Davern T, Munoz S, et al. Fulminant hepatitis A virus infection in the United States: incidence, prognosis, and outcomes. Hepatology 2006;44(6): 1589-97.
41. Sarwar S, Khan AA, Alam A, et al. Predictors of fatal outcome in fulminant hepatic failure. J Coll Physicians Surg Pak 2006;16(2):112-6.
42. Daniels D, Grytdal S, Wasley A, Centers for Disease Control and Prevention (CDC). Surveillance for acute viral hepatitis - United States, 2007. Morb Mortal Wkly Rep Surveill Summ 2009;58(3):1-27.

43. Bianco E, Stroffolini T, Spada E, et al. Case fatality rate of acute viral hepatitis in Italy: 1995-2000. An update. Dig Liver Dis 2003;35(6):404–8.
44. Detre K, Belle S, Beringer K, et al. Liver transplantation for fulminant hepatic failure in the United States: October 1987 through December 1991. Clin Transplant 1994;8(3 Pt 1):274–80.
45. Mudawi HMY, Yousif BA. Fulminant hepatic failure in an African setting: etiology, clinical course, and predictors of mortality. Dig Dis Sci 2007;52(11): 3266–9.
46. Acharya SK, Batra Y, Hazari S, et al. Etiopathogenesis of acute hepatic failure: Eastern versus Western countries. J Gastroenterol Hepatol 2002;17(Suppl 3): S268–73.
47. Aggarwal R, Jameel S. Hepatitis E. Hepatology 2011;54(6):2218–26.
48. Mansuy JM, Abravanel F, Miedouge M, et al. Acute hepatitis E in south-west France over a 5-year period. J Clin Virol 2009;44(1):74–7.
49. Fontana RJ, Engle RE, Scaglione S, et al. The role of hepatitis E virus infection in adult Americans with acute liver failure. Hepatology 2016;64(6):1870–80.
50. Dalton HR, Stableforth W, Thurairajah P, et al. Autochthonous hepatitis E in Southwest England: natural history, complications and seasonal variation, and hepatitis E virus IgG seroprevalence in blood donors, the elderly and patients with chronic liver disease. Eur J Gastroenterol Hepatol 2008;20(8):784–90.
51. Bhatia V, Singhal A, Panda SK, et al. A 20-year single-center experience with acute liver failure during pregnancy: is the prognosis really worse? Hepatology 2008;48(5):1577–85.
52. Andrade RJ, Lucena MI, Fernández MC, et al. Drug-induced liver injury: an analysis of 461 incidences submitted to the Spanish registry over a 10-year period. Gastroenterology 2005;129(2):512–21.
53. Reuben A, Koch DG, Lee WM, Acute Liver Failure Study Group. Drug-induced acute liver failure: results of a U.S. multicenter, prospective study. Hepatology 2010;52(6):2065–76.
54. Hernández N, Bessone F, Sánchez A, et al. Profile of idiosyncratic drug induced liver injury in Latin America. An analysis of published reports. Ann Hepatol 2014; 13(2):231–9.
55. Hadem J, Tacke F, Bruns T, et al. Etiologies and outcomes of acute liver failure in Germany. Clin Gastroenterol Hepatol 2012;10(6):664–9.e2.
56. Bailey RL, Gahche JJ, Lentino CV, et al. Dietary supplement use in the United States, 2003-2006. J Nutr 2011;141(2):261–6.
57. Tujios SR, Lee WM. Acute liver failure induced by idiosyncratic reaction to drugs: challenges in diagnosis and therapy. Liver Int 2018;38(1):6–14.
58. Hillman L, Gottfried M, Whitsett M, et al. Clinical features and outcomes of complementary and alternative medicine induced acute liver failure and injury. Am J Gastroenterol 2016;111(7):958–65.
59. Hoofnagle JH, Serrano J, Knoben JE, et al. LiverTox: a website on drug-induced liver injury. Hepatology 2013;57(3):873–4.
60. Björnsson E, Talwalkar J, Treeprasertsuk S, et al. Drug-induced autoimmune hepatitis: clinical characteristics and prognosis. Hepatology 2010;51(6):2040–8.
61. Stravitz RT, Lefkowitch JH, Fontana RJ, et al. Autoimmune acute liver failure: proposed clinical and histological criteria. Hepatology 2011;53(2):517–26.
62. Henrion J. Hypoxic hepatitis. Liver Int 2012;32(7):1039–52.
63. Faria L, Ichai P, Saliba F, et al. Etiology, outcome and early causes of death in 500 patients with acute liver failure: 20 year single center experience. Hepatology 2006;44:287A–390A.

64. Korman JD, Volenberg I, Balko J, et al. Screening for Wilson disease in acute liver failure: a comparison of currently available diagnostic tests. Hepatology 2008; 48(4):1167–74.

65. Khuroo MS, Kamili S. Aetiology and prognostic factors in acute liver failure in India. J Viral Hepat 2003;10:224–31.

Acute Liver Failure
Mechanisms of Disease and Multisystemic Involvement

Steven Krawitz, MD[a],*, Vivek Lingiah, MD[b],
Nikolaos T. Pyrsopoulos, MD, PhD, MBA, FACP, AGAF, FAASLD, FRCP (Edin)[c]

KEYWORDS

• Acute liver failure • Disease mechanisms • Pathophysiology • Inflammation

KEY POINTS

- Acute liver failure is a systemic syndrome that effects many downstream organ systems.
- The syndrome of acute liver failure is initiated and propagated through systemic inflammation.
- Severe liver injury leads to decreased hepatic synthetic capacity and breakdown of metabolism.
- The combined effects of liver failure and systemic inflammation lead to the clinical picture of the acute liver failure syndrome.

INTRODUCTION

The syndrome of acute liver failure (ALF) includes not only severe liver injury and resultant hepatic dysfunction, but also widespread secondary organ dysfunction, regardless of the etiology of the initial liver insult. Beyond simply a liver problem, ALF has been known for decades to have severe consequences affecting most of the major organ systems in the body. Less clear is how severe hepatic injury leads to complex, multisystemic ramifications. As the mechanisms of the underlying pathophysiology are decoded, more understanding into this devastating syndrome is accomplished providing hope for more meaningful clinical interventions in the future.

Disclosure Statement: The authors have nothing to disclose.
[a] Department of Medicine, Division of Gastroenterology and Hepatology, Rutgers New Jersey Medical School, 185 South Orange Avenue, H-534, Newark, NJ 07103, USA; [b] Department of Medicine, Division of Gastroenterology and Hepatology, Rutgers New Jersey Medical School, 185 South Orange Avenue, H-530, Newark, NJ 07103, USA; [c] Division of Gastroenterology and Hepatology, Department of Medicine, Rutgers New Jersey Medical School, 185 South Orange Avenue, H-536, Newark, NJ 07103, USA
* Corresponding author.
E-mail address: sak290@njms.rutgers.edu

Clin Liver Dis 22 (2018) 243–256
https://doi.org/10.1016/j.cld.2018.01.002

liver.theclinics.com

LIVER

ALF is a race initiated by a severe liver insult leading to competition between hepatocyte cell death and regeneration. In ALF, hepatocyte death typically proceeds along 2 well-conserved pathways: apoptosis and necrosis, depending on the etiology of ALF. As apoptosis in its pure form induces cellular shrinkage and subsequent implosion while maintaining the cellular membrane, this form of cell death tends to be silent, inducing minimal inflammation. This is opposed to necrosis, in which adenosine triphosphate (ATP) depletion triggers cell swelling and eventual rupture, inducing a significant inflammatory response.[1] Cell death is mediated by a multitude of interrelated factors and signals, including caspases, oxidative stress and antioxidants, transcription factors, cytokines, chemokines, and kinases.[2]

After hepatocyte injury leads to ATP depletion, cellular swelling results in the development of membrane bleb formation in the necrotic pathway. This is followed by mitochondrial depolarization, lysosomal breakdown, and rapid ion changes inducing more extreme volume shifting, cell swelling, and further bleb formation, culminating in cell membrane rupture.[3] Membrane rupture leads to irreconcilable destabilization of the cell and ultimately cell death. Theoretically, hepatocytes can be resurrected up until fatal membrane rupture, and this is evidenced in certain injuries, such as ischemia/reperfusion injury.[4] Cellular rupture spills intracellular contents, instigating secondary inflammation.

Hepatocyte death via the apoptotic pathway in ALF follows a cascade of several steps reliant more on paired binding interactions. Apoptosis has both an extrinsic (type 1, external to the cell) and intrinsic (type 2, internal to the cell) pathway. The intrinsic pathway starts with oxidative stress, such as DNA damage or p53 activation.[4] The extrinsic pathway begins with binding of ligands (tumor necrosis factor [TNF]-α, FasL) to their transmembrane proteins (TNF-R1, Fas), which then cleave procaspase 8 to its active form. With adequate activation, caspase 8 activates caspase 3 leading to apoptosis, and can even affect mitochondrial expression of proapoptotic signals, thus influencing the intrinsic pathway as well. More recently, there are descriptions of overlap between the apoptotic and necrotic pathways, appropriately labeled necroapoptosis.

If the liver injury is severe enough, and the rate of cell death rapid enough to outpace the regenerative capabilities of the liver, a critical mass of hepatocyte loss will develop, leading to ALF. In this setting, hepatic insufficiency develops, leading to synthetic dysfunction and breakdown of intrahepatic metabolism, which tremendously impacts downstream organ systems and processes. The necrotic burden of hepatocyte death subsequently leads to a wave of systemic inflammation that is compounded by decreased hepatic ability to clear circulating cytokines. Taken together, these consequences of severe liver injury lead to the syndrome of ALF, which has multiorgan ramifications and carries a grave prognosis (**Fig. 1**).

IMMUNE SYSTEM

The immune system plays a large role in the syndrome of ALF, both in its propagation and its consequences. The similar phenotype of the systemic inflammatory response syndrome (SIRS) and ALF belies a similar underlying pathogenesis centered around inflammatory response and immune activation. Those patients with ALF who do develop SIRS, whether secondary to infection or not, more often progress to encephalopathy and have worse prognosis, highlighting the role of the immune system and its importance in ALF.[5]

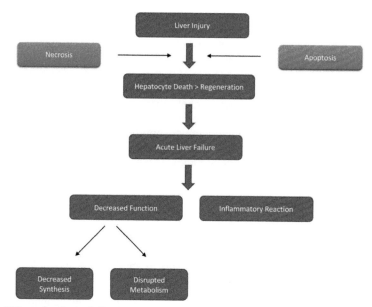

Fig. 1. ALF mechanism of disease.

Despite a strong inflammatory immune response, it has been noted for many decades that patients with ALF still have an increased incidence of both bacterial[6] and fungal infections. One study that examined 50 consecutive patients with ALF found 32% were diagnosed with fungal infections.[7] In addition to functional immunosuppression and increased risk of infection, patients with ALF often fail to mount typical responses to infection and often fail to develop fevers or leukocytosis. This might be attributed to a strong compensatory anti-inflammatory response system. Similar to other severe inflammatory conditions, such as acute pancreatitis, the syndrome of ALF involves an intense immune response that is a sum total of both proinflammatory (TNF-α, interleukin [IL]-1β, IL-6) and anti-inflammatory components (TNF-soluble receptors, IL-1 receptor antagonist, IL-4, IL-10). Just like the dynamic hemostatic process, the immune system in ALF is a balanced system dependent on the interplay of many factors, in this case cytokines and their downstream effects. An imbalance between proinflammatory and anti-inflammatory factors leads to immune dysregulation in ALF, which contributes to the poor outcomes in this patient population.

Patients with ALF have disturbed innate immunity due to several factors. Similar to most clotting factors, the liver is the primary site of complement synthesis.[8] Not only are clotting factor levels decreased in ALF, so too are complement levels decreased leading to defective opsonization[9]; a deficiency known to reverse with recovery after ALF. In a study of 27 patients with ALF, all had low levels of C3 and C5; and there was significantly decreased neutrophil stimulant activity.[10] Neutrophil function is further impaired in patients with ALF, as evidenced in decreased superoxide and hydrogen peroxide production, as well as decreased complement receptor expression.[11] The liver is also the primary site of production of fibronectin, a glycoprotein important in the opsonization process. Fibronectin helps in the clearance of pathogens via Kupffer cells and the reticuloendothelial system. Patients with ALF have been shown to have significantly lower levels of fibronectin; with lower levels linked to increased mortality.[12]

Monocytes play an important role in both the innate and the adaptive immune systems. Once activated, monocytes/macrophages produce large amounts of cytokines supporting both proinflammatory and anti-inflammatory responses, as well as stimulate T-cell activation. Several alterations of monocyte function and secretion have been documented in ALF. Elevated levels of IL-6 and associated C-reactive protein have been noted.[13] Monocyte function studied within the ALF syndrome have shown reduced ability to secrete TNF-α when challenged, a finding associated with poor prognosis.[14] Despite decreased secretion of TNF-α, there is increased secretion of IL-10, a potent anti-inflammatory and immunosuppressive cytokine, and decreased ability of monocyte antigen presentation function.[8] Taken together, monocyte function seems to have an anti-inflammatory and immunosuppressive effect on immune balance in ALF.

BRAIN

Neurologic dysfunction is a key part of ALF, with the rapid onset of hepatic encephalopathy (HE) from mild confusion and agitation, to delirium, seizures, and coma.[15] In the severe stages of HE, patients can develop cerebral edema and increased intracranial pressure, which studies have linked to reduced rates of spontaneous liver recovery (20% vs 70% in encephalopathy stages 1/2).[16]

In ALF, there is release of contents from dying hepatocytes as well as inflammatory cytokines from the splanchnic circulation that move to the systemic circulation. As a result, there is decreased systemic vascular resistance, increased cardiac output, and decreased systemic blood pressure, leading to decreased cerebral perfusion pressure (CPP). Due to impaired cerebral autoregulation in ALF, these episodes of arterial hypotension can lead to cerebral hypoperfusion, which can cause cerebral edema.[17] Conversely, despite a decreased CPP due to impaired autoregulation with decreased cerebrovascular resistance, cerebral blood flow (CBF) can be significantly increased. As a result, many deleterious substances circulating in the blood (eg, ammonia and cytokines) have increased delivery to the brain.[18]

Circulating cytokines are produced as a part of SIRS. SIRS is the clinical presentation of the systemic release of proinflammatory cytokines, including TNF-α, IL-1, and IL-6.[19] The presence of SIRS has been shown in prior studies to predict the progression of HE or elevation in intracranial pressure (ICP).[5] Aside from being transported to the brain via the systemic circulation, studies have shown that the proinflammatory cascade is activated within the brain via microglia as well. These increased brain levels of cytokines were joined by increases in the expression of the genes they encoded, suggesting that they were made within the brain itself.[20]

Cerebral edema occurs less often in patients with mild HE (stages 1 and 2); however, the incidence increases with the severity of HE, occurring in 25% of patients with stage 3 HE, and in 75% with stage 4.[21] The pathogenesis of cerebral edema has been postulated via 2 mechanisms, cytotoxic or vasogenic. Cytotoxic edema, the more compelling theory, rests on the idea that the blood-brain barrier (BBB) is intact and that intracellular swelling is occurring. Vasogenic edema alternatively posits that there is a loss of function of the BBB and that water/solutes build up in the extracellular space.[22] The pathophysiology of cytotoxic edema is discussed in this article.

The primary cell in the brain that undergoes edematous changes in ALF is the astrocyte; this has been shown both in experimental models and in humans with ALF.[23,24] Astrocytes compose approximately one-third of the brain volume, and MRI diffusion-weighted images in patients with ALF have shown a decreased size of the extracellular space, implying intracellular accumulation of fluid.[25] Although the exact cause of astrocyte edema is still unclear, there is significant evidence that ammonia is the key contributing element to the process. Ammonia is produced in the small bowel and degraded principally in the liver via the urea cycle. In ALF, this pathway is inadequate, leading to increased blood ammonia levels.[22] Prior studies have shown that elevated arterial ammonia concentrations are correlated with higher uptake in the brain, cerebral edema, and herniation.[26] Similar results have been shown in children with ornithine carbamoyl transferase deficiency, a urea cycle disorder, leading to hyperammonemia and imaging findings of cerebral edema.[27] Astrocytes are the cells in the brain that mediate ammonia detoxification, by combining it intracellularly with glutamate via the enzyme glutamine synthetase to form glutamine.[15] Studies have found elevated glutamine levels in brain tissues of patients with HE from ALF, suggesting that elevated ammonia levels caused increased production and buildup of glutamine in astrocytes, leading to edema.[22]

The osmotic gliopathy hypothesis is based on increased glutamine levels contributing as an osmotic stressor causing an influx of water into the cell. This has been tested with the use of methionine-s-sulfoximine (MSO), an inhibitor of glutamine synthetase. MSO was noted to decrease glutamine in normal brains and significantly decrease astrocyte edema in vivo and in vitro.[22] A variant to this theory proposes that rather than increased production of glutamine within the astrocyte, in ALF there is a defect/loss of expression in SNAT5, the glutamine transporter, leading to "trapping" of glutamine in the cell. Additionally, as a result of glutamine accumulation within the cell, the pool of releasable glutamate decreases, leading to diminished glutamatergic neurotransmission in the brain and increased neuroinhibition, consistent with the encephalopathy of ALF[28] (**Fig. 2**). However, additional studies have shown that glutamine levels do not necessarily correlate with the degree of cerebral edema. Evaluating studies of rat models of ALF in which hypothermia was used to combat cerebral edema reveals that whereas the edema indeed improved with hypothermia, glutamine levels did not decrease.[22]

The "Trojan Horse" hypothesis has been conceptualized as an alternative theory, whereby the excess glutamine produced within astrocytes is moved into the mitochondria and broken down by phosphate-activated glutaminase (PAG) into ammonia and glutamate (see **Fig. 2**). Glutamine, the "Trojan horse," transports ammonia into mitochondria, where ammonia buildup leads to oxidative/nitrosative stress, astrocyte edema, and cell breakdown.[29]

Oxidative stress has been shown to be a part of the pathophysiology of HE since O'Connor and colleagues[30] showed that hyperammonemic mice showed significant rates of lipid peroxidation. Ammonia also has been noted to create free radicals in rat models, as well as in cultured astrocytes.[31,32] Decreased antioxidant activity in glutathione peroxide, superoxide dismutase, and catalase was also noted in mice treated with high levels of ammonia.[33] Oxidative stress has been shown to cause astrocyte edema both in brain slices and in culture.[15] In addition, the use of antioxidants like superoxide dismutase, catalase, and vitamin E have been noted to prevent ammonia-related astrocyte edema.[34]

Nitrosative stress also contributes to ammonia-related HE. Inhibiting nitric oxide synthase with nitroarginine decreased deaths in hyperammonemic mice. Additionally, in rats with porto-caval shunts given ammonia infusions, nitric oxide levels were increased.[22]

Oxidative/nitrosative stress can lead to induction of the mitochondrial permeability transition (MPT). When initiated, the opening of the permeability transition pore (a large pore on the inner mitochondrial membrane) allows increased permeability to protons,

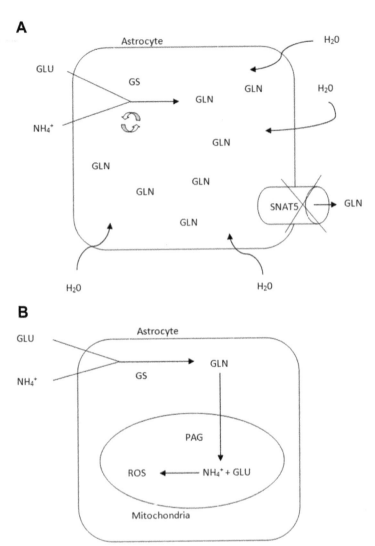

Fig. 2. (A) In the osmotic gliopathy theory, significant amounts of glutamine (GLN) are made by combining glutamate (GLU) and ammonia (NH_4^+) intracellularly via glutamine synthetase (GS) to detoxify hyperammonemic states. The increased intracellular glutamine levels lead to increased amounts of H_2O being drawn intracellularly, resulting in cell swelling. A variant to this theory proposes that downregulation of the SNAT5 glutamine transporter leads to restricted transfer of glutamine out of the cell, which, rather than overproduction of glutamine, causes cell swelling. (B) In the Trojan Horse theory, glutamine produced by GS is transported to the mitochondria, where it is broken back down to ammonia and glutamate via PAG. The ammonia produced in the mitochondria goes on to form reactive oxygen species. The resultant oxidative stress causes cell swelling.

ions, and other solutes. This reduces the inner mitochondrial membrane potential, leading to decreased oxidative phosphorylation and therefore decreased ATP production. Free radicals are produced by this process, leading to cyclic worsening of the problem.[22]

The MPT also contributes to astrocyte edema, although the mechanism is not as clear. This association is reinforced by the fact that cyclosporin, an MPT inhibitor, has been shown to prevent astrocyte edema. Other MPT-inhibiting agents, like trifluoparazome, magnesium, pyruvate, and L-histidine, have been shown to inhibit ammonia-induced astrocyte edema to different degrees.[15] Another agent that works to block PAG, 6-diazo-5-oxo-L-norleucine (DON), has been shown to reduce the generation of free radicals, MPT induction, and astrocyte edema.[22] So although its mechanism is unclear, the MPT has been shown to contribute to brain edema. Potentially this is from the production of free radicals, which contributes to oxidative stress. It also may be related to the reduction in oxidative phosphorylation and ATP production, which induces problems with the function of the ion transporters that regulate cell volume.[15]

The Na/K/Cl cotransporter-1 transporter has been noted to be involved in astrocyte edema. Jayakumar and colleagues[35] showed that ammonia contact (facilitated by oxidative/nitrosative stress) leads to activation of the channel, with ion/water influx and cell edema. Another channel, the ATP-dependent, nonselective cation channel (NCCa-ATP channel), was studied by the same group. They noted that astrocytes treated with ammonia showed significant increase in NCCa-ATP channel activation, as measured by sulfonylurea receptor 1 protein (SUR1), a regulatory protein on the channel. Increased SUR1 levels were associated with astrocyte edema, and SUR1 levels were activated only in low ATP situations.[36] Further evidence for the significance of the energy failure in ALF comes from a mouse model study of ALF evaluating glutamine and lactate. In this study, they showed a significant 2.0-fold to 4.5-fold increase in total brain glutamine and lactate in early stages of HE. However, in the later (coma) stages, there was a further significant lactate increase, but no increase in glutamine, suggesting that damaged glucose oxidative pathways rather than the buildup of intracellular glutamine played the significant role in cerebral edema.[19]

KIDNEY

Renal involvement, most commonly acute kidney injury (AKI), is another complication frequently seen in ALF. The incidence is high, between 40% and 85% depending on the etiology, and is more common in acetaminophen-related ALF.[37,38] Many articles in the past have posited that the functional renal failure present in ALF has similar pathophysiologic mechanisms to the hepatorenal syndrome seen in cirrhotic patients with portal hypertension; with splanchnic vasodilatation leading to decreased arterial circulating blood volume and decreased renal perfusion pressure. This leads to the activation of the sympathetic nervous system (SNS), renin-angiotensin-aldosterone system (RAAS), and vasopressin release, which, unable to improve the decreased renal perfusion pressure, causes further activation of the cycle leading to worsening kidney injury.[39] However the acute renal injury seen in ALF differs from that classic physiology in several ways. Clinically significant portal hypertension is not a prerequisite in patients with ALF and kidney injury. Additionally, if portal hypertension is present in ALF, it is rarely equal to that seen in patients with hepatorenal syndrome in the setting of cirrhosis. Moreover, the vasodilatation in ALF is more generalized and not primarily in the splanchnic circulation, as it is with cirrhosis. The more classic mechanism of hepatorenal AKI may be more common in patients with sub-ALF, in which there is higher likelihood of more clinically significant portal hypertension being present.[40]

Generalized vasodilatation, hypotension, and subsequent activation of the SNS and RAAS are more compatible with the concept of SIRS and sepsis. Leithead and colleagues[40] did a retrospective analysis of 308 patients with ALF and noted that age, severity of ALF, hypotension, acetaminophen-induced ALF, infection, and SIRS were all independently associated with AKI. Of patients in this study, 70% developed SIRS and 43% had AKI. Those who developed AKI had a higher systemic inflammatory response, with 78% of the patients with AKI having SIRS as compared with only 58% of those without AKI ($P<.001$). Critically, when the etiology of ALF was divided between acetaminophen and non-acetaminophen–induced AKI, SIRS was still noted to be significantly associated with AKI in the non-acetaminophen group, showing that the possible confounder of direct nephrotoxicity of the medication was not influencing results.[41]

SIRS is propagated by an inflammatory cascade from systemic cytokine release. This syndrome can occur in patients with both infectious and noninfectious conditions. The source of this cytokine release is a combination of hepatocyte breakdown in the necrotic liver, endotoxemia, or impaired hepatic cytokine metabolism.[41,42] Increased levels of cytokines (like IL-1, TNF-α, and IL-60) directly cause renal tissue inflammation and stimulate the inflammatory response to renal tubular cell apoptosis.[43] Necrosis of renal cells, as well as hepatocyte loss from the necrotic liver in ALF, leads to the release of damage-associated molecular patterns (DAMPs), which lead to renal innate immune system activation via activation of toll-like receptors and nuclear factor–Kb.[43,44] This inflammatory pathway can be further amplified in infection with the release of pathogen-associated molecular patterns. One of these DAMPs, cyclophilin A, has been studied in more depth. A recent study showed that mice lacking cyclophilin A were noted to be resistant to acetaminophen toxicity. Cyclophilin A levels also have been noted to be elevated in the urine of patients with acetaminophen-related ALF.[43]

Acute tubular necrosis (ATN) is another cause of renal injury in ALF, occurring in 22% to 50% of patients with ALF.[38] It can be classified into ischemic or toxic. Ischemic ATN occurs when the kidneys are inadequately perfused for an extended period, with subsequent loss of proximal tubule cell integrity.[43] Toxic ATN results from overdose with hepatotoxins with direct nephrotoxicity (acetaminophen ingestion, *Amanita* poisoning, trimethoprim-sulfamethoxazole) or other nephrotoxic drugs, such as aminoglycosides, nonsteroidal anti-inflammatory drugs, or amphotericin.[39,45] Acetaminophen, in particular, has been shown to have direct nephrotoxic effects, with cases of renal failure occurring in patients with acetaminophen overdose who did not develop significant liver injury.[40]

HEMOSTASIS

Liver injury, both chronic in the form of cirrhosis and acute in the setting of ALF, leads to alterations in the underlying components that contribute to the hemostatic process, including primary and secondary hemostasis and fibrinolysis. Routine blood tests of hemostasis are often abnormal in liver disease. A well-recognized complication of ALF has been hemorrhage; however, unlike chronic liver disease and portal hypertensive bleeding, acute liver failure is associated with more mild, mucosal bleeding or hematoma formation. This is despite the fact that portal hypertension is known to develop in the setting of ALF due to sinusoidal collapse.[46] More recently, evidence questions if patients with ALF are truly more prone to bleeding versus thrombosis based on thromboelastography (TEG).[47] TEG tracings in 20 patients with ALF showed a hypocoagulable profile in 20%, a normal profile in 45%, and a hypercoagulable state in 35% of patients.[48] Hemostasis in patients with ALF is unique and dependent on the net effect of the derangements specific to the pathophysiological consequences of ALF.

Platelets function to seal the initial endothelial injury to abort hemorrhage and contribute to primary hemostasis. The thrombocytopenia seen in ALF is likely multifactorial. Thrombopoietin (TPO), the primary regulator of platelet production, is synthesized in the liver. Perhaps decreased TPO production contributes to the depressed platelet number and therefore contributes to bleeding in ALF. It has been proposed that cirrhotic patients have significantly lower levels of TPO, and therefore lower levels of platelets.[49] However, other studies have shown increased levels of TPO even in advanced stages of decompensated cirrhosis despite thrombocytopenia.[50] TPO concentration was measured in 51 patients with ALF and found to be normal to elevated despite thrombocytopenia.[51] Thrombopoietin levels did not correlate with platelet counts. Therefore, although TPO is produced in the liver, its synthesis appears preserved and does not seem to contribute to thrombocytopenia, altered hemostasis, or bleeding tendency in ALF.

More likely, platelets are consumed or are dysfunctional. Indeed, thrombocytopenia has been associated with SIRS that is often confluent with the multiorgan system failure seen in ALF.[52] Moreover, SIRS leads to endothelial cell activation increasing levels of Von Willebrand Factor (VWF), which acts to help maintain platelet function.[53] Patients with ALF have been shown to have elevated levels of VWF, supporting platelet adhesion despite generally lower levels of platelet numbers.[54] SIRS also contributes to microparticle formation, cell-derived membrane fragments that have been shown to be procoagulant, and increased in numbers in ALF.[55]

Hemorrhage in ALF has been attributed to deficient clotting factor levels threatening secondary hemostasis. Most patients with liver disease have reduced levels of vitamin K–dependent clotting factors (namely II, VII, IX, X). Patients with ALF have lower levels of coagulation factors than those with advanced cirrhosis; in fact, lower levels are prognostic for poor outcomes. Decreased levels of clotting factors are likely due to a combination of decreased synthesis in a dysfunctional liver, hemodilution, short protein half-lives, and increased consumption.[56] At the same time, there is also a decrease in procoagulant factors synthesized by the liver contributing to variably altered hemostasis (eg, protein C, protein S). Both patients with cirrhosis and patients with ALF have lower levels of clotting factors, antithrombin III, prekallikrein, plasminogen, and α2-antiplasmin, with the most severe decrease seen in the ALF group.[57,58]

Hemostasis is the net product of the interplay between coagulation and fibrinolysis. Fibrinolysis is the natural dissolution of the fibrin clot central to coagulation. The liver not only synthesizes important coagulation proteins but also many important fibrinolytic ones. One possible etiology of increased bleeding in ALF is disrupted fibrinolysis. Indeed, in fulminant liver failure there are alterations in several key fibrinolytic proteins (**Fig. 3**). Both the levels of plasminogen and, to a lesser extent, α_2-antiplasmin are decreased in patients with ALF compared with healthy volunteers.[59] No change was

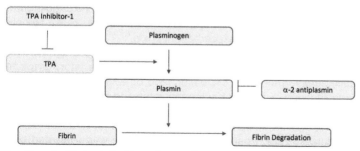

Fig. 3. Alterations in fibrinolysis. Green boxes show proteins with increased levels in ALF. Red boxes demarcate proteins with decreased levels in ALF. The orange box indicates studies have shown no change in levels.

noted in tissue plasminogen activator activity, but there was an increase in plasminogen activator inhibitor-1 levels (produced in endothelial cells). Despite the decreased activity of central proteins in the fibrinolytic pathway, adequate inhibitor presence limited bleeding proclivity.

METABOLISM

Several derangements in basic metabolism have been described in patients with the ALF syndrome. Patients have been noted to have low $Paco_2$; most commonly with an associated alkalemia. The liver is the primary site of lactate removal, and liver injury leads to a decreased rate of hepatic lactate metabolism.[60] Despite a subsequent increase in voluntary muscle lactate metabolism, lactate levels are significantly elevated in patients with ALF. Blood lactate, pyruvate, and acetoacetate concentrations are several times higher than in healthy controls, as are concentrations of free fatty acids.[61] Original reports of ALF induced by acetaminophen overdose prominently described hypoglycemia,[62,63] a derangement that also can be seen in less severe liver injury than ALF. Hypoglycemia likely results from decreased stores and mobilization of glycogen, as well as decreased gluconeogenesis. As with cirrhosis, ALF is a catabolic state with protein breakdown leading to increased levels of amino acids in the blood, as well as increased ammonia concentrations.[64]

PULMONARY

The initial pulmonary presentation of ALF includes central hyperventilation with a resultant respiratory alkalosis.[38] As ICP increases, this hyperventilation worsens and hyperventilation leads to precapillary vasoconstriction, causing a reduction in CBF and ICP.[38,65] Hypoxemia is a significant problem in ALF and is considered a contraindication to transplantation if refractory to therapy.[66] Pulmonary edema can occur as ALF progresses, and has been shown to be significantly more common in patients with cerebral edema. This overlap leads to the possibility that pulmonary edema has a central/neurogenic origin, as opposed to a common systemic physiology affecting both organs for instance elevated intracapillary pressure or elevated capillary permeability.[67] High levels of positive end-expiratory pressure (PEEP) could be another link between the 2 edematous organs, as PEEP increases the risk for cerebral edema by decreasing venous return. Intrapulmonary vasodilatation (noted by elevated amounts of intrapulmonary arteriovenous shunting) is another risk factor for pulmonary edema. Significant dilatation of pulmonary vasculature has been noted on morphometry of autopsied inflated lungs of patients who had died from ALF. Although these changes are not as severe as those seen in cirrhosis, this vasodilatation could expose the pulmonary capillaries to higher hydrostatic pressure, leading to pulmonary edema, although pulmonary artery/left atrial pressures were normal. These higher levels of intrapulmonary shunts also can exacerbate hypoxia.[67,68]

More recently, oxidative stress and cytokine release have been hypothesized as mechanisms of lung injury. Just as ALF causes proinflammatory cytokine release and oxidative stress in the liver, circulation, and other organs, this might also be a pathway inducing lung injury.[66,69] Kostopanagiotou and colleagues[69] tested this theory by giving pigs who had surgical devascularization of the liver intravenous infusions of desferrioxamine (DFX), an iron chelator, to impede hydroxyl radical production and decrease oxidative stress. Postoperative lung damage was evaluated by histology and bronchoalveolar lavage fluid (BALF) analysis. Pigs receiving DFX had significantly less BALF total protein/nitrite/nitrate levels compared with the control group (suggesting a decrease in alveolocapillary membrane disruption), as well as decreased alveolar collapse, alveolar epithelial cell necrosis, and total lung injury. These findings show that lung injury in ALF is at least partially due to oxidative stress, and that inhibiting these reactions improved lung injury.

SUMMARY

ALF is a syndrome with systemic consequences. Regardless of etiology, severe liver injury initiates massive hepatocyte death beyond the liver's ability of regeneration. Hepatic synthetic and metabolic failure combine with a dysregulated inflammatory response to impact downstream organs. The summative systemic dysfunction leads to what is recognized in clinical practice as the syndrome of ALF. Decoding the mechanisms of the disease process and multisystemic involvement of ALF offers potential for targeted treatment opportunities and improved clinical outcomes in this sick population.

REFERENCES

1. Kaplowitz N. Mechanisms of liver cell injury. J Hepatol 2000;32:39–47.
2. Riordan SM, Williams R. Mechanisms of hepatocyte injury, multiorgan failure, and prognostic criteria in acute liver failure. 2003;1(212):69–75.
3. Jaeschke H, Lemasters JJ. Apoptosis versus oncotic necrosis in hepatic ischemia/reperfusion injury. Gastroenterology 2003;125(4):1246–57.
4. Rutherford A, Chung RT. Acute liver failure: mechanisms of hepatocyte injury and regeneration. Semin Liver Dis 2008;28(2):167–74.
5. Rolando N. The systemic inflammatory response syndrome in acute liver failure. Hepatology 2000;32(4):734–9.
6. Rolando N, Harvey F, Brahm J, et al. Prospective study of bacterial infection in acute liver failure: an analysis of fifty patients. Hepatology 1990;11(1):49–53. Available at: http://www.ncbi.nlm.nih.gov/pubmed/2295471.
7. Rolando N. Fungal infection: a common, unrecognised complication of acute liver failure. J Hepatol 1991;12:1–9.
8. Antoniades CG, Berry PA, Wendon JA, et al. The importance of immune dysfunction in determining outcome in acute liver failure. J Hepatol 2008;49(5):845–61.
9. Williams R. Defective opsonisation and complement deficiency in serum from patients with fulminant hepatic failure. Gut 1980;21:643–9.
10. Wyke J, Yousif-Kadaru AG, Rajkovic IA, et al. Serum stimulatory activity and polymorphonuclear leucocyte movement in patients with fulminant hepatic failure. Clin Exp Immunol 1982;50(2):442–9.
11. Clapperton M, Rolando N, Sandoval L, et al. Neutrophil superoxide and hydrogen peroxide production in patients with acute liver failure. Eur J Clin Invest 1997;27(2):164–8. Available at: http://www.ncbi.nlm.nih.gov/pubmed/9061311.
12. Acharya SK, Dasarathy S, Irshad M. Prospective study of plasma fibronectin in fulminant hepatitis: association with infection and mortality. J Hepatol 1995;23(1):8–13.
13. Izumi S, Hughes RD, Langley PG, et al. Extent of the acute phase response in fulminant hepatic failure. Gut 1994;35(7):982–6. Available at: http://www.pubmedcentral.nih.gov/articlerender.fcgi?artid=1374848&tool=pmcentrez&rendertype=abstract.
14. Wigmore SJ, Walsh TS, Lee A, et al. Pro-inflammatory cytokine release and mediation of the acute phase protein response in fulminant hepatic failure. Intensive Care Med 1998;24(3):224–9.
15. Rama Rao KV, Jayakumar AR, Norenberg MD. Brain edema in acute liver failure: mechanisms and concepts. Metab Brain Dis 2014;29(4):927–36.

16. Vaquero J, Chung C, Cahill ME, et al. Pathogenesis of hepatic encephalopathy in acute liver failure. Semin Liver Dis 2003;23(3):259–69.

17. Bernal W, Lee WM, Wendon J, et al. Acute liver failure: a curable disease by 2024? J Hepatol 2015;62(S1):S112–20.

18. Larsen FS, Wendon J. Prevention and management of brain edema in acute liver failure. Liver Transpl 2008;14:S90–6.

19. Aldridge DR, Tranah EJ, Shawcross DL. Pathogenesis of hepatic encephalopathy: role of ammonia and systemic inflammation. J Clin Exp Hepatol 2015; 5(S1):S7–20.

20. Butterworth RF. Pathogenesis of hepatic encephalopathy and brain edema in acute liver failure. J Clin Exp Hepatol 2015;5(S1):S96–103.

21. Leventhal TM, Liu KD. What a nephrologist needs to know about acute liver failure. Adv Chronic Kidney Dis 2015;22(5):376–81.

22. Scott TR, Kronsten VT, Hughes RD, et al. Pathophysiology of cerebral oedema in acute liver failure. World J Gastroenterol 2013;19(48):9240–55.

23. Traber PG, Canto MD, Ganger DR, et al. Electron microscopic evaluation of brain edema in rabbits with galactosamine-induced fulminant hepatic failure: ultrastructure and integrity of the blood-brain barrier. Hepatology 1987;7(6):1272–7.

24. Kato M, Hughes RD, Keays RT, et al. Electron microscopic study of brain capillaries in cerebral edema from fulminant hepatic failure. Hepatology 1992;15(6):1060–6.

25. Chavarria L, Alonso J, Rovira A, et al. Neuroimaging in acute liver failure. Neurochem Int 2011;59(8):1175–80.

26. Clemmesen JO, Larsen FS, Kondrup J, et al. Cerebral herniation in patients with acute liver failure is correlated with arterial ammonia concentration. Hepatology 1999;29(3):648–53.

27. Kendall BE, Kingsley DP, Leonard JV, et al. Neurological features and computed tomography of the brain in children with ornithine carbamoyl transferase deficiency. J Neurol Neurosurg Psychiatry 1983;46(1):28–34.

28. Desjardins P, Du T, Jiang W, et al. Pathogenesis of hepatic encephalopathy and brain edema in acute liver failure: role of glutamine redefined. Neurochem Int 2012;60(7):690–6.

29. Albrecht J, Norenberg MD. Glutamine: a Trojan horse in ammonia neurotoxicity. Hepatology 2006;44(4):788–94.

30. O'Connor JE, Costello M. New Roles of Carnitine Metabolism in Ammonia Cytotoxicity. In: Grisolia S, Felipo V, Minana MD, editors. Cirrhosis, Hepatic Encephalopathy, and Ammonium Toxicity. Advances in Experimental Medicine and Biology. Boston (MA): Springer; 1990 (272). p. 183–195.

31. Kosenko E, Felipo V, Montoliu C, et al. Effects of acute hyperammonemia in vivo on oxidative metabolism in nonsynaptic rat brain mitochondria. Metab Brain Dis 1997;12(1):69–82.

32. Murthy CR, Rama Rao KV, Bai G, et al. Ammonia-induced production of free radicals in primary cultures of rat astrocytes. J Neurosci Res 2001;66(2):282–8.

33. Kosenko E, Kaminsky Y, Kaminsky A, et al. Superoxide production and antioxidant enzymes in ammonia intoxication in rats. Free Radic Res 1997;27(6):637–44.

34. Jayakumar AR, Panickar KS, Murthy CRK, et al. Oxidative stress and mitogen-activated protein kinase phosphorylation mediate ammonia-induced cell swelling and glutamate uptake inhibition in cultured astrocytes. J Neurosci 2006;26(18): 4774–84.

35. Jayakumar AR, Liu M, Moriyama M, et al. Na-K-Cl cotransporter-1 in the mechanism of ammonia-induced astrocyte swelling. J Biol Chem 2008;283(49): 33874–82.

36. Jayakumar A, Valdes V, Tong XY, et al. Sulfonylurea receptor 1 contributes to the astrocyte swelling and brain edema in acute liver failure. Transl Stroke Res 2014; 5:28–37.

37. Betrosian A-P, Agarwal B, Douzinas EE. Acute renal dysfunction in liver diseases. World J Gastroenterol 2007;13(42):5552–9.

38. Karvellas CJ, Stravitz RT. 20-acute liver failure. In: Sanyal AJ, Boyer T, Terrault N, et al, editors. Zakim and Boyer's Hepatology: a textbook of liver disease. 7th edition. Philadelphia, PA: Elsevier Inc; 2017.

39. Moore K. Renal failure in acute liver failure. Eur J Gastroenterol Hepatol 1999;11: 967–75.

40. Leithead JA, Ferguson JW, Bates CM, et al. The systemic inflammatory response syndrome is predictive of renal dysfunction in patients with non-paracetamol-induced acute liver failure. Gut 2009;58(3):443–9.

41. Donnelly MC, Hayes PC, Simpson KJ. Role of inflammation and infection in the pathogenesis of human acute liver failure: clinical implications for monitoring and therapy. World J Gastroenterol 2016;22(26):5958–70.

42. Bone R. Toward a theory regarding the pathogenesis of the systemic inflammatory response syndrome: what we do and do not know about cytokine regulation. Crit Care Med 1996;24:163–72.

43. Moore JK, Love E, Craig DG, et al. Acute kidney injury in acute liver failure: a review. Expert Rev Gastroenterol Hepatol 2013;7(8):701–12.

44. Vaure C, Liu Y. A comparative review of toll-like receptor 4 expression and functionality in different animal species. Front Immunol 2014;5:1–15.

45. Lee WM, Stravitz RT, Larson AM. Introduction to the revised American Association for the Study of Liver Diseases position paper on acute liver failure 2011. Hepatology 2012;55(3):965–7.

46. Valla D, Flejou J-F, Lebrec D, et al. Portal hypertension and ascites in acute hepatitis: clinical, hemodynamic and histological correlations. Hepatology 1989;10(4):482–7.

47. Stravitz RT, Lisman T, Luketic VA, et al. Minimal effects of acute liver injury/acute liver failure on hemostasis as assessed by thromboelastography. J Hepatol 2012; 56(1):129–36.

48. Agarwal B, Wright G, Gatt A, et al. Evaluation of coagulation abnormalities in acute liver failure. J Hepatol 2012;57(4):780–6.

49. Peck-Radosavljevic M, Zacherl J, Meng YG, et al. Is inadequate thrombopoietin production a major cause of thrombocytopenia in cirrhosis of the liver. J Hepatol 1997;27(1):127–31.

50. Temel T, Cansu DU, Temel HE, et al. Serum thrombopoietin levels and its relationship with thrombocytopenia in patients with cirrhosis. Hepat Mon 2014;14(5). https://doi.org/10.5812/hepatmon.18556.

51. Schiødt FV, Balko J, Schilsky M, et al. Thrombopoietin in acute liver failure. Hepatology 2003;37(3):558–61.

52. Stravitz RT, Ellerbe C, Durkalski V, et al. Thrombocytopenia is associated with multi-organ system failure in patients with acute liver failure. Clin Gastroenterol Hepatol 2016;14(4):613–20.e4.

53. Lisman T, Stravitz RT. Rebalanced hemostasis in patients with acute liver failure. Semin Thromb Hemost 2015;1(212):468–73.

54. Hugenholtz GCG, Adelmeijer J, Meijers JCM, et al. An unbalance between von Willebrand factor and ADAMTS13 in acute liver failure: implications for hemostasis and clinical outcome. Hepatology 2013;58(2):752–61.

55. Stravitz RT, Bowling R, Bradford RL, et al. Role of procoagulant microparticles in mediating complications and outcome of acute liver injury/acute liver failure. Hepatology 2013;58(1):304–13.
56. Munoz SJ, Stravitz RT, Gabriel DA. Coagulopathy of acute liver failure. Clin Liver Dis 2009;13(1):95–107.
57. Boks AL, Brommer EJP, Schalm SW, et al. Hemostasis and fibrinolysis in severe liver failure and their relation to hemorrhage. Hepatology 1986;6(1):79–86.
58. Kerr R, Newsome P, Germain L, et al. Effects of acute liver injury on blood coagulation. J Thromb Haemost 2003;1(4):754–9.
59. Pernambuco JRB, Langley PG, Hughes RD, et al. Activation of the fibrinolytic system in patients with fulminant liver failure. Hepatology 1993;18(6):1350–6.
60. Record CO, Chase RA, Williams R, et al. Disturbances in lactate metabolism in patients with liver damage due to paracetamol overdose. Metabolism 1981; 30(7):638–43.
61. Record CO, Iles RA, Cohen RD, et al. Acid-base and metabolic disturbances in fulminant hepatic failure. Gut 1975;16(2):144–9.
62. Clark R, Borirakchanyavat V, Davidson AR, et al. Hepatic damage and death from overdose of paracetamol. Lancet 1973;301(7794):66–70.
63. Davidson DG, Eastham WN. Acute liver necrosis following overdose of paracetamol. Br Med J 1966;2(5512):497–9.
64. Clemmesen JO, Kondrup J, Ott P. Splanchnic and leg exchange of amino acids and ammonia in acute liver failure. Gastroenterology 2000;118(6):1131–9.
65. Damm TW, Kramer DJ. The liver in critical illness. Crit Care Clin 2016;32(3): 425–38.
66. Audimoolam VK, McPhail MJW, Wendon JA, et al. Lung injury and its prognostic significance in acute liver failure. Crit Care Med 2014;42(3):592–600.
67. Trewby PN, Warren R, Contini S, et al. Incidence and pathophysiology of pulmonary edema in fulminant hepatic failure. Gastroenterology 1978;74:859–65.
68. Williams A, Trewby P, Williams R, et al. Structural alterations to the pulmonary circulation in fulminant hepatic failure. Thorax 1979;34(4):447–53.
69. Kostopanagiotou GG, Kalimeris KA, Arkadopoulos NP, et al. Desferrioxamine attenuates minor lung injury following surgical acute liver failure. Eur Respir J 2009; 33(6):1429–36.

The Pathology of Acute Liver Failure

Billie Fyfe, MD*, Francisco Zaldana, DO, Chen Liu, MD, PhD*

KEYWORDS

- Acute liver failure pathology • Massive hepatic necrosis
- Submassive hepatic necrosis • Zonal necrosis • Acetaminophen
- Hepatotropic viral hepatitis • Autoimmune hepatitis

KEY POINTS

- Acute liver failure is typically characterized pathologically by massive hepatic necrosis with extensive loss of parenchyma, variable inflammation, and bile ductular proliferation.
- Identifying zonal, nonzonal, or hepatitic patterns of submassive hepatic necrosis may help to distinguish the etiology; drug toxicity and hepatotropic viral infection are the most common causes.
- Centrilobular necrosis is the most common zonal pattern of injury, and the one associated with most diverse etiology.
- Determining prognosis based on percent viable remaining hepatic parenchyma in acute liver failure specimens is prone to sampling error owing to regional variation in necrosis and inflammation.
- Owing to the liver's capacity for recovery, regeneration and regenerative nodule formation in specimens from patients with acute liver failure may occur and should be distinguished from cirrhosis.

Acute liver failure (ALF; also called fulminant hepatic failure, fulminant hepatitis, acute hepatic failure) is an uncommon (<10 cases/million persons/year) but severe disease. It is defined by the American Association for the Study of Liver Disease as acute hepatitis in patients with no preexisting liver disease, presenting within 26 weeks of symptom onset with coagulopathy (International Normalized Ratio of $\geq$1.5) and the presence of an altered sensorium (encephalopathy). Fulminant hepatic failure historically described patients with encephalopathy within 8 weeks of symptom onset, and subfulminant hepatic failure described those with encephalopathy developing within greater than 8 but 26 weeks or less of symptoms. ALF is now the accepted terminology to encompass this entire spectrum of patients.[1] In pediatric patients, ALF is

Disclosure Statement: The authors have nothing to disclose.
Department of Pathology, Rutgers Robert Wood Johnson Medical School, One Robert Wood Johnson Place, MEB 212, New Brunswick, NJ 08903, USA
* Corresponding authors.
E-mail addresses: fyfekibs@rwjms.rutgers.edu (B.F.); cl1063@njms.rutgers.edu (C.L.)

defined with slight modification owing to difficulties diagnosing encephalopathy and also owing to frequent occult chronic liver disease.[2]

ALF in the Pediatric Population (Pediatric ALF Study Group Definition)
- Presence of liver-related illness.
- No known history of prior chronic liver disease.
- Coagulopathy not corrected by vitamin K.
  - International Normalized Ratio of 1.5 or greater or a prothrombin time of 15 or greater, plus encephalopathy.
  - International Normalized Ratio of 2.0 or greater or a prothrombin time of 20 or greater, with or without encephalopathy.

The lack of prior liver disease is important in distinguishing ALF from the more recently recognized clinical entity of acute-on-chronic liver failure.[3] The latter, although currently without a consensus definition, is characterized by acute hepatic dysfunction in patients with preexistent chronic liver disease associated with multiorgan failure and high short-term mortality.

ALF classification systems such as O'Grady, Bernuau, and Japanese have defined disease by timing of symptoms as hyperacute, acute, or subacute; fulminant or subfulminant; and fulminant or late onset disease, respectively. Such classifications may help to define the etiology and pathologic presentation, as well as likely complications and prognosis; acetaminophen (paracetamol) and viral injury are prone to hyperacute presentation, whereas idiosyncratic drug-induced liver injury, Wilson's disease, or autoimmune hepatitis may present less acutely.[4–7] Clinical features include hepatic encephalopathy, coagulopathy, systemic inflammatory response syndrome, and multiorgan failure.[4] Death occurs in up to 50% of patients, so pathologists may encounter these types of specimens at biopsy, native liver at transplantation, and also during postmortem examination. The most common causes of death in ALF are sepsis and cerebral edema.[8]

ETIOLOGY

ALF is as varied etiologically as chronic liver disease[1,8] (**Box 1**), and approximately 15% are of unknown cause in adults (higher in children, approximately 50%). In developing countries, hepatotropic viral infection (hepatitis A, E, and/or B) is the most common cause of ALF. Hepatitis A and E are responsible for most cases worldwide.[9]

Hepatitis A
- Single-stranded RNA virus (*picornaviridae*).
- Acute self-limited hepatitis common (especially in children); ALF is rare (<1%); no chronic disease.
- Approximately 31% of patients with hepatitis A-induced ALF require transplantation or expire.
- The pathogenesis of development of ALF are poorly understood.
  - Evidence is inconclusive as to whether a viral sequence specific to ALF cases exists; there is stronger evidence for the role of cytotoxic T-cell response in determining course of disease.
- Serologic studies are available for immunoglobulin (Ig)M and IgG, and polymerase chain reaction (PCR) assays to detect viral RNA.

Hepatitis E
- Small, nonenveloped positive strand RNA virus (*hepeviridae*).
- May be associated with epidemic outbreak; it accounts for 20% to 40% of ALF in developing countries.

Box 1
Etiology of acute hepatic failure

- Drug/toxin
  - Nonopioid "aniline" analgesic
    - Tylenol (Paracetamol)
  - Nonsteroidal antiinflammatory drugs
    - Ibuprofen
    - Naproxen
    - Indomethacin
  - Antituberculous agents
    - Isoniazid
    - Rifampin
  - Antibiotics
    - Sulfonamides
    - Amoxicillin
    - Nitrofurantoin
  - Disease-modifying antirheumatic agent
    - Sulfasalazine
  - Antithyroid medication
    - Prolylthiouricil
  - Anticonvulsant
    - Carbamazepine
  - Antifungal
    - Ketoconazole
  - Antialcohol
    - Disulfiram
  - Toxins/herbals/supplements
    - Toxic mushroom
    - Black cohosh
    - Ferrous sulfate

- Infections
  - Hepatotropic viruses
    - Hepatitis A and E most common
    - Hepatitis B
  - Other viral infections
    - Herpes simplex virus
    - Cytomegalovirus
    - Epstein-Barr virus
    - Varicella zoster virus
    - Parvovirus B 19
    - Adenovirus
    - Flaviviridae (dengue and yellow fever)

- Autoimmune disorders
  - Autoimmune hepatitis

- Metabolic
  - Wilson's disease
  - Mitochondriopathies
  - Galactosemia
  - Tyrosinemia type 1

- Neoplastic
  - Usually metastatic malignancy
    - Carcinoma (lung/breast)
    - Leukemia/Lymphoma
    - Melanoma

- Hemodynamic
  - Shock/ischemia
    - Hypovolemic, cardiogenic, septic
  - Acute Budd-Chiari syndrome

- Pregnancy related
  - Preeclampsia, acute fatty liver, HEELP
- Other endothelial injury
  - Sickle cell disease
- Unknown

- In developed countries, it is usually self-limited with exception: chronic disease related to genotype 3 nonepidemic infection in immunocompromised individuals (solid organ transplant recipients, human immunodeficiency virus infection, and patients with hematologic malignancies undergoing chemotherapy).
- ALF in pregnant women, especially in the third trimester, with genotype 1 and 2 infection.
- Acute-on-chronic liver disease in genotype 3 infection in patients with preexistent chronic liver disease.
- Serologic studies for IgM and IgG, and PCR to detect viral RNA.

Hepatitis B ALF is often a reactivation of subclinical chronic infection in a patient who is subsequently immunosuppressed.[9,10]

Hepatitis B
- DNA virus (*Hepadnaviridae*).
- ALF in approximately 1% of acute hepatitis cases.
- ALF in viral reactivation has increased mortality than ALF in primary infection and is seen in patients with stable subclinical infection undergoing iatrogenic immunosuppression during cancer chemotherapy.
- Serologic testing for hepatitis B surface antigen, IgM hepatitis core antigen, and hepatitis B DNA PCR.
  - In fulminant infection, hepatitis B surface antigen and hepatitis B DNA may decrease with liver failure and be negative at time of encephalopathy presentation.

Other viral infections (cytomegalovirus, herpesvirus, adenovirus, Epstein–Barr virus) generally occur in immunosuppressed patients and may be an important cause of ALF after chemotherapy, hematopoietic stem cell therapy, and solid organ transplantation.

According to the Acute Liver Failure Study Group (utsouthwestern.edu) the most common causes of ALF in the United States as of 2017 are acetaminophen (Tylenol; paracetamol) toxicity (46%), indeterminate (12%), and other drugs (11%). This finding is in concordance with published data showing that, in developed countries, drug and toxin exposure are the most common cause of ALF, with acetaminophen responsible for up to 50% of cases. However, almost any class of therapeutic agent has been implicated at least in sporadic reports. Drug toxicity may be idiosyncratic or dose related.[1,8]

Acetaminophen Hepatotoxicity
- Dose related either through intentional or accidental overdose.
  - Usually at least 10 g/d to cause hepatotoxicity, might be less with chronic alcohol use.
  - Mediated via metabolism of the drug by P450 system into the toxic metabolite N-Acetyl-p-benzoquinone imine (NAPQI).

○ In nontoxic dosing, *N*-para-aminoquinonimine is in low amount and catalyzed by intrinsic hepatocyte glutathione.

Other causes of ALF are generally uncommon. Autoimmune hepatitis may present as ALF in a small proportion of cases. Because it is more commonly a chronic disease, diagnosis requires a high index of suspicion by clinician and pathologist alike, especially because autoimmune hepatitis is a potentially reversible cause of ALF.

Malignancy as a cause of ALF has been recently reviewed from the consortium of cases complied by the Acute Liver Failure Study Group.[11]

Malignancy-Associated ALF

- Found in 1.4% of a large series of ALF cases.
- Leukemia/lymphoma and breast cancer followed by colon cancer were most frequently noted malignancies.
- Most patients with lymphoma/leukemia had no history of the malignancy before ALF presentation.
- Most breast cancer patients did have a history of the malignancy before ALF presentation.
- High mortality noted (89% within 3 weeks of presentation).

PATHOLOGY

ALF is a clinical, not a pathologic, diagnosis and the various etiologies may result in similar morphologic patterns, especially when hepatic necrosis becomes extensive. Clinical correlation with chemical, toxicologic, and virologic studies, imaging and history are imperative. In the pediatric population in particular, saving tissue for mitochondrial DNA testing or metabolic studies may be warranted and ultrastructural studies may be helpful. Quantitative analysis of tissues for metal may also be warranted in cases of suspected Wilson's disease or ferrous sulfate toxicity.[2] Because many of these biopsies are transjugular owing to the incident coagulopathy, material may be limited and prior studies have shown poor correlation between biopsy and explant for determining extent of confluent necrosis.[12]

A consensus-derived pathologic classification system for the quantitation and distribution of necrosis and regeneration encountered in ALF has not been published, likely owing to the rarity of these specimens, the varied etiologies of injury, and severity of presentation often limiting pathologic material to postmortem examination. Although not specifically quantitatively defined, most pathologists identify severe liver injury patterns as diffuse, massive, and zonal with massive hepatic necrosis, with near-complete parenchymal necrosis associated with variable inflammation and ductular reaction, as the most severe pathologic presentation of ALF. Submassive hepatic necrosis, a less severe extent of ALF pathology, may have identifiable patterns of necrosis that help to identify etiology; specifically, zonal (central, midzonal, and periportal), nonzonal, and hepatitis, as recently reviewed by Lefkowich.[13] A regenerative response may occur even in ALF specimens with massive necrosis, and this pattern needs to be distinguished from cirrhosis. A pathologic scheme that proposed to further classify degree of necrosis and regeneration identified 4 categories: multiacinar necrosis with or without regeneration, bridging necrosis with regeneration, and differential pathology (combinations of former); it was applied retrospectively in autopsy livers, was not correlated with etiology of ALF, and by the nature of the study did not impart prognostic information.[14] The King's College group defined patterns of hepatic necrosis identified at the time of auxiliary hepatic transplantation for ALF as follows.[15]

King's College ALF Classification
- Diffuse injury:
  - Confluent liver cell loss (less than complete).
  - Uniform distribution from lobule to lobule.
- Maplike injury:
  - Broad regions of complete liver cell loss.
  - Collapse of reticulin framework.
  - Marked ductular reaction.
  - Alternating areas of regeneration.
  - Uneven distribution of changes in liver.
- Complete:
  - Complete loss of parenchyma.
  - Extensive collapse of reticulin framework.
  - Extensive ductular reaction.

In this classification system, diffuse injury was characteristic of all cases of acetaminophen, hepatitis B, and drug toxicity. Idiopathic and autoimmune cases were characterized by maplike injury. Complete loss (corresponding with massive hepatic necrosis) was the least common pattern noted in only 1 idiopathic and 2 drug-induced cases.

Gross Pathology

The gross pathology of ALF depends on the extent of hepatic necrosis and the underlying etiology[13] (**Fig. 1**). Sometimes, as in cases of metastatic malignancy, the gross appearance is diagnostic. Malignancy is the unusual ALF etiology potentially associated with an enlarged liver. The liver in massive hepatic necrosis demonstrates a general decrease in weight to less than 1000 g.

Normal liver weight in adult men and women (as recently reviewed in a forensic population without liver disease) are as follows.[16,17]

- Men: mean 1561 g (range, 838–2584 g), and
- Women: mean 1288 g (range, 775–2395 g).

The capsule is often wrinkled owing to a decrease in hepatic volume, and there are areas of mottled parenchyma with a reddish appearance, sometimes having a nutmeg appearance. Large geographic areas of necrosis spanning multiple complete lobules may be seen and areas of remaining viable parenchyma may appear as nodules. Formalin fixation may help to delineate areas of necrosis. With chronicity, nodularity may develop owing to regeneration.

Microscopic Pathology

Massive hepatic necrosis

There is severe, confluent necrosis of hepatocytes with either retention of reticulin framework (very acute lesion up to 3 days) or collapse/compression of the reticulin framework (more subacute; **Fig. 2**). Variable ductular reaction in the region of portal tracts (periportal) and variable amounts of inflammation are noted, both depending on duration of disease and nature of the insult. In very acute insult, a ductular reaction may not have had time to develop. Sinusoidal congestion and hemorrhage may be present, especially in the centrilobular areas. Ceroid macrophages may be noted, usually most prominently in the centrilobular areas. Sinusoidal and portal inflammation are usually chronic in nature and composed of lymphocytes. A study of the nature of the infiltrating inflammatory cells in various etiologies of ALF including drug-induced, viral, and autoimmune hepatitis revealed that natural killer cells (CD8/56) predominate in

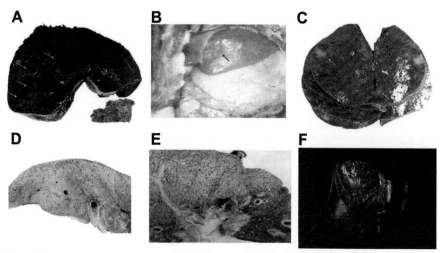

Fig. 1. (*A*) Gross appearance of liver from patient who expired with acute liver failure (ALF) as a consequence of extensive metastatic malignant melanoma. This is the rare case of potential hepatic enlargement in ALF. Virtually the entire liver is replaced by black nodules of tumor (*arrows*). The *inset* shows the microscopic appearance of darkly pigmented melanoma cells that replace virtually the entire hepatic parenchyma (hematoxylin and eosin, original magnification ×20). (*B*) A markedly shrunken liver at autopsy from patient with ALF with capsular wrinkling (*arrow*). (*C*) This liver from a patient with ALF as a consequence of shock with ischemic hepatopathy reveals red discoloration (nutmeg appearance) and large areas of necrosis (*arrows*). (*D*) Sometimes, formalin fixation can highlight areas of necrosis as noted in this liver with extensive necrosis beneath the capsule and also extending throughout the parenchyma. (*E*) With chronicity, regeneration may begin, imparting a nodular appearance to the liver (*arrow*). (*F*) Sometimes, as in this case of ALF of unknown etiology in a young patient, the liver may seem to be deceptively normal grossly, but small foci of necrosis can be identified on close inspection of the capsular surface (*arrow*). (*Courtesy of* [*B*] Dr Kenneth Klein, Rutgers New Jersey Medical School, Newark, NJ; [*E*] A. Quaglia, Institute of Liver Studies, King's College Hospital, London, UK; and [*F*] P. Russo, MD, Children's Hospital of Pennsylvania, Philadelphia, PA.)

viral hepatitis. Plasma cells were most prominent in autoimmune hepatitis, less so in drug-induced autoimmune hepatitis, and uncommon in nonautoimmune drug induced liver injury. B cells (CD20) were more prominent in viral ALF and autoimmune hepatitis than drug-induced liver injury. Cytotoxic T cells (CD8) and macrophages were prominent in all ALF etiologies.[18] Although aiding in our understanding of some aspects of the pathophysiology of different types of ALF, immunophenotypic analysis of infiltrating inflammatory cells is not currently considered of diagnostic value in ALF specimens. The exception is the need to identify plasma cells as an indicator of autoimmune injury, but this determination is usually made without the use of immunohistochemical stains or in situ hybridization.

Viable hepatocytes tend to be located in the periportal region and may demonstrate steatosis, cholestasis, and giant cell transformation.

Regeneration may occur with chronicity and can coexist with active hepatocyte necrosis. Trichrome staining is helpful in distinguishing the blue staining of type 1 collagen from the paler blue staining of newly developed connective tissue in areas of regenerative nodule formation.

Special Stains of Potential Use in the Evaluation of ALF Specimens
- Periodic acid–Schiff diastase (ceroid macrophages).
- Periodic acid–Schiff (glycogenated nuclei—possible Wilson's disease).

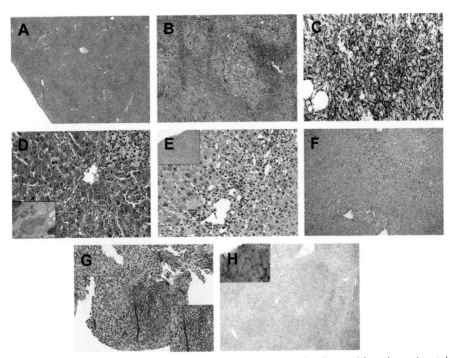

Fig. 2. (A) Almost complete hepatic necrosis is present in this liver with only periportal hepatocytes remaining (*arrows*) (hematoxylin and eosin, original magnification ×20). (*B*) Massive hepatic necrosis with marked ductular reaction and mild inflammation (hematoxylin and eosin, original magnification ×40). (*C*) Reticulin stain with marked collapse owing to loss of hepatic parenchyma (reticulin, original magnification ×100). (*D*) Necrosis in adenoviral hepatitis has an irregular distribution pattern and can involve zone 3 as demonstrated in this lobule. Note the basophilic viral inclusions (*arrows*). Diagnosis was confirmed clinically and with adenoviral immunohistochemistry (inset adenovirus immunohistochemistry, original magnification ×100) and ultrastructure demonstrating icosahedral viral particles in the nucleus (inset electron microscopy, original magnification ×55,000). (*E*) This clinically confirmed case of hepatitis E-induced ALF showed evidence of pericentral necrosis with ceroid macrophages (*arrow*), active chronic inflammation and apoptosis of hepatocytes, mild central venulitis (*black arrow*) and a brisk portal infiltrate (*inset* hematoxylin and eosin, original magnification ×100) (hematoxylin and eosin, original magnification ×400). This pattern of ALF histology requires careful clinicopathologic correlation. (*F*) This submassive necrosis with extensive inflammation in a young patient was unable to be classified as to etiology. This finding is more common in the pediatric (50%) than in the adult population (hematoxylin and eosin, original magnification ×200). (*G*) Autoimmune hepatitis may at times present as ALF. In this clinically confirmed case, there is marked portal inflammation with plasma cells and interface hepatitis (*lower right inset*) as well as central necrosis with brisk inflammation with occasional plasma cells (*upper right inset*); (hematoxylin and eosin, original magnification ×100; insets hematoxylin and eosin, original magnification ×400). (*H*) This submassive necrosis case demonstrates regenerative nodule formation. The pale gray staining around the nodules should not be mistaken for fibrous bands of collagen. Those bands have a deep blue staining pattern (*inset*); (trichrome, original magnification ×40) photo (not inset). (*Courtesy of* [*E*] Rachel Hudacko, MD, Orange Pathology Associates P.C. [*F*] P. Russo, MD, Children's Hospital of Pennsylvania, Philadelphia, PA; [*G*] L. Zhang, MD, MS, Princeton Medical Center, Princeton, NJ; and [*H*] A. Quaglia, Institute of Liver Studies, King's College Hospital, London, UK.)

- Masson trichrome (blue indicates type 1 collagen and cirrhosis; pale blue gray indicates young connective tissue and a regenerative nodule).
- Reticulin (preserved spacing of reticulin architecture indicates acute insult usually <3 days; compressed/collapsed parenchyma indicates more subacute insult).
- Prussian blue (hepatocyte and sinusoidal staining in iron toxicity).
- Rhodanine (copper indicates possible Wilson's disease).
- Victoria blue/Orcein (elastic fibers present indicates cirrhosis; absent to rare indicates a regenerative nodule).
- Cytokeratin 7/19 (highlight ductular reaction, usually not necessary).
- Viral immunohistochemistry (herpes simplex virus, cytomegalovirus, adenovirus).
- Viral in situ hybridization (Epstein-Barr encoded RNA for Epstein–Barr virus).

SUBMASSIVE HEPATIC NECROSIS WITH ZONAL PATTERN
Centrilobular Necrosis

There is extensive coagulative necrosis of hepatocytes in the central zonal region of the lobule, usually sharply demarcated from remaining lobule. This pattern is seen in ischemic injury, acetaminophen toxicity, heat stroke, and mushroom poisoning. There is little associated inflammation, with the exception of mild neutrophilic infiltrate in patients who have been maintained on vasopressors.[13] Heat stroke injury may also induce mild inflammation (macrophages and polymorphonuclear leukocytes) via activation of the systemic inflammatory response syndrome, and ischemic injury may be superimposed owing to dehydration and shunting of blood flow to skin to cool the core body temperature.[19] Innate immunity is also involved in the inflammatory response to acetaminophen toxicity. No specific pathologic features distinguish among these causes of central zonal necrosis. The extent of reticulin collapse and any regenerative response depends on the duration of the injury.

Midzonal Necrosis

This infrequently encountered pattern is identified in viral infection with flaviviridae (Dengue and yellow fever). Midzonal necrosis in autopsy livers of patients with shock was identified by Hutchins and either associated with centrilobular regeneration or on occasion with centrilobular sparing.[20] This histology was unique, but pathologists should be aware of this potential presentation. Midzonal necrosis has also been seen in experimental models of drug toxicity with high dosing of furosemide, paraquat, and beryllium not likely to be encountered clinically.[20] As its name describes, necrosis of hepatocytes in this setting is limited to the midzonal region with centrilobular and periportal sparing. Inflammatory response and reticulin collapse depend on the duration and nature of the injury.

Periportal Necrosis

Periportal necrosis is an uncommon toxin-induced pattern associated with ferrous sulfate and phosphorous intoxication.[13] The injury is felt to relate to delivery of the toxin to the periportal hepatocytes via portal blood flow.[21] In an autopsy series of ferrous sulfate poisoning, iron staining of necrotic hepatocytes and sinusoids was identified with Prussian blue staining and quantitative iron analysis on paraffin-embedded liver with absorption spectrophotometery showed elevated measurements.[21]

Nonzonal Necrosis

Confluent but nonzonal (geographic) areas of necrosis are identified in herpes simplex virus and adenoviral hepatitis. The necrosis in adenoviral hepatitis can range from spotty to massive. Nuclear inclusions are seen most frequently at the edge of necrosis and range from the classically described basophilic inclusions to some large eosinophilic inclusions.[22] Inflammation is generally scant. Immunohistochemical stains for adenovirus are generally positive in the nuclei of infected hepatocytes, although occasional cases may be negative, possibly related to antibody specificity. In suspect cases with negative immunohistochemistry, PCR may be helpful to confirm the diagnosis.[22] Ultrastructure reveals 60- to 90-nm icosahedral viral particles in a crystalline array. Focal to sometimes diffuse necrosis may be seen in herpesvirus hepatitis. Like adenovirus, herpesvirus infection may be associated with little inflammation; viral inclusions are often most prominent at the edge of necrosis and immunohistochemical stains for herpesvirus should be positive.[23] The inclusions are typical of the Cowdry type A eosinophilic, or Cowdry type B basophilic inclusions and the nucleus has a ground glass appearance. Multinucleated infected hepatocytes may be seen. Of interest, human herpesvirus 6, when reactivated in immunosuppressed liver transplant recipients, may cause acute graft hepatitis with a periportal pattern of confluent necrosis.[24]

HEPATITIS PATTERN

This pattern appears as an acute hepatitis with portal and lobular inflammation and irregularly distributed areas of hepatocyte ballooning and necrosis, often demonstrating more apoptotic cell injury. Necrosis may become confluent, bridge from lobule to lobule, and become multilobar. This pattern is seen in hepatitis viral infection and drug-induced liver injury. The diagnosis requires extensive clinical correlation as there is no specifically diagnostic feature for any of these etiologies.

Autoimmune hepatitis may on occasion be associated with ALF. The following histologic criteria have been identified as characteristic of ALF specimens in patients who fulfilled clinical criteria for autoimmune cause of ALF.[13,25]

Histologic Features of Autoimmune Hepatitis-Associated ALF
- Massive hepatic necrosis with prominent centrilobular hemorrhagic necrosis or massive hepatic necrosis with persistent portal inflammation with interface activity.
- Portal lymphoid aggregates.
- Plasma cells noted in the infiltrate.
- Central venulitis and perivenulitis.

PATHOLOGIC PREDICTION OF OUTCOME

Regeneration after massive hepatic necrosis is often not possible as identified in a study of auxiliary liver transplantation in ALF, but in lesser degrees of hepatic necrosis almost normal hepatocyte architecture could be achieved regardless of etiology of insult, being noted in paracetamol, drug-induced, hepatitis B–induced, and idiopathic cases.[15] As noted, liver core biopsy is often not a good representation of the degree of hepatic necrosis noted in explanted livers or at autopsy, and probably should not be used to predict prognosis, although it is thought that a 50% necrosis on a liver biopsy is a threshold to trigger clinical concern for possible need for liver transplantation.[12,13]

SYSTEMIC COMPLICATIONS

The systemic pathology of ALF at autopsy is generally that of multiorgan system failure. All organ systems can be affected and sepsis is often superimposed. Additionally, hemorrhagic complications related to coagulopathy and possible ensuing disseminated intravascular coagulation are common.[26]

SUMMARY

The pathologist's role in the multidisciplinary team supporting patients with ALF is vital. In the examination of both surgical pathology as well as autopsy specimens, pathologists can contribute to the team's understanding of the nature and extent of the hepatic injury, and existing or potential for regenerative response, with the understanding that in limited biopsy specimens, the pathologic data should be interpreted with caution. Pathologists who examine ALF patients at autopsy can also contribute to the team's understanding of effects of therapy and systemic complications.

REFERENCES

1. Murali AR, Narayanan Menon KV. Acute liver failure. Lyndhurst (OH): Cleveland Clinic Center for Continuing Education; 2017. Available at: http://www.clevelandclinicmeded.com/medicalpubs/diseasemanagement/hepatology/acute-liver-failure/. Accessed October 4, 2017.
2. Ruchelli E, Rand EB, Haber BA. Hepatitis and liver failure in infancy and childhood. In: Russo P, Ruchelli E, Piccoli DA, editors. Pathology of pediatric gastrointestinal and liver disease. New York: Springer; 2004. p. 255–8.
3. Hernaez R, Solà E, Moreau R, et al. Acute-on-chronic liver failure: an update. Gut 2017;66:541–53.
4. Bernal W, Wendon J. Acute liver failure. N Engl J Med 2013;369:2525–34.
5. O'Grady JG, Schalm SW, Williams R. Acute liver failure: redefining the syndromes. Lancet 1993;342:273–5.
6. Bernau J, Rueff B, Benhamou JP. Fulminant and subfulminant liver failure: definitions and causes. Semin Liver Dis 1986;6:97–106.
7. Mochida S, Nakayama N, Matsui A, et al. Re-evaluation of the guideline published by the acute liver failure study group of Japan in 1996 to determine the indications of liver transplantation in patients with fulminant hepatitis. Hepatol Res 2008;38:970–9.
8. Lee WM, Squires RH, Byberrg SL, et al. Acute liver failure: summary of a workshop. Hepatology 2008;47:1401–15.
9. Manka P, Verheyen J, Gerken G, et al. Liver failure due to acute viral hepatitis (A-E). Visc Med 2016;32:80–5.
10. Lee HC. Acute liver failure related to hepatitis B virus. Hepatol Res 2008;38: S9–13.
11. Rich NE, Sanders C, Hughes R, et al. Malignant infiltration of the liver presenting as acute liver failure. Clin Gastroenterol Hepatol 2015;13:1025–8.
12. Hanau C, Munoz SJ, Rubin R. Histopathological heterogeneity in fulminant hepatic failure. Hepatology 1995;21:345–51.
13. Lefkowich JH. The pathology of acute liver failure. Adv Anat Pathol 2016;23: 144–58.
14. Das P, Jain D, Das A. A retrospective autopsy study of histopathologic spectrum and etiologic trend of fulminant hepatic failure from North India. Diagn Pathol 2007;2:27–34.
15. Quaglia A, Portmann BC, Knisley AS, et al. Auxiliary transplantation for acute liver failure: histopathological study of native liver regeneration. Liver Transpl 2008;14: 1437–48.

16. Molina DK, DiMaio VJM. Normal organ weights in men part II- the brain, lungs, liver, spleen and kidneys. Am J Forensic Med Pathol 2012;33:368–72.

17. Molina DK, DiMaio VJM. Normal organ weights in women part II- the brain, lungs, liver, spleen and kidney. Am J Forensic Med Pathol 2015;36:182–7.

18. Foureau DM, Walling TL, Maddukuri A, et al. Comparative analysis of portal hepatic infiltrating leucocytes in acute drug-induced liver injury, idiopathic autoimmune and viral hepatitis. Clin Exp Immunol 2014;180:40–51.

19. Davis BC, Tillman H, Chung RT, et al. Heat stroke leading to acute liver injury and failure: a case series from the acute liver failure study group. Liver Int 2017;37: 509–13.

20. DeLaMonte SM, Arcidi JM, Moore GW, et al. Midzonal necrosis as a pattern of hepatocellular injury after shock. Gastroenterology 1984;86:627–31.

21. Pestaner JP, Ishak KG, Mullick FG, et al. Ferrous sulfate toxicity: a review of autopsy findings. Biol Trace Elem Res 1999;69:191–8.

22. Schabert K, Kambham N, Sibley R, et al. Adenovirus hepatitis clinicopathologic analysis of 12 consecutive cases from a single institution. Am J Surg Pathol 2017;41:810–9.

23. Kusne S, Schwartz M, Breining MK, et al. Herpes simplex hepatitis after solid organ transplantation in adults. J Infect Dis 1991;163:1001–7.

24. Buyse S, Roque-Alfonso A-M, Vagheefi P, et al. Acute hepatitis with periportal confluent necrosis associated with human herpesvirus 6 infection in liver transplant patients. Am J Clin Pathol 2013;140:403–9.

25. Stravitz RT, Lefkowich JH, Fontana RJ, et al. Autoimmune acute liver failure: proposed clinical and histological criteria. Hepatology 2011;53:517–26.

26. Hudacko R, Chiaffarano J. Acute liver failure. In: Fyfe B, Miller D, editors. Diagnostic pathology: hospital autopsy. Philadelphia: Elsevier; 2015. p. 2015. II-I-64-67.

Liver Regeneration in the Acute Liver Failure Patient

Keith M. Wirth, MD[a,*], Scott Kizy, MD[a], Clifford J. Steer, MD[b]

KEYWORDS

- Acute liver failure • Cytokines • Growth factors • Homeostasis • MicroRNAs
- Partial hepatectomy • Regeneration • Stem cells

KEY POINTS

- Liver regeneration is a tightly regulated process of coordinating cytokines, growth factors, inflammation, and cell fate.
- Emerging pathophysiologic mechanisms of this process include the gut-liver axis, micro-RNAs, the Hippo/Yap pathway, and stem cell function.
- Promising therapeutics include immunomodulation, microRNA technology, and stem cell therapy.

INTRODUCTION

The study of liver regeneration has evolved for decades, with the first experimental model of liver injury and regeneration, the two-thirds partial hepatectomy (PHx), described in 1931.[1] The majority of the understanding of liver regeneration stems from this surgical model of disease. Of interest in this review, as well as in much of the translational application of this topic, however, is liver regeneration in the setting of toxic and infectious insults as well as in the background of chronic liver dysfunction.

To understand the most recent data and findings as related to liver regeneration in acute liver failure (ALF), therefore, it is important to understand the historical context. Throughout this article, the two-thirds PHx model is referenced, providing a basis for understanding the pathways as well as a topic to contrast most recent findings as related to ALF.

BACKGROUND

The liver is an organ of homeostasis, with functions ranging from metabolism and detoxification to the balancing of glucose, lipid, and cholesterol levels as well as

Disclosure Statement: The authors have nothing to disclose.
[a] Department of Surgery, University of Minnesota Medical School, 420 Delaware Street South-East, MMC 195, Minneapolis, MN 55455, USA; [b] Departments of Medicine, and Genetics, Cell Biology and Development, University of Minnesota Medical School, 420 Delaware Street South-East, MMC 36, Minneapolis, MN 55455, USA
* Corresponding author.
E-mail address: wirth129@umn.edu

synthetic functioning. With such a far-reaching homeostatic role, it logically follows that the liver also has unique mechanisms to maintain its own normal cell function in times of injury. These unique characteristics of liver homeostasis include rapid initiation of mitosis from quiescent hepatocyte(s), a synchrony of this process, and a remarkable ability to regulate the final mass of the liver.

Early work in parabiotic models first suggested an extrahepatic, or humoral, factor initiating regeneration. In these studies, investigators found a significant increase in mitosis and DNA synthesis in the hepatocytes of a normal rat induced by cross-circulation with a recently hepatectomized rat.[2] Later work described a "synchrony" of regeneration, particularly noting a "wave" of mitoses, from periportal to pericentral regions.[3] Also, and interestingly, this synchrony was cell autonomous. Mouse hepatocytes implanted into the rat liver followed the same time course of regeneration as if they were in a mouse liver and did not take on the characteristics of the surrounding cellular millieu.[4] Early studies of the two-thirds PHx demonstrated the restoration of liver mass to preoperative weight and noted that the balance tipped toward massive necrosis and failed regeneration after a significantly greater percentage of resection.[1,5]

These findings, among many others, led to a search for the perfect mitogen, which would allow for initiation and synchronization of liver regeneration; withdrawal of this mitogen would cease regeneration when appropriate liver mass was obtained. This search has led to an ever-expanding list of contributors to this process, which has been explored in great detail in books and articles of significantly greater length and depth. This article hopes to highlight the basis of modern understanding of these mechanisms to apply them to the setting of ALF. First described is the classical pathway of cytokines and growth factors and then an alternative pathway and stem cells.

CLASSICAL PATHWAY(S)

This classical pathway of regeneration focuses on the extrahepatic and intrahepatic signaling cascades, which act rapidly and with precision on hepatocytes and the surrounding cellular milieu. This process has been described as "priming and progression," referring to the concept that regeneration is first preceded by a signal to hepatocytes priming them for mitosis and division, prompting the progression from G_0.[6] This signal alone, however, is not sufficient to direct hepatocytes through the cell cycle; a second factor, likely an extrahepatic mitogen, then tips the scales for cells to progress through G_1 and later divide. The data for this proposed mechanism are discussed throughout each topic.

IMMUNE REGULATION

The liver is the first checkpoint of portal blood returning from the gut; the gut-liver relationship is a complex balance of regulating inflammation and tolerance of this constant barrage of toxins and microbial input.[7] It is a reservoir for immune cells, notably the resident macrophages of the liver, also known as Kupffer cells. Kupffer cells make up the majority of all tissue macrophages as well as 30% of all sinusoidal cells.[8] This important interaction with portal blood makes the Kupffer cell an important signaling and filtering cell as well as an integral part of the regeneration process.

In response to liver injury, macrophage number and division are significantly up-regulated, and recruitment of circulating monocytes is increased.[9] The decisive role of Kupffer cells and recruited macrophages in liver regeneration remains controversial, with a mix of outcomes after activation and depletion studies. Depletion studies have shown delayed regeneration and loss of nuclear factor (NF)-κB activation and decreased recruitment of infiltrating macrophages, while protective effects of inactivation have also been reported.[9–12] With a recent understanding of macrophage polarization and the M1/M2 phenotype, this dual role has become more clear and likely shifts between phenotypes throughout the repair process and later fibrosis.[13]

A large proportion of the mediators discussed in this review are cytokines and signaling molecules integral to the immune system; the key mediators of this immune response are also of great interest and have evolved over time (**Fig. 1**). Early studies in germ-free, athymic, lipopolysaccharide (LPS)-resistant mice first implicated the innate inflammatory response in liver regeneration.[14] This resistance was later discovered to be a defect in Toll-like receptor (TLR)-4. Further investigation demonstrated intact regeneration with TLR4 knockout; however, downstream signaling modulated by MyD88 via knockout models showed significantly decreased regeneration.[15,16] Also, studies of liver regeneration in C3 and C5 knockout mice demonstrated impaired regeneration.[17]

ALF secondary to acetaminophen (APAP) overdose in humans also showed an altered immune response, with a depletion of circulating monocytes, infiltration of macrophages into necrotic liver tissue, and proliferating local Kupffer cells. This was accompanied by significant up-regulation of the monocyte chemoattractants CCL2 (chemokine ligand 2) and CCL3 concurrent with expression of CCR2 (chemokine receptor type 2) on all circulating monocyte subsets.[9] Macrophage colony-stimulating factor (CSF)-1 has also been correlated with increased macrophage infiltration and accelerated liver regeneration after PHx and increases proportionally to the amount of tissue resected.[18,19] Finally, in APAP overdose, serum levels of CSF-1 have been demonstrated to predict mortality, with lower levels associated with worse prognosis.[20] Immunomodulating therapies in ALF are under investigation and the utility of steroids remains controversial; however, therapeutic possibilities certainly exist.[21] A small number of pilot studies have shown improved mortality in acute on chronic liver failure patients treated with the addition of granulocyte CSF.[22,23]

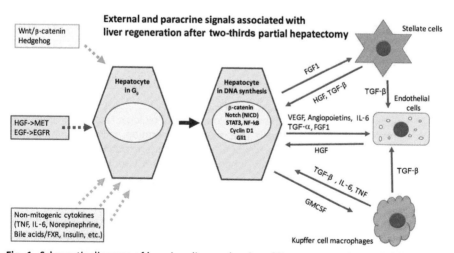

Fig. 1. Schematic diagram of key signaling molecules of liver regeneration. On the left, the quiescent hepatocyte in G_0, with priming cytokines and growth factors, is outlined. On the right is the progression phase with hepatocytes and corresponding nonparenchymal cells exchanging regulatory signals. (*From* Michalopoulos GK. Hepatostat: liver regeneration and normal liver tissue maintenance. Hepatology 2017;65:1384–92; with permission.)

INTRACELLULAR SIGNALS

Investigating the molecular mechanisms of liver regeneration has necessitated identification of signaling mechanisms swift enough to match the rapid response to insult, with an early focus on transcription factors, such as STAT3, NF-κB, and β-catenin.[24,25] With the main effects of these factors post-translational and no reliance on protein synthesis, an expedient effect on cell-cycle regulation and gene expression can be noted. Regulators of these processes will be discussed here.

CYTOKINE-MEDIATED PATHWAYS
Tumor Necrosis Factor α

Continuing with the theme of immune involvement in regeneration, tumor necrosis factor (TNF)-α plays a significant role. TNF-α serum levels are increased rapidly after PHx, potentiated by LPS treatment, and suppressed by pretreatment with Kupffer cell depletion.[26] TNF receptor-1 (TNFR-1) knockout mice demonstrated significant impairment in replication time as well as delay in weight recovery after CCL4-induced injury. Final liver weight does eventually recover in this knockout model and the delay was reversed with interleukin (IL)-6 treatment.[27] Anti-TNF treatment prior to PH resulted in significantly increased IL-6 concentration as opposed to no treatment.[28] These data place TNF-α as an effector in the priming cascade, with IL-6 likely both a downstream and concurrent signaling molecule.

Redundancy is a trend that becomes obvious when discussing signaling in regeneration, and the intracellular cascades initiated follow a similar pattern. NF-κB and STAT3 have been and continue to be well-studied pathways in TNF-α signaling. TNF-α has been demonstrated to rapidly activate NF-κB and STAT3 and significantly increased the proliferative response of hepatocytes to the growth factors HGF and transforming growth factor (TGF)-α.[29] NF-κB is crucial to liver development and integral to regulating apoptosis, with embryonic lethality and massive liver degeneration noted when NF-κB subunit ReAl is deficient.[30] NF-κB and TNF-α have been implicated in the fine balance between regeneration and massive necrosis after greater than two-thirds PHX, in this study an 85% PHX, and thought to be mediated by a balance of receptor for advanced glycation end products and myeloid differentiating factor 88 (Myd88) signaling.[31] NF-κB has several pathways controlling the cell cycle and apoptosis, with the canonical pathway involving IkB kinase, degradation the most relevant to TNF-α signaling.[32]

Interleukin 6

IL-6 is a pleiotropic cytokine involved in a wide range of biologic responses, including inflammation and the acute phase response, regeneration, and carcinogenesis. Kupffer cells are likely the main source of IL-6 in liver regeneration, as demonstrated in bone marrow transplant and macrophage-specific IL-6 knockout experiments.[33] Stimulating factors for production and secretion of this cytokine include inflammatory factors, such as LPS-induced TNF-α as well as activation of TLRs and the NF-κB pathway.[34]

IL-6 signal transduction is described in 2 separate pathways, referred to as the classical and trans-signaling pathways. In the classical pathway, after binding of IL-6 to the membrane-bound receptor IL-6 receptor (IL-6R) (also known as glycoprotein [gp]-80) of effector cells, this complex associates with 2 units of another membrane-bound protein, gp-130, leading to autophosphorylation of gp-130 by its cytoplasmic tyrosine kinase JAK1.[35] An alternative trans-signaling pathway acting through an IL-6R has provided a unique opportunity for an experimental tool in liver regeneration. Soluble IL-6R is cleaved from the cell membrane by metalloproteinase ADAM17 and shed into serum and cytoplasm. This soluble receptor protein allows for IL-6 signal transduction in cells not typically expressing an IL-6R.[36] Important downstream effects of activation of this complex include phosphorylation of STAT3 by JAK 1, gp-130 activation mitogen-activated protein kinase, and the phosphatidyli-nositide 3-kinase cascade.[34]

IL-6 levels have been demonstrated to increase within 2 hours after PHx and peak within 6 hours.[37] The first study implicating IL-6 in impaired regeneration was in IL-6–deficient mice, where a blunted DNA synthetic response, absence of STAT3 phos-phorylation, and reversal of these findings with IL-6 treatment were observed.[38] As discussed previously, IL-6 treatment also reversed the impaired regeneration of TNFR-1 knockout mice.[27] Studies of IL-6 knockout mice demonstrated a high mortal-ity after PHx, which was prevented by subcutaneous but not intravenous injection of IL-6, indicating a need for sustained activity for this effect.[39] This protective effect was proposed to be mediated at least in part by protection of Fas-mediated death. As seen in Jo-2 mAb experiments, IL-6(−/−) mice demonstrated significant hepatitis and high mortality after treatment, whereas IL-6(+/+) mice only suffered mild hepatic injury with significantly improved survival. Survival improved in IL-6(−/−) mice with pretreatment of IL-6.[40] A caveat to this, as seen with TNF-α, is the redundancy of this antiapoptotic mechanism, demonstrated in minimal effects on cell cycle and DNA synthesis after PHx in gp-130 knockout mice, the main effector molecule of IL-6.[41]

GROWTH FACTORS

Described in the classical priming and progression pathway, IL-6, TNF-α, and LPS, signal the departure from quiescence. Hepatocytes, however, must receive a second signal to progress through G_1. The most studied growth factors and mitogens are hepa-tocyte growth factor (HGF) and ligands of the epidermal growth factor receptor (EGFR).

Hepatocyte Growth Factor

One of the first mitogens isolated from the serum of hepatectomized mice, HGF, has proved essential to the process of liver regeneration.[42,43] HGF is synthesized by mesenchymal cells of the liver, notably endothelial and Kupffer cells, and is pro-posed to act in a paracrine fashion.[44] Knockout models of the receptor for HGF, tyro-sine-protein kinase Met (c-MET), fail embryologic development and have significant liver abnormalities.[45] Conditional knockouts have demonstrated a hypersensitivity to Fas-induced apoptosis and impaired recovery from centrolobular lesions.[43] c-MET has been shown to directly bind to and sequester the Fas receptor in hepatocytes, lending to this antiapoptotic hypothesis.[46]

Epidermal Growth Factor Receptor

The ligands of EGFR include EGF, TGF-α, heparin-binding (HB)-EGF, and amphire-gulin. EGFR knockout mice survive on average 8 days, with multiple developmental issues, namely in epithelial and neural development.[47] In a conditional EGFR knockout model, liver regeneration was noted significantly delayed after PHx, with increased mortality. Reduced hepatocyte proliferation and a defective cell-cycle progression at G_1–S-phase entry was accompanied by decreased cyclin D1.[48] HB-EGF is also a key ligand in cell-cycle progression, as studied in a model with varying PHx percent-ages. After one-third PHx, HB-EGF was undetectable; however, in the two-thirds PHx, an increase in serum HB-EGF preceded DNA replication. In addition, treatment of HB-EGF after one-third PHx resulted in a greater than 15-fold increase in DNA replication, providing notable evidence of HB-EGF and EGFR in cell-cycle progression after priming by those factors.[49] With acute silencing of EGFR via short hairpin RNA, hepatocyte proliferation is suppressed and, however, does eventually recover. c-MET signaling is concurrently up-regulated with this silencing, suggesting a compensatory response.[50] In a study of MET knockout mice after PHx, inhibition of EGFR via canertinib resulted in failure of liver regeneration as well as later liver failure.

A study integrating these signaling cascades in an APAP overdose reported interesting findings with incremental dosing. At a defined low dose of 300 mg/kg, the classical pathways held true as expected. Cyclin D1 expression increased at lower dose preceding the regenerative phase but, however, was completely inhibited at higher dosing (600 mg/kg). TNF-α/NF-κB and IL-6/STAT3, are all known to induce cyclin D1. This effect was lost, however, at higher dosing, despite persistence of these pathways, with even higher IL-6/STAT3 induction.[51] This study highlights the need for further investigation of these basic pathways in acute liver injury exclusive to that of surgical models.

MicroRNAs

MicroRNAs (miRNAs) are small noncoding RNAs that act to repress gene expression post-transcriptionally via obstructing translation or leading to degradation of messenger RNA (mRNA) via binding 3′-untranslated regions of mRNA.[52] They are modified from an intermediate called pre-miRNA and then modified further into mature miRNA by an endoribonuclease Dicer.[53] Mechanisms involving miRNA rearrangements have been implicated in liver regeneration and hepatic carcinogenesis and differentiation.[54] The loss of functional miRNAs via a postnatal Dicer liver knockout model demonstrated both increased apoptosis and cell proliferation in juveniles as well as progressive liver damage and inflammation in aged mice. This led to the hypothesis that, although not essential to maintaining hepatic function of the adult hepatocyte, these miRNAs play a role in regulating regeneration and inflammation.[55]

In clinical studies, serum levels of miR-122, miR-21, and miR-221 were significantly higher in patients with spontaneous recovery from ALF compared with nonrecovered patients. Additionally, miR-122 was elevated in both serum and liver tissue of those with spontaneous recovery.[56] These findings have led to a growing interest in the potential use of miRNAs as both a prognostic marker and possible therapy in ALF.

The most abundant miRNA found in hepatic tissue is miR-122, making up more than 70% of all mi-RNAs cloned, is specific to the liver and is undetectable in all other tissues.[57] As discussed previously, miR-122 has been associated with improved prognosis clinically in patients suffering from ALF, which has been recapitulated in the mouse model. Both dose-dependent and duration-dependent increases of circulating miR-122 were noted after APAP-induced liver injury in the mouse model.[58] Mechanistically, miR-122 has been demonstrated to promote hepatic differentiation as well as FoxA1 and HNF4a levels in vitro, altering the balance of the epithelial-to-mesenchymal transition and mesenchymal-to-epithelial transition (MET), suggesting a link to regeneration and carcinogenesis.[59]

Another well-studied miRNA, miR-21, has been implicated in cell proliferation after injury. miR-21 expression is significantly up-regulated during the early stages of liver regeneration, acting via Pellino-1 and inhibiting NF-κB signaling.[60] It is also up-regulated by ursodeoxycholic acid both in vitro and after PHx.[61] Decreasing cyclin D1 translation and altering AKT1/mTor signaling, knockdown models of miR-21 have demonstrated a role of miR-21 in progressing through the S phase of the cell cycle.[62] Somewhat paradoxic, however, is that antisense inhibition of miR-21 via AM21 (antisense DNA to miR-21) treatment in ethanol-fed animals completely restored regeneration and enhanced PHx-induced hepatocyte proliferation to levels comparable to those of untreated or chow-fed animals.[63]

Another antiapoptotic miRNA, miR-221, has been shown to protect from Fas-induced ALF via p53 up-regulated modulator of apoptosis.[64] Adeno-associated virus (AAV) overexpression models of miR-221 have shown rapid entry of hepatocytes into S phase in vitro as well as after PHx, via targets p27 and p57.[65] Finally, specific reconstitution of miR-221 in hepatocyte-specific Dicer knockouts rescued liver regeneration via inhibition of p27.[66] Further investigation for the role of miRNA in progenitor cell differentiation also lends to possible therapeutic targets, with the recent demonstration of miR194 as a potent inducer of differentiation via the Yes-associated protein (YAP)1 pathway.[67]

METABOLISM

The role of bile acids in liver regeneration has been documented for some time, with early studies demonstrating significantly reduced regenerative capacity after PHx, with external biliary drainage versus internal biliary drainage in the cholestatic liver.[68] Similar findings were noted after CCL4-induced injury, with restoration of regenerative capacity reported after bile acid replacement, concurrent with FOXM1 signaling alteration, a key transcription factor in cell-cycle progression.[69] In rats fed cholic acid versus cholestyramine (a bile acid sequestrant), the group fed cholestyramine had a decreased bile acid pool, delayed regeneration, decreased farsenoid X receptor (FXR) expression, and increased cytochrome P450 (CYP)7A1 expression.[70] This finding was also reflected in a clinical correlative study after hemihepatectomy; liver volume was significantly decreased in those patients with external biliary drainage.[71]

Nuclear receptor FXR is a key receptor in the mechanisms of bile acid signaling. FXR is expressed in several tissues, including the liver and ileum, and acts via multiple intracellular pathway in regulating bile acid and lipid homeostasis, among other functions.[72] FXR knockout models have suggested a molecular mechanism in hepatocytes via FoxM1b expression.[73] In enterocytes, FXR has been demonstrated to bind a response element in mouse fibroblast growth factor (FGF) 15, the analog of human FGF19, which acts to inhibit CYP7A1, a key enzyme in bile acid synthesis.[74]

The defined relationship of FXR and bile acid homeostasis in normal liver regeneration has been demonstrated in several studies. As an example, PHx in an FXR knockout mouse and varying amounts of bile acid supplementation resulted in a decrease in early liver weight during regeneration as well as prevention of its acceleration in those animals supplemented with increased bile acid diet. Elevated levels of serum and hepatic bile acids were noted in the FXR(−/−) after PHx, with transient blocking of induction of FoxM1b transcripts.[73] Similar results were also found in FXR(−/−) mice after CCL4 treatment, with increased hepatocyte death and liver injury also noted in FXR(−/−) mice.[75] Parsing out the key roles of FXR in regeneration, a study of hepatic-specific and intestine-specific FXR knockout models presented findings of hepatic FXR required for induction of FOXm1B induction in both CCL4-induced injury and PHx; this finding was not observed in the selective enterocyte FXR(−/−) mice. Furthermore, defective regeneration in the selective enterocyte knockout model was rescued with ectopic expression of FGF15 by recombinant adenovirus.[76]

The interaction of bile acid homeostasis and the gut microbiota has also received increasing attention over the past years, with important therapeutic implications.[77]

After PHx, bacterial translocation from a leaky gut is increased significantly, and exposure to byproducts of the microbiome is certainly increased.[78] The composition of the microbiome alters bile acid homeostasis via changes in primary and secondary bile acid production. In a study of cirrhotic patients, reduced diversity of the microbiome and decreased conversion of primary to secondary bile acids was significantly associated with cirrhosis.[79]

PARACRINE MEDIATORS

The Wnt/β-catenin pathway plays a critical role in liver regeneration, development, and normal physiology. Without Wnt signaling, cytosolic β-catenin is typically marked for degradation by a complex involving the tumor suppressor adenomatous polyposis coli (APC) protein. When activated, free β-catenin translocates to the nucleus and mediates target gene transcription via T-cell factor proteins.[80] Free levels of free β-catenin are tightly regulated, with a significant proportion typically bound to either the APC complex or E-cadherin at the cell membrane.[81]

Within 5 minutes after PHx, cytosolic β-catenin levels are significantly increased and translocation to the nucleus soon follows.[82] The importance of this signaling pathway in liver regeneration after PHx has been investigated in mice treated with β-catenin antisense oligonucleotide as well as conditional β-catenin knockout mice, both demonstrating a delay of proliferation and decreased liver–to–body weight ratios early during regeneration.[83,84]

This signaling pathway has also proved particularly relevant in APAP-induced liver injury in both clinical and laboratory models. A retrospective evaluation of biopsies obtained from patients after APAP overdose demonstrated a significant correlation between nuclear β-catenin localization and spontaneous liver regeneration.[85] A β-catenin–only knockout mouse model lacks the enzyme necessary for APAP-induced hepatotoxicity; therefore, this group also created a unique murine model with inducible expression of this enzyme, CYP2E1/A2. With this they demonstrated decreased proliferation in the β-catenin mice, even at equitoxic doses of APAP, despite induction of the enzyme.[85]

This pathway is also implicated in the metabolic zonation of the liver during development and likely during regeneration, via a gradient of Wnt signaling, β-catenin activation, and APC regulation. With varying signal patterns, hepatocytes express a gradient between periportal or pericentral phenotypes and their related metabolic activities.[86,87] The involvement of Wnt/β-catenin in architectural development during regeneration is also suggested by the close association with β-catenin with E-cadherin. After PHx, increased levels of β-catenin are opposite those of E-cadherin expression, suggesting a coordination with cell-cell adhesion.[82,88]

TRANSFORMING GROWTH FACTOR β

Transforming growth factor beta (TGF-β) presents a key regulator in termination of liver regeneration. Early in vitro studies demonstrated TGF-β as a robust inhibitor of DNA synthesis in mitogen-stimulated hepatocytes, an effect that notably decreased in a time-dependent fashion when hepatocytes were isolated from regenerating livers.[89,90] TGF-β mRNA expression is increased immediately after PHx and reaches peak levels after the first major wave of hepatocyte cell division has taken place.[91] This increased level of TGF-β is countered by a significant reduction in TGF-β receptor expression immediately after PHx, with type II receptors returning to preoperative levels by 120 hours after PHx.[92] Conditional TGF-βII receptor knockout models demonstrate increased hepatocyte proliferation and liver mass–to–body weight ratio compared with flx/flx mice.[93] These effects are mediated in part by inhibition of cyclin D1 and progression through G_1 of the cell cycle.[94]

Another key receptor molecule in TGF-β signaling, beta-2 spectrin (β2SP), yielded somewhat unexpected findings in liver regeneration models. Knockout models of β2SP, a Smad3/4 receptor protein, resulted in a delay in liver regeneration after PHx, induction of p53 with arrest at the G2/M checkpoint, and increased DNA damage.[95] These data suggest that TGF-β plays more of a coordinating role in regeneration as opposed to being simply a terminal signal.

HEPATOSTAT

The term, *hepatostat*, has been used more frequently in recent literature, defining the homeostatic mechanisms ensuring appropriate liver size and architecture after injury or stress.[96] As discussed previously, each species-specific regenerative model follows a typical time course, with final restoration of liver mass in 5 days to 7 days in rodents and 3 months to 4 months in humans.[97] This process of proliferation is not simply mitosis and cell division but a still developing understanding of cell fate and timing of division. It has long been appreciated that hepatocytes divide at differing rates depending on location, with periportal and zone 2 hepatocytes accounting for as much as 80% of all cell division.[98] This disparate division is also noted to be affected by nuclear ploidy.[99] Recent investigation has demonstrated that cell hypertrophy also plays a significant role in restoration of liver mass, making up all of the mass regained after 30% PHx as well as equal contribution after 70% PHx.[100]

Hippo/Yap

A substantial contributor to the regulation of liver size as well as progenitor cell fate is the Yap/Hippo pathway.[101] The transcription coactivator YAP1 is the main effector of the pathway, with nuclear localization negatively controlled by Hippo upstream signaling. Hippo activation leads to phosphorylation and activation of mammalian sterile 20-like kinases 1 and 2, which in turn phosphorylate and activate large tumor suppressors (LATSs) 1 and 2. LATS kinase phosphorylation of YAP1 prevents its translocation to the nucleus and, therefore, interactions with TEA domain (TEAD) transcription factors, the main output of the Hippo/Yap pathway (**Fig. 2**).[102]

In a transgenic inducible gene model, overexpression of YAP1, which is typically at very low levels in quiescent hepatocytes, created a greater than 4-fold increase in liver size via an increase in cell number, which was reversible on interruption of YAP1 expression.[103] Cell growth inhibition via cell-cell contact is one regulator of this pathway. Overexpression of YAP has been shown to overcome this normal inhibition and increased YAP nuclear localization has been noted in some hepatocellular carcinomas.[104] Not only influencing cell number, an AAV-mediated, hepatocyte-specific overexpression of YAP also has demonstrated both a rapid increase in liver growth mainly via growth of a progenitor-like population of hepatocytes.[105] During liver regeneration, YAP protein levels expectedly increased significantly; however, mRNA levels did not reflect this large increase as opposed to a large increase of both in hepatocellular carcinoma. This finding has suggested a mechanism of post-translational modification or inhibition of degradation during regeneration.[106]

As elucidation of the molecular mechanisms of this pathway has become more clear, the list of regulators has grown significantly, prompting some investigators to deem this an "integrator" of the many signals described throughout this article.[96] These include an increase in YAP activation and carcinogenesis with FXR knockout

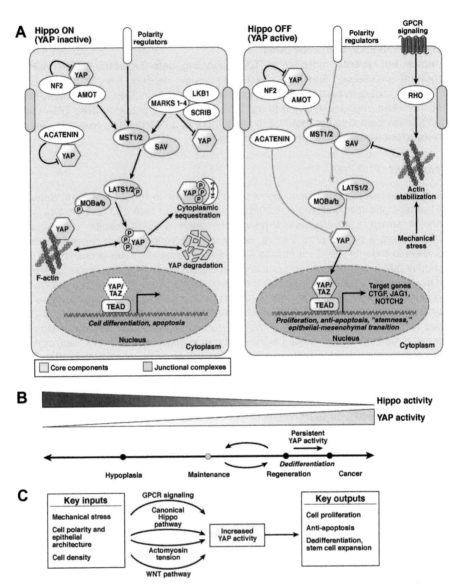

Fig. 2. Schematic of Hippo/YAP pathway in liver regeneration. (*A*) Molecular mechanisms are mapped. The Hippo ON signaling pathway is depicted on the left, with downstream effects of YAP phosphorylation and ultimately cytoplasmic sequestration and proteasomal degradation. The Hippo OFF signaling pathway is noted on the right with active YAP interacting with TEAD transcription factors, promoting cell growth and regeneration. (*B*) Correlation of cell cycle and phenotype with varying YAP activity levels is illustrated. (*C*) Diagram of key inputs, signaling pathways, and key outputs of Hippo/YAP activity. (*From* Patel SH, Camargo FD, Yimlamai D, et al. Hippo signaling in the liver regulates organ size, cell fate, and carcinogenesis. Gastroenterology 2017;152:533–45; with permission.)

and altered bile acid homeostasis as well as the Wnt/β-catenin pathway.[107,108] YAP has also been implicated in the transduction of mechanosensing signals, a key regulator of extracellular matrix remodeling and architectural changes during regeneration.[109] One final element to mention in the regulation of the hepatostat is the point that the final size of the liver is not static. Recent investigation of the diurnal changes of liver size and hepatocyte metabolism has demonstrated distinct changes in ribosomal assembly and correlations with light-dark and the fasting-fed cycles.[110]

STEM CELLS

Stem cell biology has become an increasingly studied topic in the past decade; however, simply the existence of stem cells in normal liver physiology and regeneration has stirred significant controversy.[111] One topic of less controversy among hepatic stem cells is the role of hepatocytes as facultative stem cells for cholangiocytes. In bile duct ligation studies, labeled hepatocytes were injected into rat livers prior to bile duct ligation, and the rats were then treated with diaminodiphenylmethane (DAPM), a biliary toxin, or sham. In both experiments, a number of regenerated cholangiocytes were labeled, indicating a transdifferentiation from hepatocytes, and these labeled cells made a significantly higher contribution after DAPM treatment.[112] One mechanism of inducing this transition is the Notch pathway, as demonstrated with an inducible Notch signaling model. In an in vivo model, Cre-induced hepatocyte-specific Notch signaling resulted in a significant percentage of hepatocytes expressing a biliary epithelial cell markers, with the exception of zone 3 hepatocytes.[113] Blockade of the Notch cascade via a downstream effector RBPJ transcription factor resulted in significantly impaired hepatocyte to a biliary epithelial cell transition as well as repressed YAP levels, implicating a cross-talk of Notch and Hippo/YAP in transdifferentiation.[114]

The existence of a true liver progenitor cell (LPC) or the ability of hepatocytes and cholangiocytes to dedifferentiate into LPCs is, in contrast, much more controversial. The varying terms used across species and fields can make the translation of the literature somewhat difficult. Most studies have focused on a population of cells adjacent to the canal of Hering, or terminal bile ductular system. In rats, these cells are termed *oval cells*, or cells that express both a hepatocyte and cholangiocyte phenotype, which are only present in the damaged liver.[115] In humans, this is termed a *ductular reaction*, as seen in fulminant hepatic failure.

One limitation to the study of oval cells and LPCs is the extreme conditions necessary to make these cell populations develop. Early studies of oval cells were performed by a combination of a liver insult, such as PHx or CCL4, in combination with acetylaminofluorene (AAF), a chemical that causes hepatocyte cell-cycle arrest. After PHx, this protocol in combination with thymidine labeling did demonstrate that oval cells labeled with thymidine went on to migrate and become small hepatocytes.[116] Later studies into the mechanism of AAF pointed toward an increase of p21 and lack of cyclin E halting cell-cycle progression in hepatocytes.[117] In mice, this experimental protocol does not produce an oval cell population. A mouse model mimicking the hepatocyte cell death and senescence induced by AAF as in rats was developed in mice; using a hepatocyte-specific, inducible Mdm2 inactivation Cre mouse, the hepatocytes demonstrated significantly up-regulation of p53 and p21, inducing hepatocyte senescence. Despite an arrested cell cycle of hepatocytes, the liver was repopulated with Mdm2-positive hepatocytes. After tagging cholangiocytes, the investigators concluded that these were the main source of progenitors in this population.[118]

Although these conditions provide some confidence that an LPC population may exist and contribute to regeneration, several recent lineage studies have provided varying evidence. With an osteopontin-labeled promoter, 0.75% to 2.45% of biliary or LPC-derived cells were labeled after CCL4 administration or PHx.[119] Using a variety of fate-tracing strategies, including Sox-9, other investigators have not been able to definitively identify a contribution of a progenitor cell population to hepatocyte proliferation.[120,121] Most recently, a study modeling chronic liver disease, a state in which regenerative capacity is thought to be lost, along with an up-regulation of p21, suggests that such extreme situations are necessary for a progenitor-mediated regeneration. With an AAV-derived fate tracing, these investigators studied a β-integrin knockout model as well as p21 AAV-vector and found up to 25% of cells from biliary origin.[122]

When regeneration fails, the only current viable option is liver transplantation. Although outcomes continue to improve, the waitlist for solid organ transplantation continues to outnumber those organs available, with a significant number of patients dying while on the waitlist.[123] Stem cell therapy continues to be investigated, albeit with a significant number of challenges. The current options for sources of stem cells include human pluripotent stem cells and mesenchymal stem cells (MSCs), with the latter in much more abundant supply.[124] Although differentiation into hepatocytes from MSCs in vitro has proved effective, differentiation in vivo remains a challenge.[124,125] Promising studies of MSC treatment via injection and exosomal treatment in mouse models have demonstrated improved survival and more efficient regeneration in drug-induced ALF.[126] Use of MSCs in patients has also improved safe and effective in preliminary human trials with an improvement of liver function and ascites seen in decompensated cirrhosis.[127]

ACUTE-ON-CHRONIC LIVER FAILURE

This discussion focuses on regeneration after an acute insult to a previously healthy and functional liver, either surgical or chemical. Recent literature has also begun to explore regeneration in the setting of acute-on-chronic liver failure (ACLF), when functional reserve of the liver is already diminished. Aside from the diminished functional capacity, this population also demonstrates a significantly altered immune milieu, a state of chronic inflammation. Serum studies have shown significantly elevated levels on several inflammatory markers in this patient population, with a paradoxic associated immune dysfunction. Although levels of inflammatory markers, such as IL-6 are lower only than those patients with sepsis, the induction of TNF-α production and HLA-DR expression is significantly diminished in patients with ACLF.[128] In addition to the cytokines and signaling, function of regulatory monocytes and macrophages also seem dysfunctional.[129] An analysis of single nucleotide polymorphisms among patients with ACLF found protective effects of specific IL-1 single nucleotide polymorphisms against progression of ACLF.[130] As might be imagined, an alteration of immune function and cytokines may have a significant effect on regenerative capacity. This inherent dysfunction of immune system in ACLF is the main driver behind emerging therapies to enhance recovery and regeneration. One example discussed previously, granulocyte CSF therapy, aims to mobilize endogenous bone marrow–derived stem cells in an effort to enhance tissue repair and reduce inflammation after injury.[22,23]

SUMMARY

With notable heterogeneity of both insult and recovery, the study of regeneration in ALF will certainly continue to evolve, with identification of predisposing factors and pathophysiology helping to guide future therapies. Factors of regeneration highlighted here, including immunomodulation and stem cell therapy, continue to be explored in the clinical setting with some positive results, whereas more recent discoveries, such as the Hippo/Yap pathway and miRNA, hold promising avenues for future intervention. The authors hope that a deeper understanding of the interplay of these elements and the host, as in the microbiome, bile acid homeostasis, and mechanosensing, will aid in the development of novel prevention strategies and patient optimization.

REFERENCES

1. Higgins GM. Experimental pathology of the liver. I. Restoration of the liver in the white rat following partial surgical removal. Arch Pathol 1931;12:186–202.
2. Moolten FL, Bucher NL. Regeneration of rat liver: transfer of humoral agent by cross circulation. Science 1967;158:272–4.
3. Rabes HM. Kinetics of hepatocellular proliferation as a function of the microvascular structure and functional state of the liver. Ciba Found Symp 1977;31–53.
4. Weglarz TC, Sandgren EP. Timing of hepatocyte entry into DNA synthesis after partial hepatectomy is cell autonomous. Proc Natl Acad Sci U S A 2000;97:12595–600.
5. Panis Y, McMullan DM, Emond JC. Progressive necrosis after hepatectomy and the pathophysiology of liver failure after massive resection. Surgery 1997;121:142–9.
6. Fausto N, Laird AD, Webber EM. Liver regeneration. 2. Role of growth factors and cytokines in hepatic regeneration. FASEB J 1995;9:1527–36.
7. Balmer ML, Slack E, de Gottardi A, et al. The liver may act as a firewall mediating mutualism between the host and its gut commensal microbiota. Sci Transl Med 2014;6:237ra66.
8. Bouwens L, Baekeland M, De Zanger R, et al. Quantitation, tissue distribution and proliferation kinetics of Kupffer cells in normal rat liver. Hepatology 1986;6:718–22.
9. Antoniades CG, Quaglia A, Taams LS, et al. Source and characterization of hepatic macrophages in acetaminophen-induced acute liver failure in humans. Hepatology 2012;56:735–46.
10. Abshagen K, Eipel C, Kalff JC, et al. Loss of NF-κB activation in Kupffer cell-depleted mice impairs liver regeneration after partial hepatectomy. Am J Physiol Gastrointest Liver Physiol 2007;292:G1570–7.
11. You Q, Holt M, Yin H, et al. Role of hepatic resident and infiltrating macrophages in liver repair after acute injury. Biochem Pharmacol 2013;86:836–43.
12. Ju C, Reilly TP, Bourdi M, et al. Protective role of Kupffer cells in acetaminophen-induced hepatic injury in mice. Chem Res Toxicol 2002;15:1504–13.
13. Sica A, Invernizzi P, Mantovani A. Macrophage plasticity and polarization in liver homeostasis and pathology. Hepatology 2014;59:2034–42.
14. Cornell RP, Liljequist BL, Bartizal KF. Depressed liver regeneration after partial hepatectomy of germ-free, athymic and lipopolysaccharide-resistant mice. Hepatology 1990;11:916–22.
15. Poltorak A, He X, Smirnova I, et al. Defective LPS signaling in C3H/HeJ and C57BL/10ScCr mice: mutations in Tlr4 gene. Science 1998;282:2085–8.
16. Seki E, Tsutsui H, Iimuro Y, et al. Contribution of Toll-like receptor/myeloid differentiation factor 88 signaling to murine liver regeneration. Hepatology 2005;41:443–50.
17. Markiewski MM, DeAngelis RA, Strey CW, et al. The regulation of liver cell survival by complement. J Immunol 2009;182:5412–8.
18. Matsumoto K, Miyake Y, Umeda Y, et al. Serial changes of serum growth factor levels and liver regeneration after partial hepatectomy in healthy humans. Int J Mol Sci 2013;14:20877–89.

19. Sauter KA, Waddell LA, Lisowski ZM, et al. Macrophage colony-stimulating factor (CSF1) controls monocyte production and maturation and the steady-state size of the liver in pigs. Am J Physiol Gastrointest Liver Physiol 2016;311: G533–47.

20. Stutchfield BM, Antoine DJ, Mackinnon AC, et al. CSF1 Restores innate immunity after liver injury in mice and serum levels indicate outcomes of patients with acute liver failure. Gastroenterology 2015;149:1896–909.

21. Possamai LA, Thursz MR, Wendon JA, et al. Modulation of monocyte/macrophage function: a therapeutic strategy in the treatment of acute liver failure. J Hepatol 2014;61:439–45.

22. Garg V, Garg H, Khan A, et al. Granulocyte colony-stimulating factor mobilizes $CD34^+$ cells and improves survival of patients with acute-on-chronic liver failure. Gastroenterology 2012;142:505–12.

23. Saha BK, Mahtab MA, Akbar SMF, et al. Therapeutic implications of granulocyte colony stimulating factor in patients with acute-on-chronic liver failure: increased survival and containment of liver damage. Hepatol Int 2017;11:540–6.

24. Cressman DE, Diamond RH, Taub R. Rapid activation of the Stat3 transcription complex in liver regeneration. Hepatology 1995;21:1443–9.

25. Cressman DE, Greenbaum LE, Haber BA, et al. Rapid activation of post-hepatectomy factor/nuclear factor κB in hepatocytes, a primary response in the regenerating liver. J Biol Chem 1994;269:30429–35.

26. Iwai M, Cui TX, Kitamura H, et al. Increased secretion of tumour necrosis factor and interleukin 6 from isolated, perfused liver of rats after partial hepatectomy. Cytokine 2001;13:60–4.

27. Yamada Y, Fausto N. Deficient liver regeneration after carbon tetrachloride injury in mice lacking type 1 but not type 2 tumor necrosis factor receptor. Am J Pathol 1998;152:1577–89.

28. Akerman P, Cote P, Yang SQ, et al. Antibodies to tumor necrosis factor-α inhibit liver regeneration after partial hepatectomy. Am J Physiol Gastrointest Liver Physiol 1992;263:G579–85.

29. Webber EM, Bruix J, Pierce RH, et al. Tumor necrosis factor primes hepatocytes for DNA replication in the rat. Hepatology 1998;28:1226–34.

30. Beg AA, Sha WC, Bronson RT, et al. Embryonic lethality and liver degeneration in mice lacking the RelA component of NF-κB. Nature 1995;376:167–70.

31. Zeng S, Zhang QY, Huang J, et al. Opposing roles of RAGE and Myd88 signaling in extensive liver resection. FASEB J 2012;26:882–93.

32. Sun B, Karin M. NF-κB signaling, liver disease and hepatoprotective agents. Oncogene 2008;27:6228–44.

33. Aldeguer X, Debonera F, Shaked A, et al. Interleukin-6 from intrahepatic cells of bone marrow origin is required for normal murine liver regeneration. Hepatology 2002;35:40–8.

34. Schaper F, Rose-John S. Interleukin-6: biology, signaling and strategies of blockade. Cytokine Growth Factor Rev 2015;26:475–87.

35. Schmidt-Arras D, Rose-John S. IL-6 pathway in the liver: from physiopathology to therapy. J Hepatol 2016;64:1403–15.

36. Mackiewicz A, Schooltink H, Heinrich PC, et al. Complex of soluble human IL-6-receptor/IL-6 up-regulates expression of acute-phase proteins. J Immunol 1992;149:2021–7.

37. Trautwein C, Rakemann T, Niehof M, et al. Acute-phase response factor, increased binding, and target gene transcription during liver regeneration. Gastroenterology 1996;110:1854–62.

38. Cressman DE, Greenbaum LE, DeAngelis RA, et al. Liver failure and defective hepatocyte regeneration in interleukin-6-deficient mice. Science 1996;274:1379–83.
39. Blindenbacher A, Wang X, Langer I, et al. Interleukin 6 is important for survival after partial hepatectomy in mice. Hepatology 2003;38:674–82.
40. Kovalovich K, Li W, DeAngelis R, et al. Interleukin-6 protects against Fas-mediated death by establishing a critical level of anti-apoptotic hepatic proteins FLIP, Bcl-2, and Bcl-xL. J Biol Chem 2001;276:26605–13.
41. Wuestefeld T, Klein C, Streetz KL, et al. Interleukin-6/glycoprotein 130-dependent pathways are protective during liver regeneration. J Biol Chem 2003;278: 11281–8.
42. Nakamura T, Nawa K, Ichihara A. Partial purification and characterization of hepatocyte growth factor from serum of hepatectomized rats. Biochem Biophys Res Commun 1984;122:1450–9.
43. Huh CG, Factor VM, Sánchez A, et al. Hepatocyte growth factor/c-met signaling pathway is required for efficient liver regeneration and repair. Proc Natl Acad Sci U S A 2004;101:4477–82.
44. Noji S, Tashiro K, Koyama E, et al. Expression of hepatocyte growth factor gene in endothelial and Kupffer cells of damaged rat livers, as revealed by in situ hybridization. Biochem Biophys Res Commun 1990;173:42–7.
45. Schmidt C, Bladt F, Goedecke S, et al. Scatter factor/hepatocyte growth factor is essential for liver development. Nature 1995;373:699–702.
46. Wang X, DeFrances MC, Dai Y, et al. A mechanism of cell survival: sequestration of Fas by the HGF receptor Met. Mol Cell 2002;9:411–21.
47. Miettinen PJ, Berger JE, Meneses J, et al. Epithelial immaturity and multiorgan failure in mice lacking epidermal growth factor receptor. Nature 1995;376: 337–41.
48. Natarajan A, Wagner B, Sibilia M. The EGF receptor is required for efficient liver regeneration. Proc Natl Acad Sci U S A 2007;104:17081–6.
49. Mitchell C, Nivison M, Jackson LF, et al. Heparin-binding epidermal growth factor-like growth factor links hepatocyte priming with cell cycle progression during liver regeneration. J Biol Chem 2005;280:2562–8.
50. Paranjpe S, Bowen WC, Tseng GC, et al. RNA interference against hepatic epidermal growth factor receptor has suppressive effects on liver regeneration in rats. Am J Pathol 2010;176:2669–81.
51. Bhushan B, Walesky C, Manley M, et al. Pro-regenerative signaling after acetaminophen-induced acute liver injury in mice identified using a novel incremental dose model. Am J Pathol 2014;184:3013–25.
52. Lim LP, Lau NC, Garrett-Engele P, et al. Microarray analysis shows that some microRNAs downregulate large numbers of target mRNAs. Nature 2005;433: 769–73.
53. Bartel DP. MicroRNAs: genomics, biogenesis, mechanism, and function. Cell 2004;116:281–97.
54. Lauschke VM, Vorrink SU, Moro SML, et al. Massive rearrangements of cellular MicroRNA signatures are key drivers of hepatocyte dedifferentiation. Hepatology 2016;64:1743–56.
55. Hand NJ, Master ZR, Le Lay J, et al. Hepatic function is preserved in the absence of mature microRNAs. Hepatology 2009;49:618–26.
56. John K, Hadem J, Krech T, et al. MicroRNAs play a role in spontaneous recovery from acute liver failure. Hepatology 2014;60:1346–55.
57. Lagos-Quintana M, Rauhut R, Yalcin A, et al. Identification of tissue-specific microRNAs from mouse. Curr Biol 2002;12:735–9.

58. Wang K, Zhang S, Marzolf B, et al. Circulating microRNAs, potential biomarkers for drug-induced liver injury. Proc Natl Acad Sci U S A 2009;106:4402–7.

59. Deng XG, Qiu RL, Wu YH, et al. Overexpression of miR-122 promotes the hepatic differentiation and maturation of mouse ESCs through a miR-122/FoxA1/HNF4a-positive feedback loop. Liver Int 2014;34:281–95.

60. Marquez RT, Wendlandt E, Galle CS, et al. MicroRNA-21 is upregulated during the proliferative phase of liver regeneration, targets Pellino-1, and inhibits NF-κB signaling. Am J Physiol Gastrointest Liver Physiol 2010;298:G535–41.

61. Castro R, Ferreira D, Zhang X, et al. Identification of microRNAs during rat liver regeneration after partial hepatectomy and modulation by ursodeoxycholic acid. Am J Physiol Gastrointest Liver Physiol 2010;299:G887–97.

62. Ng R, Song G, Roll GR, et al. A microRNA-21 surge facilitates rapid cyclin D1 translation and cell cycle progression in mouse liver regeneration. J Clin Invest 2012;122:1097–108.

63. Juskeviciute E, Dippold RP, Antony AN, et al. Inhibition of miR-21 rescues liver regeneration after partial hepatectomy in ethanol-fed rats. Am J Physiol Gastrointest Liver Physiol 2016;311:G794–806.

64. Sharma AD, Narain N, Händel EM, et al. MicroRNA-221 regulates FAS-induced fulminant liver failure. Hepatology 2011;53:1651–61.

65. Yuan Q, Loya K, Rani B, et al. MicroRNA-221 overexpression accelerates hepatocyte proliferation during liver regeneration. Hepatology 2013;57:299–310.

66. Oya Y, Masuzaki R, Tsugawa D, et al. Dicer-dependent production of microRNA221 in hepatocytes inhibits p27 and is required for liver regeneration in mice. Am J Physiol Gastrointest Liver Physiol 2017;312:G464–73.

67. Jung KH, McCarthy RL, Zhou C, et al. MicroRNA regulates hepatocytic differentiation of progenitor cells by targeting YAP1. Stem Cells 2016;34:1284–96.

68. Suzuki H, Iyomasa S, Nimura Y, et al. Internal biliary drainage, unlike external drainage, does not suppress the regeneration of cholestatic rat liver after partial hepatectomy. Hepatology 1994;20:1318–22.

69. Naugler WE. Bile acid flux is necessary for normal liver regeneration. PLoS One 2014;9:1–10.

70. Dong X, Zhao H, Ma X, et al. Reduction in bile acid pool causes delayed liver regeneration accompanied by down-regulated expression of FXR and c-Jun mRNA in rats. J Huazhong Univ Sci Technolog Med Sci 2010;30:55–60.

71. Otao R, Beppu T, Isiko T, et al. External biliary drainage and liver regeneration after major hepatectomy. Br J Surg 2012;99:1569–74.

72. Sinal CJ, Tohkin M, Miyata M, et al. Targeted disruption of the nuclear receptor FXR/BAR impairs bile acid and lipid homeostasis. Cell 2000;102:731–44.

73. Huang W. Nuclear receptor-dependent bile acid signaling is required for normal liver regeneration. Science 2006;312:233–6.

74. Inagaki T, Choi M, Moschetta A, et al. Fibroblast growth factor 15 functions as an enterohepatic signal to regulate bile acid homeostasis. Cell Metab 2005;2:217–25.

75. Meng Z, Wang Y, Wang L, et al. FXR regulates liver repair after CCl_4 -induced toxic liinjury. Mol Endocrinol 2010;24:886–97.

76. Zhang L, Wang YD, Chen WD, et al. Promotion of liver regeneration/repair by farnesoid X receptor in both liver and intestine in mice. Hepatology 2012;56:2336–43.

77. Liu HX, Keane R, Sheng L, et al. Implications of microbiota and bile acid in liver injury and regeneration. J Hepatol 2015;63:1502–10.

78. Wang XD, Soltesz V, Andersson R, et al. Bacterial translocation in acute liver failure induced by 90 per cent hepatectomy in the rat. Br J Surg 1993;80:72–4.
79. Kakiyama G, Pandak WM, Gillevet PM, et al. Modulation of the fecal bile acid profile by gut microbiota in cirrhosis. J Hepatol 2013;58:949–55.
80. Cadigan KM, Waterman ML. TCF/LEFs and Wnt signaling in the nucleus. Cold Spring Harb Symp Quant Biol 2012;4:1–22.
81. Monga SPS, Mars WM, Pediaditakis P, et al. Hepatocyte growth factor induces Wnt-independent nuclear translocation of β-catenin after Met-β-catenin dissociation in hepatocytes. Cancer Res 2002;62:2064–71.
82. Monga SPS, Pediaditakis P, Mule K, et al. Changes in wnt/β-catenin pathway during regulated growth in rat liver regeneration. Hepatology 2001;33: 1098–109.
83. Sodhi D, Micsenyi A, Bowen WC, et al. Morpholino oligonucleotide-triggered β-catenin knockdown compromises normal liver regeneration. J Hepatol 2005; 43:132–41.
84. Tan X, Behari J, Cieply B, et al. Conditional deletion of β-catenin reveals its role in liver growth and regeneration. Gastroenterology 2006;131:1561–72.
85. Apte U, Singh S, Zeng G, et al. β-catenin activation promotes liver regeneration after acetaminophen-induced injury. Am J Pathol 2009;175:1056–65.
86. Gougelet A, Torre C, Veber P, et al. T-cell factor 4 and β-catenin chromatin occupancies pattern zonal liver metabolism in mice. Hepatology 2014;59: 2344–57.
87. Leibing T, Géraud C, Augustin I, et al. Angiocrine Wnt signaling controls liver growth and metabolic maturation in mice. Hepatology 2017;1–36. https://doi.org/10.1002/hep.29613.
88. Nelson WJ, Nusse R. Convergence of Wnt, β-catenin, and cadherin pathways. Science 2004;303:1483–7.
89. Nakamura T, Tomita Y, Hirai R, et al. Inhibitory effect of transforming growth factor-β on DNA synthesis of adult rat hepatocytes in primary culture. Biochem Biophys Res Commun 1985;133:1042–50.
90. Strain AJ, Hill DJ. Changes in sensitivity of hepatocytes isolated from regenerating rat liver to the growth inhibitory action of transforming growth factor β. Liver 1990;10:282–90.
91. Braun L, Mead JE, Panzica M, et al. Transforming growth factor β mRNA increases during liver regeneration: a possible paracrine mechanism of growth regulation. Proc Natl Acad Sci U S A 1988;85:1539–43.
92. Chari RS, Price DT, Sue SR, et al. Down-regulation of transforming growth factor β receptor type I, II, and III during liver regeneration. Am J Surg 1995;169: 126–31, 131–2.
93. Romero-Gallo J, Sozmen EG, Chytil A, et al. Inactivation of TGF-β signaling in hepatocytes results in an increased proliferative response after partial hepatectomy. Oncogene 2005;24:3028–41.
94. Ko TC, Yu W, Sakai T, et al. TGF-β1 effects on proliferation of rat intestinal epithelial cells are due to inhibition of cyclin D1 expression. Oncogene 1998;16: 3445–54.
95. Thenappan A, Shukla V, Abdul Khalek FJ, et al. Loss of transforming growth factor β adaptor protein β-2 spectrin leads to delayed liver regeneration in mice. Hepatology 2011;53:1641–50.
96. Michalopoulos GK. Hepatostat: liver regeneration and normal liver tissue maintenance. Hepatology 2017;65:1384–92.

97. Taub R. Liver regeneration: from myth to mechanism. Nat Rev Mol Cell Biol 2004;5:836–47.

98. Grisham JW. A morphologic study of deoxyribonucleic acid synthesis and cell proliferation in regenerating rat liver; autoradiography with thymidine-H3. Cancer Res 1962;22:842–9.

99. Gerlyng P, Abyholm A, Grotmol T, et al. Binucleation and polyploidization patterns in developmental and regenerative rat liver growth. Cell Prolif 1993;26:557–65.

100. Miyaoka Y, Ebato K, Kato H, et al. Hypertrophy and unconventional cell division of hepatocytes underlie liver regeneration. Curr Biol 2012;22:1166–75.

101. Dong J, Feldmann G, Huang J, et al. Elucidation of a universal size-control mechanism in Drosophila and mammals. Cell 2007;130:1120–33.

102. Patel SH, Camargo FD, Yimlamai D. Hippo signaling in the liver regulates organ size, cell fate, and carcinogenesis. Gastroenterology 2017;152:533–45.

103. Camargo FD, Gokhale S, Johnnidis JB, et al. YAP1 increases organ size and expands undifferentiated progenitor cells. Curr Biol 2007;17:2054–60.

104. Zhao B, Wei X, Li W, et al. Inactivation of YAP oncoprotein by the Hippo pathway is involved in cell contact inhibition and tissue growth control. Genes Dev 2007;21:2747–61.

105. Yimlamai D, Christodoulou C, Galli GG, et al. Hippo pathway activity influences liver cell fate. Cell 2014;157:1324–38.

106. Wang C, Zhang L, He Q, et al. Differences in Yes-associated protein and mRNA levels in regenerating liver and hepatocellular carcinoma. Mol Med Rep 2012;5:410–4.

107. Anakk S, Bhosale M, Schmidt VA, et al. Bile acids activate YAP to promote liver carcinogenesis. Cell Rep 2013;5:1060–9.

108. Azzolin L, Panciera T, Soligo S, et al. YAP/TAZ incorporation in the β-catenin destruction complex orchestrates the Wnt response. Cell 2014;158:157–70.

109. Song Z, Gupta K, Ng IC, et al. Mechanosensing in liver regeneration. Semin Cell Dev Biol 2017;71:153–67.

110. Sinturel F, Gerber A, Mauvoisin D, et al. Diurnal oscillations in liver mass and cell size accompany ribosome assembly cycles. Cell 2017;169:651–63.

111. Michalopoulos GK, Khan Z. Liver stem cells: experimental findings and implications for human liver disease. Gastroenterology 2015;149:876–82.

112. Michalopoulos GK, Barua L, Bowen WC. Transdifferentiation of rat hepatocytes into biliary cells after bile duct ligation and toxic biliary injury. Hepatology 2005;41:535–44.

113. Yanger K, Zong Y, Maggs LR, et al. Robust cellular reprogramming occurs spontaneously during liver regeneration. Genes Dev 2013;27:719–24.

114. Lu J, Zhou Y, Hu T, et al. Notch signaling coordinates progenitor cell-mediated biliary regeneration following partial hepatectomy. Sci Rep 2016;6:22754.

115. Dollé L, Best J, Mei J, et al. The quest for liver progenitor cells: a practical point of view. J Hepatol 2010;52:117–29.

116. Evarts RP, Nagy P, Nakatsukasa H, et al. In vivo differentiation of rat liver oval cells into hepatocytes. Cancer Res 1989;49:1541–7.

117. Trautwein C, Will M, Kubicka S, et al. 2-acetaminofluorene blocks cell cycle progression after hepatectomy by p21 induction and lack of cyclin E expression. Oncogene 1999;18:6443–53.

118. Lu WY, Bird TG, Boulter L, et al. Hepatic progenitor cells of biliary origin with liver repopulation capacity. Nat Cell Biol 2015;17:971–83.

119. Español-Suñer R, Carpentier R, Van Hul N, et al. Liver progenitor cells yield functional hepatocytes in response to chronic liver injury in mice. Gastroenterology 2012;143:1564–75.

120. Schaub JR, Malato Y, Gormond C, et al. Evidence against a stem cell origin of new hepatocytes in a common mouse model of chronic liver injury. Cell Rep 2014;8:933–9.

121. Tarlow BD, Finegold MJ, Grompe M. Clonal tracing of Sox9+ liver progenitors in mouse oval cell injury. Hepatology 2014;60:278–89.

122. Raven A, Lu WY, Man TY, et al. Cholangiocytes act as facultative liver stem cells during impaired hepatocyte regeneration. Nature 2017;547:350–4.

123. Kim WR, Lake JR, Smith JM, et al. OPTN/SRTR 2015 annual data report: liver. Am J Transplant 2017;17(Suppl 1):174–251.

124. Lee CW, Chen YF, Wu HH, et al. Historical perspectives and advances in the mesenchymal stem cell research for the treatment of liver diseases. Gastroenterology 2018;154:46–56.

125. Lee K-D, Kuo TK-C, Whang-Peng J, et al. In vitro hepatic differentiation of human mesenchymal stem cells. Hepatology 2004;40:1275–84.

126. Tan C, Lai R, Wong W, et al. Mesenchymal stem cell-derived exosomes promote hepatic regeneration in drug-induced liver injury models. Stem Cell Res Ther 2014;5:76.

127. Zhang Z, Lin H, Shi M, et al. Human umbilical cord mesenchymal stem cells improve liver function and ascites in decompensated liver cirrhosis patients. J Gastroenterol Hepatol 2012;27:112–20.

128. Wasmuth HE, Kunz D, Yagmur E, et al. Patients with acute on chronic liver failure display "sepsis-like" immune paralysis. J Hepatol 2005;42:195–201.

129. Bernsmeier C, Pop OT, Singanayagam A, et al. Patients with acute-on-chronic liver failure have increased numbers of regulatory immune cells expressing the receptor tyrosine kinase MERTK. Gastroenterology 2015;148:603–15.

130. Alcaraz-Quiles J, Titos E, Casulleras M, et al. Polymorphisms in the IL-1 gene cluster influence systemic inflammation in patients at risk for acute-on-chronic liver failure. Hepatology 2017;65:202–16.

Viral Hepatitis and Acute Liver Failure: Still a Problem

Daniel Sedhom, MD[a],*, Melroy D'Souza, MD[a], Elizabeth John, MD[a], Vinod Rustgi, MD, MBA[b]

KEYWORDS

• Viral • Hepatitis • ALF • Reactivation • HBV • HDV • HEV • Problem

KEY POINTS

• Acute liver failure (ALF) is a syndrome rather than a specific disease with several possible causes, including drug overdose, viral hepatitis, ischemia, trauma, and other causes.
• Each cause has a different clinical course and outcomes.
• The liver has the capacity to often recover after such insults; however, predicting outcomes is often a challenge.
• Understanding the cause of ALF is important for clinical management.

INTRODUCTION

Viral hepatitis remains a major cause of acute liver failure (ALF) in the world. ALF is an unpredictable and severe condition associated with high mortality in the absence of intensive care, treatment, and often liver transplantation. ALF is defined by the American Association for the Study of Liver Disease as the presence of encephalopathy and evidence of coagulopathy with international normalized ratio (INR) of greater than or equal to 1.5 without evidence of preexisting cirrhosis and with duration of symptoms for less than 26 weeks. There are various classification systems that are used to grade ALF (**Table 1**).

ALF is a syndrome rather than a specific disease with several possible causes, including drug overdose, viral hepatitis, ischemia, trauma, and other causes. Each cause has a different clinical course and outcomes. The liver has the capacity to often recover after such insults; however, predicting outcomes is often a challenge. Understanding the cause of ALF is important for clinical management. This article focuses on viral hepatitis as a cause of ALF.

Disclosure Statement: The authors have nothing to disclose.
Contributorship: All authors contributed equally in the writing of this article.
[a] Department of Internal Medicine, Rutgers Robert Wood Johnson Medical School, 1 Robert Johnson Place, New Brunswick, NJ 08903, USA; [b] Division of Gastroenterology and Hepatology, Rutgers Robert Wood Johnson Medical School, 1 Robert Johnson Place, New Brunswick, NJ 08903, USA
* Corresponding author.
E-mail address: ds1369@rwjms.rutgers.edu

Clin Liver Dis 22 (2018) 289–300
https://doi.org/10.1016/j.cld.2018.01.005
1089-3261/18/© 2018 Elsevier Inc. All rights reserved.

liver.theclinics.com

Table 1
Three classification systems used to grade acute liver failure

Variables	Clichy	King's College	Japanese
Age	✔	✔	✔
Cause	—	✔	—
Encephalopathy	✔	✔	✔
Bilirubin	—	—	✔
Coagulopathy	✔	✔	✔

VIRAL HEPATITIS: EPIDEMIOLOGY AND PATHOGENESIS

The primary cause of ALF has rapidly changed worldwide. Historically, hepatitis A and B were regarded as the most common causes of ALF.[1,2] In the 1960s, hepatitis A and B were responsible for nearly three-quarters of all cases of ALF. Over the last 3 decades, there has been a decline in viral hepatitis in the developed world, especially hepatitis A and B, as causes of ALF.[3,4] Currently, according to the US ALF Group Registry, drug-induced liver injury (DILI), particularly acetaminophen, account for more than 50% of ALF cases in this country. Indeterminate causes account for 14% of cases, with autoimmune, viral, and other rare causes accounting for the remaining cases[5] (**Fig. 1**). Northern Europe and the United Kingdom have similar statistics as the United States.[2] This dramatic change is a reflection of the impact of public health initiatives that have reduced the incidence of new cases of acute viral hepatitis. In addition, improved vaccination programs as well as better control of blood products have impacted this change.[5]

Despite the trend, hepatitis A and B are still responsible for nearly 10% of all cases of ALF in the United States.[4] An additional 2% of cases are thought to be secondary to hepatitis E, with rare cases including Epstein-Barr, herpes simplex and zoster, cytomegalovirus (CMV), and adenovirus.[3,4] Globally, viral causes of ALF remain a major contributor. Viral hepatitis infections are responsible for most ALF cases worldwide, with high incidence in Asian countries, several European countries, and the developing world. Hepatitis E, for example, is responsible for nearly one-half of all cases of ALF reported in India, with similar numbers in Bangladesh.[5] Greater than 40% of ALF cases in Japan are due to hepatitis B. Hepatitis B virus (HBV) also remains the most common

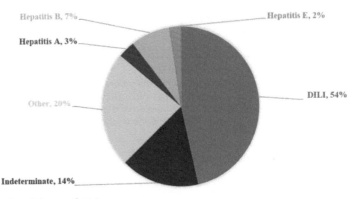

Fig. 1. The breakdown of ALF causes.

cause of ALF in Spain.[4,5] Studies also predict that underdiagnosis of certain viral causes is contributing to the high number of indeterminate cases.[4]

VIRUS SPECIFIC KEY POINTS
Hepatitis A

Liver disease caused by hepatitis A virus (HAV) ranges from mild to severe without causing chronic liver disease. The transmission of HAV is more common in developing countries with poor sanitation.[6] The World Health Organization (WHO) estimates nearly 1.4 million people are infected with HAV yearly.[7] Most patients with HAV recover fully; however, a small proportion develops ALF[8] (**Table 2**). About 3% of all cases of ALF are caused by HAV.[4] Young patients are generally asymptomatic.[8] In contrast, 70% of adults infected with HAV develop symptoms with less than 1% resulting in ALF.[9]

Hepatitis A virus prognosis

HAV-related ALF has a good overall prognosis. HAV-related ALF has a spontaneous resolution rate of about 70% with the remaining 30% requiring liver transplant or dying.[8] Certain features play a role in prognostication of HAV infections, including creatinine greater than 2, alanine aminotransferase (ALT) greater than 2600, and need for pressors or intubation.[10] The presence of these features is associated with poor outcomes. In addition, patients with nonalcoholic fatty liver disease, an increasing rising global problem, or alcoholic steatohepatitis are more susceptible to developing acute on chronic liver failure (ACLF) from HAV.[6] Studies on the difference between patients with a benign course of HAV and those with fulminant courses

Table 2
Viruses that cause acute liver failure and key points about each virus

Virus	Transmission	ALF Incidence	Risk Factors	Leads to Chronic Liver Disease
Hepatitis A	Fecal-oral	3%	Age >50, underlying liver disease, residence or travel to areas with poor sanitation, illicit drug use	No
Hepatitis B	Mother-to-child, sexual, percutaneous, nosocomial	7%	Piercings, tattoos, IV drug use, health care providers	Yes
Hepatitis D	Coinfection or superinfection with HBV	Coinfection:20% Superinfection: 5%	Endemic regions	
Hepatitis E	Sexual, undercooked meat, oral-fecal	2%	Pregnancy, underlying liver disease, areas with contaminated water	Yes
Other viruses less commonly implicated	Cytomegalovirus, Epstein-Barr virus, herpes simplex virus, adenovirus, HCV, HDV			

have not yielded clear results. Low viral loads and high rates of substitutions in the 5'-untranslated region of the viral genome are proposed to increase the likelihood of developing ALF from HAV.[11]

Hepatitis B

HBV is responsible for about 7% of all cases of ALF in the United States.[12] According to the WHO, about one-quarter of the world's population has experienced HBV and about 3% are chronically infected, with adults less likely to develop chronic infection.[7] About 1% of patients infected with HBV will develop ALF (see **Table 2**).[12] HBV may be spread via sexual transmission and perianally, although transmission can also occur via reuse of needles, transmission in medical and dental settings, tattooing, and reuse of contaminated razors with infected blood.[13]

HBV-related ALF is still a worldwide problem. De novo infections still represent a large portion of cases in the United States.[4,13,14] Furthermore, the subset of HBV incidence secondary to reactivation of stable subclinical infection without chronic disease characteristics is steadily increasing, making this a problem still worth investigating.[15–17]

Moreover, the incidence of ALF from HBV may be underestimated for various reasons. In cases of ALF from HBV, HBV DNA and hepatitis B surface antigen (HBsAg) levels decrease rapidly, and some patients are HBsAg negative at time of presentation.[18] In addition, precore and pre-S mutant HBV can produce infection without the production of hepatitis B virus e antigen (HBeAg) or HBsAg. These cases are often inaccurately attributed to indeterminate causes.[4,17] This was studied in a subset of 17 patients who went for liver transplantation for suspected non-HBV-related ALF and later were found to have 6 with a positive polymerase chain reaction (PCR) for HBV.[19]

HBV core promoter mutations are implicated in the pathogenesis of ALF. These phenotypes have enhanced viral replication, leading to stronger immune response and a fulminant course. Activation of humoral immunity is also proposed to be involved in the pathogenesis of HBV-related ALF.[4] An accumulation of immunoglobulin G and immunoglobulin M secreting plasma cells and complement components were found in necrotic areas of livers affected by HBV-related ALF.[14,18] These underlying mechanisms need further investigation.

Reactivation of latent hepatitis B virus: still a problem

Reactivation of HBV infection is possible in the setting of a chronic HBV infection or in a previously eradicated infection.[20] Chronic HBV infection is the result of an intricate balance between the virus, the integrity of the immune system, and the capabilities of the liver[21] (**Fig. 2**). Patients suffering from a chronic HBV infection have a higher risk of undergoing a reactivation of the virus.[22] In addition, reactivation is possible in patients who have a resolved HBV infection, defined by the seroprevalence of HBsAg(−), hepatitis B core antigen (+), and/or HBsAb(+).[20] Regardless of whether there is HBsAg in the serum, there are hepatocytes that contain HBV DNA, which can begin replicating with suppression of the host's immune system.[23]

The definition of hepatitis B virus reactivation (HBVR) is not standard, and various studies have used different criteria for characterizing HBVR. However, all definitions are centered on the increasing presence of HBV DNA. HBVR can be defined by the following:

- The presence of HBV DNA in a patient who previously had undetectable levels of DNA[21]
- A 10- to 100-fold increase of the baseline level of HBV DNA[24]

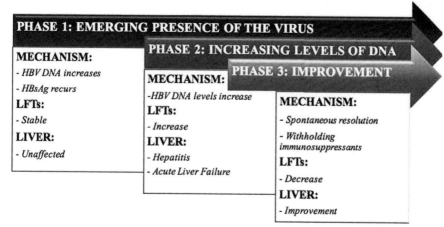

Fig. 2. The 3 phases of hepatitis B reactivation and the specific mechanisms involved in each phase.

- The de novo appearance of HBV DNA to a level at or greater than 100 IU/mL[23]
- A 3-fold increase in the baseline ALT or an ALT absolute level of 100 IU/mL[24]

The de novo appearance of HBV DNA is characterized by the presence of the genetic material in the absence of HBV antigen, HBsAg(−).[23]

Causes and mechanism of hepatitis B virus reactivation

During chronic (HBsAg+) and resolved (HBsAg−) HBV infections, the host's immune system prevents clinically significant symptoms. In the setting of immunosuppressive medication, for the treatment of various types of malignancies, inflammatory conditions, and autoimmune diseases, the risk of HBVR increases significantly.[21] The probability of an HBVR depends on a series of factors, including serologic status, viral load, type of immunosuppressive medication used, and duration of treatment.[21]

Reactivation typically occurs in 3 distinct phases. The first phase consists of an emerging presence of the virus, in either the form of increasing HBV DNA or the recurrence of HBsAg[23]; liver function tests (LFTs) remain stable and the liver remains unaffected. The second stage is characterized by increasing levels of DNA that are now accompanied by an increase in LFT. Symptoms of acute hepatitis may or may not be present.[23] It is at this second stage that a rapid progression to ALF is possible. The third stage involves an improvement of the hepatic injury secondary to either a spontaneous resolution or withholding of immunosuppressant medications.[23]

Risk factors for hepatitis B virus reactivation

As highlighted above, there are several factors that increase the risk of the development of HBVR. Detectable levels of HBV DNA, HBsAg and HBeAg positivity, and mutated viral antigens all confer a risk for the development of HBVR.[21,22]

One study that analyzed the HBsAg in HBVR found that in most cases, antigens possessed mutations that allowed them to evade detection by the humoral and cell-mediated immune systems.[25] It is likely that these mutated viruses possess an enhanced ability to reactivate in the setting of iatrogenic immunosuppression.[21]

The risk attributed to immunosuppressive medications depends on the drug class and mechanism of action. The American Gastroenterology Association has compiled the data from several studies to estimate the risk of various immunosuppressive and chemotherapeutic agents.[21] The highest risk was associated with the use of B-cell-depleting agents, anthracyclines, and corticosteroids. Numerous studies have documented the increased incidence of HBVR with the use of prednisone in a dose- and duration-dependent manner.[26,27] Corticosteroids promote the replication of HBV DNA and inhibit T-cell function.[27]

Other anti-inflammatory agents also have a significant role in HBVR. In a review assessing the use of tumor necrosis factor-α inhibitors for inflammatory conditions, it was found that HBVR occurred in up 39% of patients who were not prescribed antiviral prophylaxis.[26] Leflunomide can damage the liver and cause elevations in transaminases, an insult that can then lead to HBVR.[26] The role of methotrexate (MTX) in HBVR is still unclear; one study showed no HBVR in all chronically infected patients, whereas another saw reactivation with the conjunctive use of MTX and steroids.[26]

As the authors highlight here, the use of immunosuppressive and chemotherapeutic medications portends a significant risk of reactivation in chronically infected HBV patients. The recognition of this risk is vital in the prevention of HBVR and its progression to ALF.

Hepatitis B virus prognosis
HAV-related ALF demonstrates an overall better prognosis than that associated with HBV. HBV-related ALF has a poor rate of spontaneous resolution with about one-quarter of patients resolving and the remaining three-quarters requiring liver transplantation or dying.[4,12] The cause of ALF from HBV in some patients is not well understood. Older age or coinciding alcohol, acetaminophen, or methamphetamine usage may possibly contribute to progression of ALF.[13,14] Identifying the HBV genotype is also important because genotype D, which is more prevalent in Caucasians, has a higher prevalence in HBV-related ALF. Despite having high rates of HBV infection, Asians are often infected at birth, which is less likely to lead to ALF.[4,5]

Strategies to prevent hepatitis B virus reactivation
Screening There are several recommendations to provide HBV screening to patients in high-risk populations or if the immunosuppressive burden is expected to be high.[28] One study recommended screening all patients who will undergo treatment of hematologic malignancies.[23] A systematic review illustrated that in HBsAg + patients who underwent treatment with Rituximab, but did not receive viral prophylaxis, the rate of HBVR, liver failure, and death was 32%, 13%, and 7%, respectively.[23] Tsutsumi[28] recommends monitoring HBcAb + patients with either monthly HBV DNA PCR or following HBsAb trends, and initiating antiviral treatment when reactivation is suspected.

Antiviral prophylaxis Consideration must be given to initiating prophylactic antiviral therapy (PAT) before chemotherapy versus at the onset of HBVR.[21] In a systematic review in patients receiving chemotherapy for solid tumors, PAT reduced the risk for HBVR (odds ratio [OR] 0.12; 95% confidence interval [CI], 0.06–0.22), HBV-related hepatitis (OR 0.18; 95% CI, 0.10–0.32), and chemotherapy disruption (OR 0.10; 95% CI, 0.04–0.27).[21] The benefits of PAT are well documented, and the consequence of HBVR is dire; therefore, initiating PAT is recommended in all patients who are at risk for HBVR.

Lamivudine and entecavir, nucleoside analogues, have been effective in reducing the incidence of HBVR in immunosuppressed patients.[28] Although receiving lamivudine prophylaxis during chemotherapy, patients experienced an 87% decrease in HBVR compared with patients not given prophylaxis.[21]

Entecavir is emerging as a superior PAT agent because several studies have associated it with lower rates of HBVR as compared with lamivudine.[21] In a study of HBsAg-positive patients who received PAT, HBVR was observed in 0% of the 70 patients on entecavir compared with 7% of the 143 patients in the lamivudine group ($P = .02$)[21] The results from one randomized control trial indicated that the PAT with entecavir was associated with relative risk of 0.22 (0.08–0.61) for HBVR and had significantly fewer chemotherapy interruptions (1.6% vs 18.3%).[21]

Of note, one case series demonstrated the use of tenofovir as a PAT agent was associated with 0% HBVR in a group of 25 patients undergoing chemotherapy, and HBV DNA was undetectable in the follow-up period.[21]

As discussed, the prophylactic use of antivirals in high-risk patients makes a significant difference in the prevention of HBVR. The current guidelines suggest that PAT should be continued for 6 months after the cessation of chemosuppressive or immunosuppressive therapy and for 12 months after the use of B-cell-depleting agents.[21] After the discontinuation of PAT, patients should be monitored for at least 12 months for HBVR.[21]

Management of hepatitis B virus reactivation In the setting of HBVR, a few case series have demonstrated the efficacious use of entecavir and tenofovir to lower HBV DNA levels.[21] On the other hand, one cohort study and various case reports indicate that lamivudine is not effective in treating HBVR, and patients have died of liver failure despite receiving lamivudine at the onset of HBVR.[21]

Treatment of acute liver failure caused by hepatitis B virus
Nucleos(t)ide analogues Nucleos(t)ide analogues (NA), entecavir and lamivudine, significantly suppressed viral growth but did not improve overall survival compared with a group with no treatment.[29] Although NA have not proven to improve mortality in HBV ALF, the guidelines recommend their use in order to prevent further liver injury and progression to hepatocellular carcinoma or cirrhosis.[30]

Immune system modulating therapy The rapid deterioration seen in ALF is, in part, due to the expansive activation of the immune system, and several studies have analyzed the effects of curtailing this immune dysregulation on the progression of ACLF.[29]

Corticosteroid use is controversial. The use of steroids has been shown to be beneficial during the development of ACLF. One study from Japan detailed that the combination of NA and corticosteroids reversed the decompensation of patients during CHB exacerbations.[30] The premise behind the discovered effect is that entecavir induced viral suppression while the corticosteroid minimized the inflammatory response.[30] Various other researchers have also noted that steroids have a significant benefit in preventing the progression of liver failure, improving liver function after the onset of ACLF and improving overall survival.[29]

Hepatitis C Although a major factor in chronic hepatitis, hepatitis C virus (HCV) is not thought to be a significant cause of ALF.[4] HCV appears to only play a role with coinfection with HBV. One study showed that in 11 patients with HCV who developed ALF, 9 had concurrent HBV infection.[31] There is little evidence that HCV alone causes ALF.

Hepatitis D Hepatitis D virus (HDV) is a rare cause of ALF (see **Table 2**). HDV pathogenesis depends on coexistence with HBV.[32] HDV functions as an altered RNA virus that consists of one circular RNA strand that replicates independently of HBV. The HDV antigen, however, requires the HBsAg for encapsidation of its own genome, and in order to facilitate the assembly of the HDV genome, it depends on sharing of the envelope proteins. HDV is endemic in Mediterranean countries, the Middle East, South America and Amazonian regions, Central Asia, and Central Africa.[4,6]

HDV infection in the setting of HBV increases the risk of ALF in patients. One percent of patients infected with HBV alone will develop ALF; however, in the setting of coinfection of HDV and HBV, rates of ALF can reach about 20%.[32,33] In 2 separate studies from Europe and the United States, a more likely progression to ALF in the setting of coinfection was noted.[4,34] Most cases of coinfection lead to viral clearance.

Superinfection can also lead to ALF in about 5% of patients. Unlike coinfection, this more often leads to chronic infection estimated to be about 80% of all cases.[6] There is no approved therapy targeting HDV. HDV pathogenesis is limited to the liver because it only replicates in the liver.[33]

Changes in HDV incidence have been attributed to increased migration of people from HDV endemic nations.[35] In a study from Spain, immigrant members of the cohorts experienced the highest prevalence of HDV (10.1%).[36] Studies highlight that although the global trends of HDV prevalence have been declining over the last 30 years, the disease remains of significant concern because of immigration from endemic regions.

Hepatitis D virus prognosis

HDV-related ALF in the setting of coinfection or superinfection with HBV is considered a severe form of viral ALF. As mentioned, up to 20% of patients with coinfection can advance to have ALF, often with a poor prognosis.[35] The Baseline Event Activity score determined that older age, male gender, Mediterranean origin, elevated INR, hyperbilirubinemia, and thrombocytopenia were all associated with worse outcomes in the setting of HDV.[37]

Treatment of hepatitis D virus

Interferon-α (IFN-α) is the only medication studied extensively for treatment against HDV, and it has yielded a broad range of results. Several trials have documented that IFN-α is only marginally successful at eradicating HDV, with SVR documented in only 25% to 30% of patients, and relapse of the virus was significant.[38]

Myrcludex B, another studied agent, is a peptide that mimics regions of the HBsAg and has been developed in order to compete with intact virions for entry into cells.[39] One study found benefit in patients who received a combination of Myrcludex and IFN-α compared with Myrcludex B alone, with relapse still a major concern.[40] A scheduled phase 2 trial is underway to assess the optimal dose, duration, and frequency for the use of Myrcludex B in HBV and HDV infections.[37]

Lonafarnib is a farnesyltransferase inhibitor, a necessary enzyme for HDV production, and has been shown to be effective in vitro and in vivo. Trials indicated that lonafarnib was effective in reducing HDV RNA count and improve LFT in a dose-dependent manner.[40]

Hepatitis E

Hepatitis E virus (HEV) is a major contributor of virus-related ALF worldwide (see **Table 2**). Transmission of HEV is through contaminated water, cattle, undercooked meat, including boar, deer, and pigs, as well as sexual transmission.[41] Responsible for up to 40% of cases of ALF in developing countries, HEV is still widely thought to be underdiagnosed in cases of ALF.[39] A study in Germany demonstrated that half of cases of HEV-related ALF were initially diagnosed as DILI.[42] Similarly, studies in the United States demonstrated 3% to 22% misdiagnosis rate of patients initially thought to have DILI but later found have HEV after reassessment. Idiopathic causes of ALF have also been later found to be related to HEV.[4,43]

The manifestations of HEV infection in endemic areas range from clinically silent to ALF.[44,45] HEV infections in developed countries carry a worse prognosis, especially among middle-aged and elderly men, indicating that host factors have a role in determining the extent of the disease's course. HEV infection has been known to cause ALF in pregnant women, particularly in the third trimester.[45]

HEV prognosis is variable depending on the host. Case fatality rate for HEV is estimated at 3% in the general population.[29] However, among pregnant women, the mortality is estimated as high as 25%. The pathogenicity of HEV in the pregnant population is not well understood. Theories propose that hormonal imbalances and inadequate activation of innate immunity during pregnancy are responsible for the worse outcomes of HEV in women who are pregnant.[4,42,46]

After HEV RNA has been present in the serum for 3 months, spontaneous recovery is unlikely and antiviral therapy is indicated.[47] Ribavirin has emerged as the first-line therapy for patients with acute or chronic HEV infection.[42,46] The use of PEGylated IFN-α has also demonstrated efficacy in acute HEV in eradicating HEV RNA and reducing LFT.[44,47]

A safe and effective vaccine has been developed as prophylaxis against HEV.[44,47] The vaccine has been approved in China and will be available for use in endemic areas and in patients at high risk of infection, particularly pregnant women.

Rare viral agents

Other rare viral causes of ALF include herpes simplex and zoster, CMV, Epstein-Barr virus, and adenovirus.[4,48–51] These rare occurrences often occur in the setting of immunosuppression. Activation of such latent viruses is on the increase secondary to immunosuppressive therapy and chemotherapy.[4] In addition, advanced HIV-infected individuals are reported to have ALF from these rare cases, particularly herpes zoster infection even in the absence of a rash.[48,52] Adenovirus, especially subgroup C type 5, can lead to ALF and is often preceded by a diarrheal illness.[33] Although exceedingly rare, these viruses can be considered in the diagnostic approach of ALF in the appropriate setting of an immunocompromised host.

SUMMARY

Although its incidence is on the decline overall in the Western countries, viral hepatitis is still a key player in ALF.[4] Maintaining a high index of suspicion is critical in patients with ALF in order to quickly triage patients to the appropriate treatment setting and begin the proper management.[1] Hepatitis A, B, D, and E each are responsible for cases of ALF and are important to consider in the clinical workup in the developed and developing world.[4,5] Prompt diagnosis is important to begin early interventions in cases of virally induced ALF. Finally, testing for increasing infections such as HEV should be considered in cases where a clear diagnosis is difficult to yield.[47] Current research is investigating new treatment options in ALF, including extracorporeal devices. Such devices when medically optimized will serve a great benefit for patients suffering from ALF.

REFERENCES

1. Lee W, Squires R, Nyberg S, et al. Acute liver failure: summary of a workshop. Hepatology 2007;47:1401–15.
2. Gill R, Sterling R. Acute liver failure. J Clin Gastroenterol 2001;33:191–8.
3. Lee W. Etiologies of acute liver failure. Semin Liver Dis 2008;28:142–52.
4. Manka P, Verheyen J, Gerken G, et al. Liver failure to to acute viral hepatitis (A-E). Visc Med 2016;32:80–5.

5. Bernal W, Wendon J. Acute liver failure. N Engl J Med 2013;369:2525–34.
6. Kemmer NM, Miskovsky EP. Hepatitis A. Infect Dis Clin North Am 2000;14:605.
7. World Health Organization. WHO|Hepatitis.
8. Taylor RM, Davern T, Munoz S, et al. Fulminant hepatitis A virus infection in the United States: incidence, prognosis, and outcomes. Hepatology 2006;44:1589–97.
9. Jacobsen KH, Wiersma ST. Hepatitis A virus seroprevalence by age and world region, 1990 and 2005. Vaccine 2010;28:6653–7.
10. Ajmera V, Xia G, Vaughan G, et al. What factors determine the severity of hepatitis A-related acute liver failure? J Viral Hepat 2011;18:e167–174.
11. Fujiwara K, Yokosuka O, Ehata T, et al. Association between severity of type A hepatitis and nucleotide variations in the 5′ non-translated region of hepatitis A virus RNA: strains from fulminant hepatitis have fewer nucleotide substitutions. Gut 2002;51:82–8.
12. Liang TJ. Hepatitis B: the virus and disease. Hepatology 2009;49:S13–21.
13. Lavanchy D. Hepatitis B virus epidemiology, disease burden, treatment, and current and emerging prevention and control measures. J Viral Hepat 2004;11:97–107.
14. Wright TL, Mamish D, Combs C, et al. Hepatitis B virus and apparent fulminant non-A, non-B hepatitis. Lancet 1992;339:952.
15. Gupta S, Govindarajan S, Fong TL, et al. Spontaneous reactivation in chronic hepatitis B: patterns and natural history. J Clin Gastroenterol 1990;12:562.
16. Hoofnagle JH. Reactivation of hepatitis B. Hepatology 2009;49:S156–65.
17. Jindal A, Kumar M, Sarin SK. Management of acute hepatitis B and reactivation of hepatitis B. Liver Int 2013;33(suppl 1):164–75.
18. Baumert TF, Yang C, Schürmann P, et al. Hepatitis B virus mutations associated with fulminant hepatitis induce apoptosis in primary Tupaia hepatocytes. Hepatology 2005;41:247–56.
19. Rehermann B, Ferrari C, Pasquinelli C, et al. The hepatitis B virus persists for decades after patients' recovery from acute viral hepatitis despite active maintenance of a cytotoxic T-lymphocyte response. Nat Med 1996;2:1104–8.
20. Yamada T, Nannya Y, Suetsugu A, et al. Late reactivation of hepatitis B virus after chemotherapies for hematological malignancies: a case report and review of the literature. Intern Med 2017;56(1):115–8.
21. Pattullo V. Prevention of hepatitis B reactivation in the setting of immunosuppression. Clin Mol Hepatol 2016;22(2):219–37.
22. Yeo W, Zee B, Zhong S, et al. Comprehensive analysis of risk factors associating with hepatitis B virus (HBV) reactivation in cancer patients undergoing cytotoxic chemotherapy. Br J Cancer 2004;90:1306–11.
23. Law M, Ho R, Cheung C, et al. Prevention and management of hepatitis B virus reactivation in patients with hematological malignancies treated with anticancer therapy. World J Gastroenterol 2016;22:6484.
24. Yeo W, Chan PK, Zhong S, et al. Frequency of hepatitis B virus reactivation in cancer patients undergoing cytotoxic chemotherapy: a prospective study of 626 patients with identification of risk factors. J Med Virol 2000;62:299–307.
25. Salpini R, Colagrossi L, Bellocchi MC, et al. HBsAg genetic elements critical for immune escape correlate with HBV-reactivation upon immunosuppression. Hepatology 2015;61:823–33.
26. Sebastiani M, Atzeni F, Milazzo L, et al. Italian consensus guidelines for the management of hepatitis B virus infections in patients with rheumatoid arthritis. Joint Bone Spine 2017;84:525–30.

27. Tur-Kaspa R, Shaul Y, Moore DD, et al. The glucocorticoid receptor recognizes a specific nucleotide sequence in hepatitis B virus DNA causing increased activity of the HBV enhancer. Virology 1988;167:630–3.
28. Tsutsumi Y. Hepatitis B virus reactivation with a rituximab-containing regimen. World J Hepatol 2015;7(21):2344.
29. Liu X, Peng F, Pan Y, et al. Advanced therapeutic strategies for HBV-related acute-on-chronic liver failure. Hepatobiliary Pancreat Dis Int 2015;14:354–60.
30. Wu Y, Li X, Liu Z, et al. Hepatitis B virus reactivation and antiviral prophylaxis during lung cancer chemotherapy: a systematic review and meta-analysis. PLoS One 2017;12(6):e0179680.
31. Maheshwari A, Ray S, Thuluvath PJ. Acute hepatitis C. Lancet 2008;372:321–32.
32. Smedile A, Farci P, Verme G, et al. Influence of delta infection on severity of hepatitis B. Lancet 1982;2:945.
33. Pascarella S, Negro F. Hepatitis D virus: an update. Liver Int 2011;31:7–21.
34. Alves C, Branco C, Cunha C. Hepatitis delta virus: a peculiar virus. Adv Virol 2013;2013:560105.
35. Polson J, Lee WM, American Association for the Study of Liver Disease. AASLD position paper: the management of acute liver failure. Hepatology 2005;41: 1179–97.
36. Ordieres C, Navascués C, González-Diéguez M, et al. Prevalence and epidemiology of hepatitis D among patients with chronic hepatitis B virus infection. Eur J Gastroenterol Hepatol 2017;29:277–83.
37. Calle Serrano B, Großhennig A, Homs M, et al. Development and evaluation of a baseline-event-anticipation score for hepatitis delta. J Viral Hepat 2014;21(11): e154–63.
38. Noureddin M, Gish R. Hepatitis delta: epidemiology, diagnosis and management 36 years after discovery. Curr Gastroenterol Rep 2013;16:365.
39. Manka P, Bechmann L, Coombes J, et al. Hepatitis E virus infection as a possible cause of acute liver failure in Europe. Clin Gastroenterol Hepatol 2015;13: 1836–42.
40. Elazar M, Glenn J. Emerging concepts for the treatment of hepatitis delta. Curr Opin Virol 2017;24:55–9.
41. Chau TN, Lai ST, Tse C, et al. Epidemiology and clinical features of sporadic hepatitis E as compared with hepatitis A. Am J Gastroenterol 2006;101:292.
42. Arends J, Ghisetti V, Irving W, et al. Hepatitis E: an emerging infection in high income countries. J Clin Virol 2014;59:81–8.
43. Donnelly M, Scobie L, Crossan C, et al. Review article: hepatitis E-a concise review of virology, epidemiology, clinical presentation and therapy. Aliment Pharmacol Ther 2017;46(2):126–41.
44. Mirazo S, Ramos N, Mainardi V, et al. Transmission, diagnosis, and management of hepatitis E: an update. Hepat Med 2014;6:45–59.
45. Ahmed A, Ali I, Ghazal H, et al. Mystery of hepatitis E virus: recent advances in its diagnosis and management. Int J Hepatol 2015;2015:1–6.
46. Sharma S, Kumar A, Kar P, et al. Risk factors for vertical transmission of hepatitis E virus infection. J Viral Hepat 2017;24(11):1067–75.
47. Marano G, Vaglio S, Pupella S, et al. Hepatitis E: an old infection with new implications. Blood Transfus 2015;13:6–20.
48. Cvjetković D, Jovanović J, Hrnjaković-Cvjetković I, et al. Reactivation of herpes zoster infection by varicella-zoster virus. Med Pregl 1999;52:125.
49. Ronan BA, Agrwal N, Carey EJ, et al. Fulminant hepatitis due to human adenovirus. Infection 2014;42:105.

50. Devereaux CE, Bemiller T, Brann O. Ascites and severe hepatitis complicating Epstein-Barr infection. Am J Gastroenterol 1999;94:236.
51. Cohen JI, Corey GR. Cytomegalovirus infection in the normal host. Medicine (Baltimore) 1985;64:100–14.
52. Pinna AD, Rakela J, Demetris AJ, et al. Five cases of fulminant hepatitis due to herpes simplex virus in adults. Dig Dis Sci 2002;47:750.

Nonacetaminophen Drug-Induced Acute Liver Failure

Arul M. Thomas, MD[a], James H. Lewis, MD[b],*

KEYWORDS

- Drug-induced liver injury • Acute liver failure
- Nonacetaminophen drug-induced liver injury

KEY POINTS

- Nonacetaminophen drug injury represents 11% of all acute liver failure cases in a large acute liver failure dataset in the United States.
- Females and African Americans are disproportionally affected, with the latter having worse outcomes.
- Nearly all drugs implicated in global registries of non–acetaminophen-induced acute liver failure are older compounds that have been available for decades, but remain on the market owing to their clinical efficacy and the lack of alternative agents.
- N-Acetylcysteine has shown some benefit for non–acetaminophen-induced acute liver failure, particularly if given when patients have early stage coma grades.
- Future work is poised to elucidate potential host genetic factors that make drug-induced acute liver failure more likely and discover biomarkers that can diagnose it earlier.

INTRODUCTION

Acute liver failure (ALF) of all causes is diagnosed in between 2000 and 2500 patients annually in the United States. Although multiple etiologies are responsible, drug-induced ALF (DI-ALF) is the leading cause of ALF, accounting for more than 50% of cases overall. Even though acetaminophen (APAP), both from intentional self-harm as well as unintentional overdose, is the cause in most instances of drug-related cases, non-APAP drug injury represents 11% of all cases in the latest registry from the US ALF Study Group (US ALF SG).[1] Although rare, the development of ALF is clinically dramatic when it occurs, and requires a multidisciplinary approach to

The authors have nothing to disclose.

[a] MedStar Georgetown Transplant Institute, MedStar Georgetown University Hospital, 3800 Reservoir Road NW, Washington, DC 20007, USA; [b] Division of Gastroenterology, MedStar Georgetown University Hospital, 3800 Reservoir Road Northwest, Room M2408, Washington, DC 20007, USA
* Corresponding author.
E-mail address: lewisjh@gunet.georgetown.edu

Clin Liver Dis 22 (2018) 301–324
https://doi.org/10.1016/j.cld.2018.01.006

management. In contrast with APAP ALF, non-APAP DI-ALF has a more ominous prognosis with a lower transplant-free survival and a higher rate of chronic liver disease. DI-ALF also has had an important influence on the drug development process, with several agents having been withdrawn after approval, abandoned in the United States or not approved at all owing to the risk of ALF (**Table 1**).[2] No specific antidote is available to treat or reverse the hepatic injury from these agents, although NAC may have a role in those with early grade coma and liver support devices, such as the molecular adsorbent reticulating system (MARS; Baxter International, Deerfield, IL), have been used in some cases. Liver transplant remains the definitive therapy, but its availability remains an issue.

In this article, we summarize the recent advances in the diagnosis and management of non-APAP DI-ALF. APAP ALF is discussed in Chalermrat Bunchorntavakul and K. Rajender Reddy's article, "Acetaminophen (APAP or N-Acetyl-p-Aminophenol) and Acute Liver Failure," and ALF owing to nondrug causes is reviewed in Pavan Patel and colleagues' article, "Future Approaches and Therapeutic Modalities for Acute Liver Failure," both in this issue.

GLOBAL EPIDEMIOLOGY

In the United States, the US ALF SG has prospectively collected cases of all forms of ALF since 1998. In the initial decade of the study, 133 of 1198 subjects (11%) were suspected to have drug-induced liver injury (DILI), by expert opinion.[1] This dataset found that 70% of the subjects were female, and minorities were overrepresented (**Table 2**). Whereas APAP caused almost one-half of all cases, non-APAP DILI was the second largest group, on par with ALF owing to viral hepatitis.

In the US Drug-Induced Liver Injury Network (US DILIN), a prospective registry of patients with DILI beginning in 2004, 107 of 1089 patients died within 2 years of onset of DILI.[3] Analysis of these 107 patients who died showed that DILI had a primary role in 68 (64%) patients. Nearly three-quarters of these patients fulfilled criteria for ALF. Thirteen percent had either acute-on-chronic liver failure or acute cholestatic failure.

In an analysis of Kaiser Permanente Northern California (KPNC) admissions from 2004 to 2010, 669 patients had diagnostic and laboratory criteria suggesting ALF.[4]

Table 1
Drugs withdrawn, abandoned, or not approved in the United States owing to hepatotoxicity

Withdrawn	Abandoned	Not Approved
Iproniazid	Chloroform	Benoxaprofen
Ticrynafen	Cinchophen	Oxmetidine
Ibufenac	Phenurone	Ebrotidine
Suprofen	Phenindione	Dilevalol
Zoxazolamine	Fenclozic acid	Ajmaline
Chenodeoxycholic acid	Isoxepac	Ximelagatran
Pemoline	Thorium dioxide	Clometacine
Oxyphenisatin	Suprofen	Nimesulide
Troglitazone	Carbutamide	Lumiracoxib
Bromfenac	Metahexamide	
	Halothane (limited use elsewhere)	
	Erythromycin estolate (limited use elsewhere)	
	Phenylbutazone	

Adapted from Lewis JH. The art and science of diagnosing and managing drug-induced liver injury in 2015 and beyond. Clin Gastroenterol Hepatol 2015;13:2173–89; with permission.

Table 2
Clinical features of different ALF etiologies

	Non-APAP DI (N = 220)	APAP DI (N = 916)	Indeterminate (N = 245)	Hepatitis A/B (N = 36/142)	All Others (N = 441)
Age (median in y)	46	37	39	49/43	45
Gender (% female)	69	76	59	44/44	71
Jaundice (d)	11.5	1.0	11.0	4.0/8.0	7.0
Coma grade ≥3 (%)	35	53	48	56/52	38
Transplant (%)	40	9	42	33/39	32
Spontaneous survival (%)	24	63	22	50/21	31
Overall survival (%)	58	70	60	72/55	58

Abbreviations: ALF, acute liver failure; APAP, acetaminophen; DI, drug induced.
Adapted from Lee WM. Drug induced acute liver failure. Clin Liver Dis 2013;17:575–586; with permission.

On review of records, 62 patients had definite or possible ALF, and 32 of these patients (52%) had a drug-induced etiology. Slightly more than one-half of the patients had APAP implicated as the cause, with 14 patients having a non-APAP etiology.

Retrospective data from Denmark showed 15 of 43 patients (35%) diagnosed with DILI in a 5-year time span developed severe ALF.[5] The most common agents were disulfiram and antibiotics. In reports of suspected DILI given to the Swedish Adverse Drug Reaction Advisory Committee between 1970 and 2004, there were 784 cases. The mortality/transplantation rate was 9.2% overall.[6] A separate Swedish analysis of fulminant drug-induced hepatic failure from 1966 to 2002 demonstrated that 103 patients died or required liver transplant.[7] Data from a population-based cohort in Iceland from 2010 to 2011 showed 96 individuals diagnosed with DILI. Five of these patients developed severe DILI, using the DILI severity score.[8,9] One patient died from liver-related death.[8] In India, Devarbhavi and colleagues[10] reported a 17.3% overall mortality from severe DILI among 313 patients, with antituberculosis agents, anticonvulsants, and sulfonamides leading the list of ALF fatal causes.

A nationwide survey in Japan found that ALF from all causes was seen in 1554 patients and late-onset hepatic failure in 49 patients between 2010 and 2015.[11] The majority of patients had viral hepatitis (mostly hepatitis B). Compared with patients seen between 1998 and 2009, patients were older, and causes other than viral hepatitis were more frequent, including DI-ALF. Liver transplant was performed in 10.6% of the cohort. DI-ALF was present in 248 (15.5%) of the total, 220 cases of allergic-type reactions and 28 cases of toxic-type reactions. Specific agents were not named. Survival for the DILI groups were 86.8% overall without coma, 55.6% with ALF and 42.5% with subacute ALF.

Table 2 displays clinical features of non-APAP DI-ALF compared with different ALF etiologies.

COMMON AGENTS OF DRUG-INDUCED ACUTE LIVER FAILURE

The majority of non-APAP drugs causing ALF in the United States and around the world are from a relatively small number of chemical classes. **Table 3** lists the leading causes of adult non-APAP DI-ALF from various global registries. **Box 1** lists the leading causes of pediatric non-APAP DI-ALF. Antibiotics remain the most important causes of non-APAP DI-ALF, with specific drug classes varying geographically, and

Table 3
Leading causes of adult, nonacetaminophen DI-ALF in various registries

US ALF SG[1]	US DILIN[3]	KPNC[4]	Sweden[6,7]	India[96]
Isoniazid	Isoniazid	Isoniazid	Isoniazid	Isoniazid
Isoniazid with 2 of 3: rifampin, pyrazinamide, ethambutol	Nitrofurantoin	Amoxicillin/clavulanic acid	Trimethoprim/Sulfamethoxazole	Rifampin
Trimethoprim/sulfamethoxazole	Amoxicillin/clavulanic acid	Ibuprofen + orlistat	Flucloxacillin	Pyrazinamide
Nitrofurantoin	Azithromycin	Cytarabine + idarubicin	Halothane	Phenytoin
Phenytoin	Herbal/dietary supplements	Saw palmetto	Diclofenac	Valproic acid
Propylthiouracil		Imatinib	Naproxen	Zidovudine
Statins and ezetimibe		Leflunomide + herbals (unspecified) + lovastatin + proton pump inhibitor	Disulfiram	Stavudine
Antifungal agents		Chinese herbals	Chlorpromazine	Nevirapine
Complementary and alternative medicines and illicit substances		Nicotinic acid	Ciprofloxacin	Atorvastatin
		Tenofovir + lamivudine + zidovudine	Enalapril	
		Simvastatin + losartan		
		Pine needle tea		
		Cisplatin + herbals (unspecified)		

Abbreviations: DI-ALF, drug-induced acute liver failure; KPNC, Kaiser Permanente Northern California; US ALF SG, United States Acute Liver Failure Study Group; US DILIN, United States Drug Induced-Liver Injury Network.

Box 1
Leading causes of pediatric, nonacetaminophen DI-ALF

Isoniazid

Valproic acid

Carbamazepine

Phenobarbital

Phenytoin

Amiodarone

Minocycline

Pemoline

Pyrrolizidine alkaloids

Abbreviation: DI-ALF, drug-induced acute liver failure.
Data from Squires RH Jr. Acute liver failure in children. Semin Liver Dis 2008;28:153–66.

---

are related to the prevalence of tuberculosis, leprosy, and other acute and chronic infections. Dapsone was identified as the cause of DILI in 5.2% of 850 patients with hepatotoxicity in India, with 7 of 44 patients (16%) presenting with ALF, 2 of whom died.[12] APAP is rarely seen as a cause in India, in contrast with the United States and the European Union.[10]

In Germany, Hadem and colleagues[13] found that, among 46 patients from 11 university medical centers analyzed from 2008 to 2009, non-APAP ALF was the most common cause (32%), followed by indeterminate (24%) and viral (21%) etiologies. Interestingly, APAP was the cause of ALF in only 9% of their cases.

Within the antimicrobial classes, the incidence of ALF has been changing. For example, flucloxacillin has overtaken sulfonamides as the leading cause of DI-ALF in Sweden.[7] In India, antituberculosis drugs account for nearly three-quarters of all DI-ALF cases.[14]

RISK FACTORS FOR DRUG-INDUCED ACUTE LIVER FAILURE

Analysis of risk factors for DILI leading to ALF requires consideration of host, pharmacologic, and environmental factors. Classic host risk factors for DILI are age, female gender, preexisting liver disease, alcohol consumption, and obesity.[15–17] Recent studies, however, have started to examine these risk factors more closely with regard to developing DI-ALF.

Age

Traditionally, older age (>55 years) has been considered a risk factor for DILI, although this does not always hold for DI-ALF. In the US ALF SG, the average age was 43.8 years (range, 17–73 years; **Table 4**).[1] In the US DILIN (which included patients without ALF), the mean age was 49 years.[18] In the KPNC dataset of patients with ALF, the mean age was 65 years (range, 45–84) for herbal etiologies, 43 years (range, 39–47 years) for antimicrobial etiologies, and 49 years (range, 45–72 years) for other etiologies.[4] Retrospective data from Denmark demonstrated a mean age of 54 years (which included patients without ALF).[5] In data from Sweden, the median age was 64 years, and in data from Iceland, median age was 55 years (the Icelandic data included patients without ALF).[7,8] In a case series of 128 patients with ALF (including 21 children <18 years old) from Bangalore, India, the mean age was 38 years.[19]

Table 4
Age and gender of adult DI-ALF in various registries

	US ALF SG[1]	US DILIN[3,a]	KPNC[4]	Sweden[7,b]
Age (mean, y)	43.8	53.1	43–65 depending on etiology	64
Age, range (y)	17–73	—	39–84	47–77
Gender				
Female (%)	70	53	33–100 depending on etiology	57
Male (%)	30	47	50–66 depending on etiology	43

Abbreviations: DI-ALF, drug-induced acute liver failure; KPNC, Kaiser Permanente Northern California; US ALF SG, United States Acute Liver Failure Study Group; US DILIN, United States Drug Induced-Liver Injury Network.
ᵃ Those that died or required liver transplant 2 years after drug-induced liver injury.
ᵇ Those that died or required liver transplant between 1970 and 2004.

In the US ALF SG, there were 20 subjects greater than 60 years old, and 8 subjects greater than 65 years old.[1] Transplant-free survival was similar to the whole cohort (6 of 20 patients greater than 60 years old, 2 of 8 greater than 65 years old). A small number of patients underwent liver transplant when older than 60 years, and all survived. The older patients had higher nontransplant death rates compared with the whole cohort. In the US DILIN, those who died from DILI were younger (mean of 53.1 years vs 48.5 years) and more likely to be female.[3]

Children are also at risk for DI-ALF. It is estimated that 19% of pediatric ALF is due to a drug etiology.[20] The majority of these cases are due to APAP, with 5% of pediatric ALF attributed to a non-APAP etiology.[21,22] Mitochondrial dysfunction may explain nearly one-half of pediatric DILI, with valproate as an example.[23] Other agents include minocycline (often used to treat acne), antiepileptics, attention deficit hyperactivity disorder medications, and antidepressants[24] (see **Box 1**). Herbal and dietary supplements have also been identified to cause DILI, with increasing frequency as seen in the adult population.[25]

Gender

Female gender has been reported across many studies to have higher incidences of DILI.[15,26–31] For instance, in the US ALF SG, females accounted for 70% of patients (see **Table 4**).[1] In the US DILIN, females accounted for 59% of patients.[18] In the smaller KPNC dataset, females accounted for 50% to 100% of patients in the antimicrobial and other drug class etiologies. Among the herbal etiologies of ALF, only 2 of 6 patients were females.[4] Retrospective data from Denmark showed females accounted for 58% of patients.[5] In data from Sweden, of those with fulminant drug-induced hepatic failure from 1966 to 2002, 57% of patients were male.[7] In India, 53% of ALF cases were seen in females.[19] The higher female incidence could be attributed to a higher likelihood of hepatotoxicity from drugs.[6,28,32–35] It could also be because females use prescription (and possibly hepatotoxic) drugs more frequently.[31]

Race

The US ALF SG data showed that black patients were more likely to have DI-ALF than whites (24% vs 15%, respectively; $P = .015$).[36] The US DILIN data also have demonstrated that African Americans were more prone to develop DILI in a higher percentage or from different drugs compared with Caucasians (**Table 5**).[37] African American

Table 5
Drugs commonly implicated in idiosyncratic DILI in African Americans versus Caucasians, from US DILIN data

African Americans (N = 144)	Caucasians (N = 841)
Trimethoprim-sulfamethoxazole (7.6%)	Amoxicillin-clavulanic acid (13.4%)
Isoniazid (6.2%)	Nitrofurantoin (5.5%)
Phenytoin (4.8%)	Anabolic steroids (4.2%)
Amoxicillin-clavulanic acid (4.1%)	Isoniazid (3.6%)
Methyldopa (4.1%)	Trimethoprim-sulfamethoxazole (3.6%)
Nitrofurantoin (3.5%)	Minocycline (3%)
Unspecified herbal (3.5%)	Unspecified herbal (3%)
Allopurinol (2.7%)	Cefazolin (2.6%)
Anabolic steroids (2.7%)	Azithromycin (2%)
Diclofenac (2.7%)	Atorvastatin (1.8%)

Abbreviations: DILI, drug-induced liver injury; US DILIN, United Stated Drug Induced-Liver Injury Network.

Adapted from Chalasani N, Reddy KRK, Fontana RJ, et al. Idiosyncratic drug induced liver injury in African-Americans is associated with greater morbidity and mortality compared to Caucasians. Am J Gastroenterol 2017;112:1382–8; with permission.

individuals were overrepresented in cases caused by phenytoin, sulfamethoxazole-trimethoprim, allopurinol, and methyldopa, and underrepresented in instances of amoxicillin-clavulanate injury. Indeed, the frequency of HLA alleles reported to be higher among whites with amoxicillin-clavulanate injury has been found to be much lower in African Americans. These data also showed that African Americans with DILI had higher rates of cutaneous reactions compared with Caucasians (2.10% vs 0.36%, respectively; $P = .048$), suggesting they were more susceptible to allergic-type drug reactions, although the reason for this difference remains unclear, and they did not have more severe cutaneous reactions. However, the overall frequency of severe liver injury leading to death or liver transplantation was higher in African Americans compared with Caucasians (10% vs 6%, respectively) in the US DILIN registry.

Pharmacologic Factors

Pharmacologic risk factors for DILI include daily dosage, extent of hepatic metabolism, and degree of lipophilicity.[2,38–40] Chen and colleagues[41] have proposed a "rule of two" that states that drugs with high lipophilicity given in daily doses exceeding 100 mg were more likely to be hepatotoxic. This rule has been shown to be highly accurate when analyzing drugs that were withdrawn owing to hepatoxicity (see **Table 1**).[42] However, the sensitivity of these pharmacologic risk factors specifically for DI-ALF is not well-known. Still, it is likely that the same rules will apply to DI-ALF because the drugs involved (eg, isoniazid, trimethoprim-sulfamethoxazole, nitrofurantoin, phenytoin, and propylthiouracil, among others) are all common single agent causes of DI-ALF in the US ALF SG registry—and all are given in doses of more than 100 mg/d.

Host Genetic Factors

Genome-wide association study analyses offer the possibility of linking drugs to certain alleles that could cause DILI.[43,44] Although several causes of DILI are associated with specific HLA genotypes (eg, flucloxacillin), there have not been clear associations linking host alleles with the development of DI-ALF. Analysis of keratins, which are a major epithelial-specific subgroup of intermediate filament proteins, has found that adult hepatocytes express keratin polypeptides 8/18.[45] These polypeptides protect hepatocytes from apoptosis and necrosis. During acute liver injury (ALI), variants of natural human keratins can become pathogenic, allowing apoptosis.[46] In the US DILIN database, novel K8/18 variants were identified in 2 patients associated with fatal DI-ALF.[47]

Risk Factors of Progression to Drug-Induced Acute Liver Failure

Generally, non-APAP DI-ALF presents with a slower tempo in terms of clinical disease evolution, compared with APAP DI-ALF (see **Table 2**).[48] Poor survival with DI-ALF is associated with a longer time period from jaundice to the onset of hepatic encephalopathy.[1] In the KPNC analysis, non-APAP DI-ALF had a longer median duration from jaundice to hepatic encephalopathy than did APAP DI-ALF (8 days vs 2 days; $P<.001$).[4] In the US ALF SG, 386 patients who presented with severe ALI, but without hepatic encephalopathy (and thus no "ALF"), were analyzed from 2008 to 2013.[49] Twenty-three of the 386 patients had an etiology related to DILI (6%). Ninety of 386 patients (23%) progressed to poor outcomes, including progression to ALF, undergoing a liver transplant, or death within 21 days of study enrollment. A non-APAP etiology was at fault in most of those with poor outcomes (79%). A random Forest procedure allowed the creation of a model to predict poor outcomes. Predictors of a poor outcome were a non-APAP DI-ALF etiology, longer duration from onset of jaundice to study admission, higher APAP levels, higher bilirubin levels, and a prolonged INR.

Drug Use Past Stopping Criteria

Continuing to take a drug past the established stopping criteria may put patients at risk for more severe DILI. This pattern has been observed with isoniazid in data derived from the US DILIN from 2004 to 2013.[50] Among 69 cases of isoniazid DILI, 33 patients (55%) continued taking the drug for 7 days or more past the American Thoracic Society clinical stopping criteria. These criteria include a serum alanine aminotransferase (ALT) level of greater than 3 times the upper limit of normal, or developing clinical symptoms such as nausea, abdominal pain, jaundice, or unexplained fatigue.[51] This delay in stopping the drug was associated with more severe liver injury. In the 13 patients who died or underwent liver transplant, 9 (70%) took isoniazid for 7 days or more past stopping criteria, indicating the serious consequences of doing so.[50]

Underlying Chronic Liver Disease

Zimmerman[15] observed that underlying liver disease was rarely an independent risk factor for most cases of acute DILI. However, he did note that ALI from a drug in this setting could be more serious, and even fatal, and was prescient in predicting the current concept of acute-on-chronic liver failure.[15,52,53] In the US DILIN registry, 89 patients (10%) had chronic underlying liver disease.[18] DILI was more severe in this group, although this factor did not reach statistical significance. Mortality, however, was significantly higher (16% vs 5.2%; $P<.01$), although it is not clear how many patients died of liver-related versus other causes. Azithromycin was the only drug that seemed to be of greater risk of causing DILI in those with chronic liver disease. The literature provides evidence that a few other agents are more likely to be associated with acute DILI in the setting of chronic liver disease, including antituberculosis medications in chronic viral hepatitis.[54–56] Not all investigators have confirmed these associations with chronic liver disease, however.[57,58] Human immunodeficiency virus infection has also been implicated as a risk factor for isoniazid DILI.[59–61] Anecdotal case reports suggest that leflunomide use can be hepatotoxic in those with chronic liver disease, especially if given in combination with methotrexate.[62,63]

In a recent Italian study, nonalcoholic fatty liver disease was compared with chronic hepatitis C infection as a risk factor for DILI.[64] Fatty liver was found to increase the DILI risk by nearly 4-fold, with central obesity being a relevant factor in all patients. The number of patients with acute DILI, however, was small, being only 6 of 248 individuals (2.4%). The agents implicated in "certain" DILI by the authors included omeprazole, ticlopidine, losartan, fosinopril, piperacillin-tazobactam, and telithromycin, with only telithromycin being a well-recognized hepatotoxin.[65] Although DI-ALF did not develop in these individuals, others have also suspected nonalcoholic fatty liver disease as a possible risk factor for DILI, possibly through activation of the inflammasome.[66,67]

DIAGNOSING DRUG-INDUCED ACUTE LIVER FAILURE (VERSUS SEVERE ACUTE LIVER INJURY)

Recognition of severe ALI that can progress to ALF is critical. ALF, as defined by the US ALF SG, is any degree of hepatic encephalopathy within 26 weeks of the first symptoms, along with coagulopathy (INR >1.5) and no history of preexisting liver disease.[49] Although hepatic encephalopathy and coagulopathy certainly are keystones of the ALF diagnosis, severe ALI should also be recognized, because it can lead to ALF. This can be defined as an INR of greater than 2, ALT greater than 10 times the upper limit of normal, and total bilirubin greater than 3 times the upper limit of normal, without encephalopathy, for non-APAP etiologies. In US ALF SG data, for non-APAP etiology, 1 of 5 patients with severe ALI progressed to ALF, transplant, or death (some in combination).[49] Recognizing a drug-induced etiology requires a careful history of drug and herbal exposures over the last 6 to 12 months.[16] Latency of more than 12 months is rarely a cause of de novo DI-ALF, with the exception of agents such as nitrofurantoin, minocycline, fluoxetine, and divalproic acid.[1] A complete drug history taking is often limited owing to coma or respiratory failure when patients present with ALF. The LiverTox database is a helpful resource to review information on possible drug culprits (https://livertox.nih.gov).

The Peak of Alanine Aminotransferase in Acute Liver Failure Depends on the Etiology

In the US ALF SG, idiosyncratic DILI had a median peak ALT of 574 IU/L at presentation (range, 257–1423 IU/L; **Table 6**).[1] This value is much lower in comparison with etiologies that can cause towering elevations of aspartate aminotransferase (AST) or ALT, above 7500 IU/L, such as hypoxic hepatitis (shock liver), APAP overdose, or toxic mushroom or other chemical poisoning, and is lower than most cases of acute

Table 6
Biochemical differences of different ALF etiologies

	Non-APAP DI (N = 220)	APAP DI (N = 916)	Indeterminate (N = 245)	Hepatitis A/B (N = 36/142)	All Others (N = 441)
Alanine aminotransferase, IU/L (mean peak)	639.5	3773	865	2775/1649	681
Bilirubin, mg/dL (median peak)	20	4.3	21	12.3/18.4	14

Abbreviations: ALF, acute liver failure; APAP, acetaminophen; DI, drug-induced.
Adapted from Lee WM. Drug induced acute liver failure. Clin Liver Dis 2013;17:575–86; with permission.

fulminant viral hepatitis or even acute presentations of autoimmune hepatitis.[15,17] Certainly, some causes of acute non-APAP DILI, can present with such very high AST and ALT values.[68] However, in the presence of ALF associated with multiorgan failure, hypoxic hepatitis can supervene, and can confound the search for the etiology of the initial DILI[69] (see **Table 6**).

Acute viral hepatitis testing should initially include hepatitis A (IgM), hepatitis B (surface antigen, hepatitis B core IgM, and HBV-DNA), and hepatitis C (HCV-RNA). Acute hepatitis E virus has been diagnosed (via hepatitis E virus IgM antibody) in 3% of patients with suspected acute DILI among 318 individuals tested in the US DILIN,[70] but in only 0.4% of adults in the United States with ALF.[71] In contrast, in Europe, 10% to 15% of patients with ALF had evidence of hepatitis E virus infection, with hepatitis E virus RNA being the most sensitive marker.[72] Older patients and patient with human immunodeficiency virus infection were more likely to have hepatitis E IgM antibody positivity in the US DILIN.[70] Immunocompromised patients should be checked for Epstein-Barr virus, cytomegalovirus, and herpes simplex virus, preferably with viral load testing. Imaging should be obtained to rule out biliary processes, hepatic vascular abnormalities, and intrahepatic lesions. Ultrasound examination with Doppler can be obtained quickly, and without regard to renal function, in the critically ill patient.

Autoantibody testing should be done to rule out autoimmune diseases, which is the cause of at least 7% of ALF cases in the United States.[73] In the US ALF SG, autoantibodies were detected in 50 of 79 patients of all etiologies who were tested.[1] Nineteen patients had titers of greater than 1:40; 2 patients had anti–smooth muscle antibodies and 17 had a positive antinuclear antibody (ANA) titers. Liver histology was available in 13 of these 19 patients with high titers of anti–smooth muscle antibodies or ANA, but none of the biopsies showed typical autoimmune features. Twelve had massive or submassive necrosis and one had extensive microvascular steatosis. Nitrofurantoin and sulfasalazine were linked to smooth muscle antibody positivity in this registry. Ma-huang, nefazodone, fluoxetine, propylthiouracil, bromfenac, cerivastatin, simvastatin, troglitazone, and hydralazine were linked to high ANA titers. Antituberculosis drugs, nitrofurantoin, and ketoconazole were associated in some cases with high ANA titers. There was no rash or eosinophilia in patients with autoantibodies.

Rash did occur in 11 other patients, and was associated with phenytoin, antituberculosis medications, or sulfur drugs, and also with abacavir, allopurinol, atorvastatin, and diclofenac.[1] Eosinophilia occurred in 11 patients, and was most common with antituberculosis drugs, but also abacavir, phenytoin, disulfiram, interferon beta, and divalproic acid. Two patients had both rash and eosinophilia. Stevens-Johnson syndrome was caused by sulfasalazine or phenytoin. In the US DILIN, 9 patients had severe cutaneous drug reactions, which can be a harbinger of ALI and ALF. Drugs associated with Stevens-Johnson syndrome and toxic epidermal necrolysis were lamotrigine, azithromycin, carbamazepine, moxifloxacin, cephalexin, diclofenac, and nitrofurantoin.[18]

Liver biopsy does not have a definitive role in diagnosing DI-ALF. From the US DILIN data of 249 patients, there was no single or combination of histologic features that were pathognomonic for non-APAP DILI.[74] However, liver biopsy can be helpful to rule out other causes of liver injury, such as autoimmune diseases. Nitrofurantoin and minocycline DILI commonly has histologic features similar to autoimmune hepatitis, without an association with typical HLA alleles. Methyldopa and hydralazine DILI also has such features, although only about one-half of the time.[75] Up to 9% of well-established autoimmune hepatitis cases can be linked to a drug-induced cause.[76] This finding has implications for the duration of immunosuppressive therapy, because patients with drug-induced AIH are more likely to tolerate withdrawal of immunosuppression without relapse.[76] Liver biopsy can also evaluate for advanced fibrosis and cirrhosis, which suggest chronicity. This finding influences transplant listing, because patients with chronic liver disease cannot be listed as United Network for Organ Sharing (UNOS) status 1A, which supersedes the Model for End-stage Liver Disease (MELD) score, putting the patient at highest priority for donor organ allocation. Patients with acute-on-chronic liver failure do not qualify for UNOS status 1A listing.

APAP–cysteine adducts can be detected in the serum of patients with APAP hepatotoxicity.[77,78] According to data from the US ALF SG, one-fifth of patients with an indeterminate ALF diagnosis had positive serum testing for APAP–cysteine adducts.[79] The routine use of this assay is thought to identify APAP DILI earlier in its course and allow for quicker therapeutic intervention with N-acetylcysteine (NAC). This finding could be applicable to patients who present with ALF of an indeterminate cause, because non-APAP DI-ALF is often on the differential diagnosis when patients deny a history of APAP exposure (or cannot give a history). A new point-of-care assay, AcetaSTAT (Acetaminophen Toxicity Diagnostics, Little Rock, AR), seems to be able to identify APAP-associated ALI with a high sensitivity and specificity, and may prove useful in directing more specific treatment.[80]

TREATMENT OF ACUTE LIVER FAILURE

The treatment of DI-ALF involves the same considerations as other causes of ALF. The suspected drug must be identified and withdrawn. This process can sometimes mean that certain drugs are stopped that turn out not to be the cause of DI-ALF. Patients should be admitted to an intensive care unit at a liver transplant center. The plan of care should be devised with a critical care specialist, and must include airway protection and mechanical ventilation if respiratory failure is present, renal replacement if appropriate, and frequent neurologic examinations. Patients should be worked up promptly for a potentially life-saving liver transplant, including serology for acute and chronic liver disease, abdominal imaging, cardiac testing, and a psychosocial evaluation.[81] Patients with ALF who are critically ill qualify for UNOS status 1A liver transplant listing, which is the highest priority class for organ allocation. This status ensures very short wait times, often on the order of hours to days. The treatment of ALF, including the management of acute hepatic encephalopathy is reviewed in Pavan Patel and colleagues' article, "Future Approaches and Therapeutic Modalities for Acute Liver Failure," in this issue.

Corticosteroid use has not been proven to have benefit in ALF. Retrospective data from the US ALF SG, which included 131 patients with DI-ALF, did not find that steroid use was associated with an overall improved survival.[82] Indeed, steroids were associated with a worse survival in patients in the highest MELD score quartile. Univariate analysis showed a marginal benefit for steroids in spontaneous survival (35% vs 23%; $P = .047$), but this benefit did not persist in a multivariate analysis. Retrospective data from China suggested that steroids improved spontaneous survival in patients with ALF, up to 6 months after study admission.[83] The prior US ALF SG data had only considered patients up to 3 weeks after admission, to be labeled as spontaneous survivors.[82] In the Chinese study, patients with coma grade IV and a MELD score of greater than or equal to 35 had much lower spontaneous survival.[83] At our center, corticosteroid therapy is usually only used as a last resort, particularly if liver biopsy findings demonstrate acute inflammation.

The use of NAC has been advocated for possible use in non-APAP DI-ALF in both adults and children.[84,85] According to US ALF SG observational cohort data, NAC use has increased significantly in patients with ALF not owing to APAP between 1998 and

2013 (16% vs 49%; P<.001).[86] Lee and colleagues[87] showed significant improvements in spontaneous survival (52% vs 30%) with the use of NAC in non-APAP ALF, among patients with early coma grade I or II as compared with placebo. These data arose from a study of 173 patients with ALF of 4 etiologies: DILI, autoimmune hepatitis, hepatitis B, and indeterminate. In the subgroup of DILI patients, there was higher overall survival (79% vs 65%), and higher transplant-free survival (58% vs 27%) with NAC use. Although the primary outcome of improvement in overall survival was not achieved, no safety issues were observed with NAC use in these patients. In addition, data from the prospective US ALF SG showed significant improvements in total bilirubin and ALT values in patients with early coma grade given NAC.[88]

Darweesh and colleagues[84] from Egypt performed a prospective, multicenter, observational study of 155 adults with ALF (85 of whom were treated with NAC). They noted a liver transplant-free survival rate of 96.4% in the NAC group versus 23.3% in the control group. Liver transplant was required in 37 of 53 in the non–NAC-treated patients and the remaining 16 patients who failed to recover in the non-NAC group died. A smaller study from India of patients with ALF (some with DI-ALF) also showed a decreased mortality rate with the use of NAC.[89] The efficacy of NAC in the setting of non-APAP ALF may be related to a reduction in interleukin-17 cytokine levels.[90]

NAC is more controversial in pediatric patients with ALF. Kortsalioudaki and colleagues[85] from the Pediatric Liver Center at King's College Hospital in London studied the safety and efficacy of NAC retrospectively over 15 years in 170 children with non-APAP ALF between 1989 and 2004. The most common etiology for ALF was "indeterminate" causes (35.3%), followed by metabolic and infectious causes. Drug or toxin causes amounted to only 11 cases (6.5% of the total), of whom only 4 received NAC. Although no specifics were provided for the small number of DI-ALF cases, the authors demonstrated that NAC was safe and led to improved outcomes in children (median age, 2.0–3.5 years) with a shorter duration of stay, higher transplant-free survival, and better posttransplant survival.

In contrast, data from the Pediatric ALF SG did not show a major difference in the 1-year overall survival for children from the United States, Canada and England (median age, 3.7–4.5 years) given NAC (n = 92) or placebo (n = 92).[91] Indeed, the 1-year transplant-free survival was significantly lower with NAC, especially among those less than 2 years of age, leading the authors to conclude that their results did not support the broad use of NAC in this setting. The majority of cases were due to indeterminate causes, with only 4 patients having a non-APAP DILI etiology (1 randomized to NAC).

OUTCOMES OF DRUG-INDUCED ACUTE LIVER FAILURE

Like other forms of ALF, liver transplantation substantially decreases the risk of death in patients who do not survive without advanced interventions. In a recent mathematical model derived from the US ALF SG, the grade of hepatic encephalopathy at admission, the ALF etiology, vasopressor use, and log transformations of bilirubin and INR were significantly associated with transplant-free survival.[92] ALF etiologies could be classified as "favorable" or "unfavorable." DI-ALF was considered an unfavorable etiology.

In the US ALF SG, 36 of 133 patients recovered spontaneously.[1] In the remaining 97 patients, 56 underwent liver transplantation (58%), 17 were listed for transplantation but died waiting, and 24 were not listed. Of the patients transplanted, 4 died within the 3-week study period. The overall nontransplant mortality was 30.8%. In univariate analysis, better outcomes were associated with lower coma grades, and with lower bilirubin, INR, creatinine, and MELD scores. Age, gender, body mass index, blood pressure, drug class, type of DILI reaction, and elevations in liver enzymes were not associated with worse outcomes. Transplant-free survival was greater with NAC use than without, and coma grade was not related. The outcome was not affected by stopping the drug before or after symptoms occurred (or before or after jaundice occurred). Those who survived without transplant had shorter intervals between the onset of symptoms and stage 1 coma. The interval between jaundice and stage 1 coma was also shorter in this transplant-free survivor group.

In the multivariate logistic regression analysis, only 2 factors predicted poor outcomes: higher severity of coma and a higher MELD score. Over 2 years of follow-up, there was a statistically significant survival advantage in liver transplant recipients (92.4% surviving), compared with APAP spontaneous survivors (89.5%), and non-APAP spontaneous survivors (75.5%).[93] An analysis of the US ALF SG data did not show a difference in survival or the rate of liver transplantation between racial groups, except for transplantation being higher among Hispanics.[36]

Reddy and colleagues[94] for the US ALF SG analyzed the 21-day outcomes of 617 patients with ALF (representing about one-third of the entire cohort in the registry since 2000), of whom 95 (15.5%) were due to non-APAP DI-ALF. Overall, 117 (19%) survived without liver transplant, 108 (17.5%) died without liver transplant, and 392 (63.5%) underwent liver transplantation. Thirty-six percent of patients with APAP-induced ALF required liver transplant compared with 66% of the non-APAP DI-ALF group. With specific regard to the 95 non-APAP DI-patients with ALF, spontaneous survival was seen in only 11 patients (9%), and 21 (20%) died without liver transplant, compared with 40.5% and 23.7%, respectively, among the 173 patients in the APAP-ALF group.

An analysis of the US DILIN registry was undertaken to characterize fatal outcomes (or the need for liver transplantation) within 2 years of onset of DILI.[3] Among the 1089 patients enrolled between September 2004 and April 2015 who met criteria for severe acute DILI (ALT or AST >5× the upper limit of normal and/or alkaline phosphatase >2× the upper limit of normal on ≥2 consecutive occasions, total bilirubin of >2.5 mg/dL, or INR of >1.5 accompanied by any elevation in liver tests; excluding APAP overdose, autoimmune hepatitis, and primary biliary cholangitis), 107 (9.8%) died of any cause within 2 years from the time of the diagnosis. It was determined that DILI was the primary cause of death in nearly two-thirds of these cases (64%), contributed to death in 14%, and played no role in the death of the patient in 21%. Overall, severe acute DILI was the primary or contributory cause of death in 7.6% of patients enrolled in the US DILIN, and increased to 9.5% for patients presenting with bilirubin greater than 2.5 mg/dL, figures that validate the early observations of Hyman Zimmerman, which came to be known as Hy's law.[2] The drugs most commonly implicated in fatal ALF were herbal/dietary supplements, isoniazid, nitrofurantoin, amoxicillin/clavulanic acid, and azithromycin.[3] Herbal/dietary supplements were also the leading causes of acute-on-chronic liver failure and chronic liver failure, although the total numbers of patients was much smaller.[3]

In the US DILIN cases where DILI was the primary cause of death, the injury was ALF in 74%, acute-on-chronic liver failure in 7%, chronic liver failure in 13%, and acute cholestatic failure in 6%, with death occurring within 26 weeks of onset.[3] Malignancy was cited as the leading cause of death (55%) in the 21% of fatalities where DILI was not considered to have played a role. Patients in whom DILI was the primary cause of death (or required liver transplantation) were younger compared with those where DILI played no role (mean age, 50.7 vs 57.9 years), more likely to be female (62% vs 27%), more likely to be hepatocellular (74% vs 36%), and more likely to have met Hy's law (40.3% vs 13.6%) or the new ratio Hy's law criteria (65.6% vs 9.1%).[95] They were more likely to have had a drug reaction with eosinophilia and systemic symptoms or Stevens-Johnson syndrome, worsening of underlying liver disease, and sepsis or malignancy contribute to their death.[3] The MELD score was the best predictor of death within 26 weeks, especially when greater than 19.

African Americans were found to generally have a more severe illness in the US DILIN database, as measured by total bilirubin, INR, and DILIN severity score. There was also a higher association of severe cutaneous reactions, as compared with Caucasians. African Americans were more likely to be hospitalized, require liver transplantation, or have a liver-related death by 6 months.[37]

A retrospective analysis of the KPNC admissions data (which included APAP ALF) demonstrated that of 32 patients with drug-induced ALF, 18 were APAP related, and only 1 patient with APAP-related toxicity died.[4] Fourteen of the 32 patients were non-APAP related, and 3 died in this group. Of the 32 patients, 12 were transferred to a liver transplant center, 6 were transplanted, and 6 survived without transplant. Twenty patients were not transferred to a liver transplant center—4 died in hospital and 16 were discharged alive.

In Mumbai, India, 82 cases of acute DILI were diagnosed in 2014 and 2015, and 49% were from antituberculosis agents.[96] Other causes included anticonvulsants (12%), complementary and alternative medicines (10%), antiretrovirals (9%), and nonsteroidal antiinflammatory drugs (6%). Deaths were recorded in 10% of those with hepatocellular injury, 17% with cholestatic injury, and 24% with mixed injury. A liver-related death (with presumed ALF) was present in more than one-half of these patients. Death rates owing to the leading individual agents included 9 of 40 antituberculosis agents (22.5%), 2 of 10 anticonvulsants (20%), none of 8 complementary and alternative medicines, 1 of 7 (14.3%) from antiretrovirals, and none of 5 nonsteroidal antiinflammatory drugs. As with other series, mortality was correlated with higher MELD scores compared with survivors (28.7 vs 11.7), higher levels of hyperbilirubinemia (11.9 mg/dL vs 4.6 mg/dL), and a prolonged INR (2.5 vs 1.2).

In a related series from Bangalore, India, Devarbhavi and colleagues[97] analyzed the outcomes of 269 patients with antituberculosis DILI. Without the availability of liver transplantation, the overall 90-day mortality was 22.7%, similar to that reported by Rathi and colleagues.[96,97] When acute DILI was accompanied by jaundice, encephalopathy, or ascites, mortality increased to 30%, 69.6%, and 50.7%, respectively. An antituberculosis medication DILI model using bilirubin, INR, encephalopathy, creatinine, and albumin predicted mortality with a C-statistic of 97%, compared with a MELD score with an 88% mortality prediction. These investigators have previously reported high mortality rates for other drug classes as well from their center, before the availability of liver transplantation.[10]

A retrospective cohort study analyzing liver transplantation for DI-ALF between 1987 and 2006 using the UNOS database found that 661 patients underwent liver transplantation for DI-ALF.[98] The 4 major drug etiologies were APAP (n = 265 [40%]), antituberculosis drugs (n = 50 [8%]), antiepileptics (n = 46 [7%]), and antibiotics (n = 39 [6%]). The 1-year estimated survival probabilities were 76%, 82%, 52%, 82%, and 79% for APAP, antituberculosis drugs, antiepileptics, antibiotics, and other agents, respectively. The lower survival probability for antiepileptics was seen primarily in children. The difference in overall survival after liver transplantation, between APAP-related and non–APAP-related DI-ALF, was not significant.

There is some risk for chronic liver to develop after acute DILI, although specific data on chronicity after DILI with ALF without transplantation are lacking. Data from the US DILIN showed that 19% of patients with definite, probably, or very likely DILI had persistent AST, ALT, or alkaline phosphatase abnormalities after 6 months, and 75% of these patients still had abnormalities 12 months after DILI onset, most of which were only minor enzyme elevations.[99] On multivariable analysis, these patients were more likely to be older and to have had cholestatic DILI at onset, which historically has led to a longer recovery period and a risk of developing a vanishing bile duct syndrome.[100–102] In the Spanish DILI registry, 273 of 298 patients normalized their liver tests, imaging findings, or hepatic histology within 1 year of DILI recognition.[103] Twenty-five patients (8.4%) had ongoing signs of liver injury. Independent risk factors were older age, dyslipidemia, and severe DILI at initial presentation. In the 9 cases who underwent liver biopsy, 2 patients had ductal lesions and 7 patients had cirrhosis. Insofar as non-APAP DI-ALF is largely hepatocellular in nature, the risk of chronic injury persisting more than 1 year after spontaneous recovery is likely to be quite low.

Table 2 displays overall survival of non-APAP DI-ALF compared with other ALF etiologies.

FUTURE DIRECTIONS IN DRUG-INDUCED ACUTE LIVER FAILURE: DIAGNOSIS

The measurement of serum aminotransferases and clinical observation have been the hallmarks of DILI diagnosis for decades. There is substantial ongoing interest in identifying novel diagnostic and prognostic markers, both for acute DILI as well as progression to DI-ALF. Mechanisms involving mitochondrial dysfunction, oxidative stress, and alterations in bile acid homeostasis have been defined in intrinsic DILI, and may be important in idiosyncratic DILI and ALF as well.[104] Adaptive immune responses also play a part in idiosyncratic DILI.[104] Work in metabolomics and proteomics have identified potential targets of DILI that might identify DILI at an earlier time. Biomarkers such as high mobility group box 1 (HMGB1) and keratin-18 have been linked to APAP ALI.[105,106] HMGB1 could be a therapeutic target in ALF.[107] Mitochondrial RNAs (miRNAs) are nonencoding RNAs involved in the posttranscription regulation of gene expression.[108] They are released in organ damage. MiR-122 and MiR-192 levels are increased after toxic APAP exposure in mice.[108] Further testing is needed to determine if this is significant in idiosyncratic DILI. Testing multiple different miRNAs in profiles may have higher diagnostic value.[109]

Kupffer cells have received attention in DI-ALF, owing to their role in mediating liver inflammation. Data from the US ALF SG showed that galectin-9, which is produced by Kupffer cells, was measured in significantly higher concentrations in patients with ALF.[110] The study group was overrepresented by APAP ALF, but the levels did not vary significantly between APAP DILI and non-APAP DILI. Higher levels of galectin-9 had significant associations with the risk of mortality and need for liver transplantation. Patients could potentially be stratified into high-, intermediate-, and low-risk DI-ALF groups based on the level of this biomarker. Galectin-9 may also improve the accuracy of MELD score in predicting outcomes in DI-ALF.

Osteopontin is another novel phosphoglycoprotein expressed in Kupffer cells that may hold promise in diagnosing DI-ALF. It helps to activate natural killer cells, neutrophils, and macrophages. Data from the US ALF SG showed that, in comparison with controls, patients with ALF had very high levels of osteopontin.[111] Levels were the highest in hyperacute causes of ALF, namely, ischemic hepatitis and APAP, and were lower in etiologies such as non-APAP DILI, viral hepatitis, and autoimmune hepatitis. Despite being lower in these latter etiologies, the levels were still much higher than in control patients. Interestingly, the control group included patients with rheumatoid arthritis and patients who were postoperative from spinal fusion surgery, to allow for baseline inflammation levels. There remains a question as to whether osteopontin might actually be protective in liver injury, because the etiologies with the highest levels had a tendency to resolve with good outcomes.

FUTURE DIRECTIONS IN DRUG-INDUCED ACUTE LIVER FAILURE: TREATMENT

Artificial and bioartificial liver support systems may gain traction in the treatment of patients with ALF in the years ahead. MARS is approved in the United States for acute poisoning and hepatic encephalopathy.[112] It uses albumin dialysis as a form of artificial liver support. Uncontrolled clinical trials implementing MARS for APAP DILI have shown improved clinical parameters in treated patients, possibly owing to the accelerated clearance of APAP.[113,114] Other clinical trials have shown improvements in short-term liver recovery, but not in 6-month survival.[115,116] It should be noted that most of these trials enrolled small groups of heterogenous patients with ALF, with an unclear proportion of DI-ALF cases. The role of early liver transplantation and spontaneous recovery of liver function also limit conclusions about the short-term benefits of MARS and other artificial liver support systems. A retrospective, case-controlled study showed improved short-term response in ALI, but the 28-day mortality was not improved with MARS, compared with standard medical therapy.[117] This study examined only 20 patients with MARS, with 15 of the 20 having acute DILI. The standard medical therapy group included 30 patients, 12 of whom had DILI. Other studies show similar results. For example, a single-center, retrospective study of 27 patients with severe ALF of multiple etiologies showed that MARS could be a successful bridge to transplantation.[118] However, it was not clear how many patients had a non-APAP DILI etiology, although 5 were classified as having a toxic ingestion. A case series of 4 patients with biopsy-proven anabolic steroid-induced cholestasis showed that liver function could be improved using MARS, and avoided liver transplantation.[119]

Other artificial liver support systems include single-pass albumin dialysis, fractionated plasma and adsorption, and high-volume plasma exchange. These technologies do not yet have significant data on their usefulness in DI-ALF.[120–122] Bioartificial liver support systems, including extracorporeal liver assist devices, also will require more experience in the treatment of patients with ALF, although a modified extracorporeal liver assist system showed a decrease in mortality in pigs with APAP-induced ALF.[123]

Stravitz and colleagues[124] from the US ALF SG analyzed the safety and efficacy of L-ornithine phenylacetate in 47 patients with hyperammonemia from ALF and ALI. The initial subjects were APAP DI-ALF, although entry was opened later to other etiologies. Ornithine phenylacetate decreases serum ammonia and the risk of cerebral edema by increasing its renal excretion as phenylacetylglutamine. It was well-tolerated in this preliminary study, with headache and nausea/vomiting reported as nonserious adverse events, and may offer an additional pharmacologic tool for managing hepatic encephalopathy in these patients.

SUMMARY

Non-APAP DILI is implicated in more than 1 in 10 cases of ALF in the United States. It has a high mortality without liver transplantation, as seen in datasets from the US ALF SG, the US DILIN, and other registries. Females and African Americans are disproportionately affected, with the latter having worse outcomes. Of interest is the fact that nearly all of the drugs implicated in global registries of non-APAP DI-ALF are older compounds that have been available for decades, but remain on the market owing to their clinical efficacy and the lack of alternative agents. Fortunately, the risk of ALF from these drugs is low compared with their overall use. The diagnosis of DI-ALF can be difficult owing to challenges in obtaining a proper medication exposure history, as well as confounding results, such as the presence of autoantibodies. Treatment, like that for all forms of ALF, requires a multidisciplinary approach to care, preferably at a liver transplant center. NAC has shown some benefit for non-APAP DILI, particularly if given when patients have early stage coma grades. Future work is poised to elucidate potential host genetic factors that make DI-ALF more likely to occur, as well as to discover biomarkers that can diagnose DI-ALF at an earlier timepoint. Galectin-9 may become a useful such biomarker to stratify patients with DI-ALF by risk of severity. As with all etiologies of ALF, an increase in transplant-free survival is the primary goal, especially in this era of donor organ shortages.

REFERENCES

1. Reuben A, Koch DG, Lee WM, the Acute Liver Failure Study Group. Drug induced acute liver failure: results of a U.S. multicenter, prospective study. Hepatology 2010;52:2065–76.
2. Lewis JH. The art and science of diagnosing and managing drug-induced liver injury in 2015 and beyond. Clin Gastroenterol Hepatol 2015;13:2173–89.
3. Hayashi PH, Rockey DC, Fontana RJ, et al. Death and liver transplantation within 2 years of onset of drug-induced liver injury. Hepatology 2017;66:1275–85.
4. Goldberg DS, Forde KA, Carbonari DM, et al. Population-representative incidence of drug-induced acute liver failure based on an analysis of an integrated health care system. Gastroenterology 2015;148:1353–61.
5. Baekdal M, Ytting H, Skalshoi Kjaer M. Drug-induced liver injury: a cohort study on patients referred to the Danish transplant center over a five year period. Scand J Gastroenterol 2017;52:450–4.
6. Björnsson E, Olsson R. Outcome and prognostic markers in severe drug-induced liver disease. Hepatology 2005;42:481–9.
7. Björnsson E, Jerlstad P, Berggvist A, et al. Fulminant drug-induced hepatic failure leading to death or liver transplantation in Sweden. Scand J Gastroenterol 2005;40:1095–101.
8. Björnsson ES, Bergmann OM, Björnsson HK, et al. Incidence, presentation, and outcomes in patients with drug-induced liver injury in the general population of Iceland. Gastroenterology 2013;144:1419–25.
9. Aithal GP, Watkins PB, Andrade RJ, et al. Case definition and phenotype standardization in drug-induced liver injury. Clin Pharmacol Ther 2011;89:806–15.
10. Devarbhavi H, Dierkhising R, Kremers WK, et al. Single-center experience with drug-induced liver injury from India: causes, outcome, prognosis, and predictors of mortality. Am J Gastroenterol 2010;105:2396–404.
11. Nakao M, Nakayama N, Uchida Y, et al. Nationwide survey for acute liver failure and late-onset hepatic failure in Japan. J Gastroenterol 2017. [Epub ahead of print].
12. Devarbhavi H, Raj S, Joseph T, et al. Features and treatment of dapsone-induced hepatitis, based on analysis of 44 cases and literature review. Clin Gastroenterol Hepatol 2017;15:1805–7.
13. Hadem J, Tacke F, Bruns T, et al, Acute Liver Failure Study Group Germany. Etiologies and outcomes of acute liver failure in Germany. Clin Gastroenterol Hepatol 2012;10:664–9.
14. Devarbhavi H. Acute liver failure induced by anti-infectious drugs: causes and management. Curr Hepatol Rep 2017. https://doi.org/10.1007/s11901-017-0367-5.
15. Zimmerman HJ. Hepatotoxicity: the adverse effects of drugs and other chemicals on the liver. Philadelphia: Lippincott, William & Wilkins; 1999.

16. Chalasani NP, Hayashi PH, Bonkovsky HL, et al. ACG clinical guideline: the diagnosis and management of idiosyncratic drug-induced liver injury. Am J Gastroenterol 2014;109:950–66.

17. Lewis JH. Drug-induced liver disease. Med Clin North Am 2000;84:1275–311.

18. Chalasani N, Bonkovsky HL, Fontana R, et al. Features and outcomes of 899 patients with drug-induced liver injury: the DILIN prospective study. Gastroenterology 2015;148:1340–52.

19. Devarbhavi H, Patil M, Reddy VV, et al. Drug-induced acute liver failure in 128 patients including children: implicated drugs, outcomes, predictors of mortality, - results from a single-center drug-induced liver injury registry. Hepatology 2017;66(S1):674–5A, [abstract: 1249].

20. Amin MD, Harpavat S, Leung DH. Drug-induced liver injury in children. Curr Opin Pediatr 2015;27:625–33.

21. Squires RH Jr. Acute liver failure in children. Semin Liver Dis 2008;28:153–66.

22. Murray KF, Hadzic N, Wirth S, et al. Drug-related hepatotoxicity and acute liver failure. J Pediatr Gastroenterol Nutr 2008;47:395–405.

23. Hunt CM, Yuen NA, Stirnadel-Farrant HA, et al. Age-related differences in reporting of drug-associated liver injury: data-mining of WHO Safety Report Database. Regul Toxicol Pharmacol 2014;70:519–26.

24. Molleston JP, Fontana RJ, Lopez MJ, et al. Characteristics of idiosyncratic drug-induced liver injury in children: results from the DILIN prospective study. J Pediatr Gastroenterol Nutr 2011;53:182–9.

25. Wu CH, Wang CC, Kennedy J. The prevalence of herb and dietary supplement use among children and adolescents in the United States: results from the 2007 National Health Interview Survey. Complement Ther Med 2013;21:358–63.

26. Russo MW, Galanko JA, Shrestha R, et al. Liver transplantation for acute liver failure from drug induced injury in the United States. Liver Transpl 2004;10: 1018–23.

27. Ostapowicz G, Fontana RJ, Schiødt FV, et al, U.S. Acute Liver Failure Study Group. Results of a prospective study of acute liver failure at 17 tertiary care centers in the United States. Ann Intern Med 2002;137:947–54.

28. Andrade RJ, Lucena MI, Fernández MC, et al, Spanish Group for the Study of Drug-Induced Liver Disease. Drug-induced liver injury: an analysis of 461 incidences submitted to the Spanish Registry over a 10-year period. Gastroenterology 2005;129:512–21.

29. Rakela J, Lange SM, Ludwig J, et al. Fulminant hepatitis: Mayo Clinic experience with 34 cases. Mayo Clin Proc 1985;60:289–92.

30. Schilsky ML, Scheinberg IH, Sternlieb I. Hepatic transplantation for Wilson's disease: indications and outcome. Hepatology 1994;19:583–7.

31. Centers for Disease Control and Prevention. National Center for Health Statistics. National health and nutrition examination survey. Patterns of prescription drug use in the United States, 1988-94. Available at: http://www.cdc.gov/nchs/data/nhanes/databriefs/preuse.pdf. Accessed January 31, 2018.

32. Chalasani N, Fontana RJ, Bonkovsky HL, et al, Drug Induced Liver Injury Network (DILIN). Causes, clinical features, and outcomes from a prospective study of drug induced liver injury in the United States. Gastroenterology 2008; 135:1924–34.

33. Bjornsson E, Olsson R. Suspected drug-induced liver fatalities reported to the WHO database. Dig Liver Dis 2006;38:33–8.

34. Navarro VJ, Senior JR. Drug-related hepatotoxicity. N Engl J Med 2006;354: 731–9.

35. Kaplowitz N. Drug-induced liver disease. Chapter 1. In: Kaplowtiz N, DeLeve LD, editors. Drug-induced liver disease. 2nd edition. New York: Informa Healthcare; 2007. p. 1–11.

36. Forde KA, Reddy KR, Troxel AB, et al, Acute Liver Failure Study Group. Racial and ethnic differences in presentation, etiology, and outcomes of acute liver failure in the United States. Clin Gastroenterol Hepatol 2009;7:1121–6.

37. Chalasani N, Reddy KRK, Fontana RJ, et al. Idiosyncratic drug Induced liver injury in African-Americans is associated with greater morbidity and mortality compared to Caucasians. Am J Gastroenterol 2017;112:1382–8.

38. Corsini A, Bortolini M. Drug-induced liver injury: the role of drug metabolism and transport. J Clin Pharmacol 2013;53:463–74.

39. Vuppalanchi R, Gotur R, Reddy KR, et al. Relationship between characteristics of medications and drug-induced liver disease phenotype and outcome. Clin Gastroenterol Hepatol 2014;12:1550–5.

40. Lewis JH. Drug-induced liver injury, dosage, and drug disposition: is idiosyncrasy really unpredictable? Clin Gastroenterol Hepatol 2014;12:1556–61.

41. Chen M, Borlak J, Tong W. High lipophilicity and high daily dose of oral medications are associated with significant risk for drug induced liver injury. Hepatology 2013;58:388–96.

42. Chen M, Tung CW, Shi Q, et al. A testing strategy to predict risk for drug-induced liver injury in humans using high-content screen assays and the 'rule-of-two' model. Arch Toxicol 2014;88:1439–49.

43. Daly AK, Day CP. Genetic association studies in drug-induced liver injury. Drug Metab Rev 2012;44:116–26.

44. Daly AK. Are polymorphisms in genes relevant to drug disposition predictors of susceptibility to drug-induced liver injury? Pharm Res 2017;34:1564–9.

45. Ku NO, Strnad P, Bantel H, et al. Keratins: biomarkers and modulators of apoptotic and necrotic cells death in the liver. Hepatology 2016;64:966–76.

46. Strnad P, Zhou Q, Hanada S, et al. Keratin variants predispose to acute liver failure and adverse outcome: race and ethnic associations. Gastroenterology 2010;139:828–35.

47. Usachov V, Urban TJ, Fontana RJ, et al, Drug-Induced Liver Injury Network. Prevalence of genetic variants of keratins 8 and 18 in patients with drug-induced liver injury. BMC Med 2015;13:196.

48. Lee WM. Drug-induced acute liver failure. Clin Liver Dis 2013;17:575–86.

49. Koch DG, Speiser JL, Durkalski V, et al. The natural history of severe acute liver injury. Am J Gastroenterol 2017;112:1389–96.

50. Hayashi PH, Fontana RJ, Chalasani NP, et al, the US Drug-Induced Liver Injury Network Investigators. Under-reporting and poor adherence to monitoring guidelines for severe cases of isoniazid hepatotoxicity. Clin Gastroenterol Hepatol 2015;13:1676–82.

51. Saukonnen JJ, Cohn DL, Jasmer RM, et al, ATS (American Thoracic Society) Hepatotoxicity of Antituberculosis Therapy Subcommittee. An official ATS statement: hepatotoxicity of antituberculosis therapy. Am J Respir Crit Care Med 2006;174:935–52.

52. Jalan R, Williams R. Acute-on-chronic liver failure: pathophysiological basis of therapeutic options. Blood Purif 2002;20:252–61.

53. Olson JC. Acute-on-chronic and decompensated chronic liver failure: definitions, epidemiology, and prognostication. Crit Care Clin 2016;32:301–9.

54. Kaneko Y, Nagayama N, Kawabe Y, et al. Drug-induced hepatotoxicity caused by anti-tuberculosis drugs in tuberculosis patients complicated with chronic hepatitis. Kekkaku 2008;83:13–9.

55. Chang KC, Leung CC, Yew WW, et al. Hepatotoxicity of pyrazinamide: cohort and case-control analyses. Am J Respir Crit Care Med 2008;177:1391–6.

56. Fernández-Villar A, Sopeña B, García J, et al. Hepatitis C virus RNA in serum as a risk factor for isoniazid hepatotoxicity. Infection 2007;35:295–7.

57. Bliven EE, Podewils LJ. The role of chronic hepatitis in isoniazid hepatotoxicity during treatment for latent tuberculosis infection. Int J Tuberc Lung Dis 2009; 13:1054–60.

58. Sadaphal P, Astemborski J, Graham NM, et al. Isoniazid preventive therapy, hepatitis C virus infection, and hepatotoxicity among injection drug users infected with Mycobacterium tuberculosis. Clin Infect Dis 2001;33:1687–91.

59. Nader LA, de Mattos AA, Picon PD, et al. Hepatotoxicity due to rifampicin, isoniazid and pyrazinamide in patients with tuberculosis: is anti-HCV a risk factor? Ann Hepatol 2010;9:70–4.

60. Walker NF, Kliner M, Turner D, et al. Hepatotoxicity and antituberculosis therapy: time to revise UK guidance? Thorax 2009;64:918.

61. Yimer G, Aderaye G, Amogne W, et al. Anti-tuberculosis therapy-induced hepatotoxicity among Ethiopian HIV-positive and negative patients. PLoS One 2008; 3:e1809.

62. Alcorn N, Saunders S, Madhok R. Benefit-risk assessment of leflunomide: an appraisal of leflunomide in rheumatoid arthritis 10 years after licensing. Drug Saf 2009;32:1123–34.

63. Lee SW, Park HJ, Kim BK, et al. Leflunomide increases the risk of silent liver fibrosis in patients with rheumatoid arthritis receiving methotrexate. Arthritis Res Ther 2012;14:R232.

64. Tarantino G, Conca P, Basile V, et al. A prospective study of acute drug-induced liver injury in patients suffering from non-alcoholic fatty liver disease. Hepatol Res 2007;37:410.

65. Brinker AD, Wassel RT, Lyndly J, et al. Telithromycin-associated hepatotoxicity: clinical spectrum and causality assessment of 42 cases. Hepatology 2009;49: 250–7.

66. Massart J, Begriche K, Moreau C, et al. Role of nonalcoholic fatty liver disease as risk factor for drug-induced hepatotoxicity. J Clin Transl Res 2017; 3(suppl 1):212.

67. Szabo G, Petrasek J. Inflammasome activation and function in liver disease. Nat Rev Gastroenterol Hepatol 2015;12:387.

68. Vuppalanchi R, Hayashi PH, Chalasani N, et al, Drug-Induced Liver Injury Network. Duloxetine hepatotoxicity: a case-series from the Drug-Induced Liver Injury Network. Aliment Pharmacol Ther 2010;32:1174–83.

69. Aboelsoud MM, Javaid AI, Al-Qadi MO, et al. Hypoxic hepatitis - its biochemical profile, causes and risk factors of mortality in critically-ill patients: a cohort study of 565 patients. J Crit Care 2017;41:9–15.

70. Davern T, Chalasani N, Fontana RJ, et al, Drug-Induced Liver Injury Network. Acute hepatitis E infection accounts for some cases of suspected drug-induced liver injury. Gastroenterology 2011;141:1665–72.

71. Fontana RJ, Engle RE, Scaglione S, et al, US Acute Liver Failure Study Group. The role of hepatitis E virus infection in adult Americans with acute liver failure. Hepatology 2016;64:1870–80.

72. Manka P, Bechmann LP, Coombes JD, et al. Hepatitis E virus infection as a possible cause of acute liver failure in Europe. Clin Gastroenterol Hepatol 2015;13:1836–42.

73. Tujios SR, Lee WM. Acute liver failure induced by idiosyncratic reaction to drugs: challenges in diagnosis and therapy. Liver Int 2018;38(1):6–14.

74. Kleiner DE, Chalasani NP, Lee WM, et al, Drug-Induced Liver Injury Network. Hepatic histological findings in suspected drug-induced liver injury: systematic evaluation and clinical associations. Hepatology 2014;59:661–70.

75. de Boer YS, Kosinski AS, Urban TJ, et al, Drug-Induced Liver Injury Network. Features of autoimmune hepatitis in patients with drug-induced liver injury. Clin Gastroenterol Hepatol 2017;15:103–12.

76. Björnsson E, Talwalkar J, Treeprasertsuk S, et al. Drug-induced autoimmune hepatitis: clinical characteristics and prognosis. Hepatology 2010;51:2040–8.

77. Roberts DW, Bucci TJ, Benson RW, et al. Immunohistochemical localization and quantification of the 3-(cystein-S-yl)-acetaminophen protein adduct in acetaminophen hepatotoxicity. Am J Pathol 1991;138:359–71.

78. Frey SM, Wiegand TJ, Green JL, et al. Confirming the causative role of acetaminophen in indeterminate acute liver failure using acetaminophen-cysteine adducts. J Med Toxicol 2015;11:218–22.

79. Khandelwal N, James LP, Sanders C, et al, Acute Liver Failure Study Group. Unrecognized acetaminophen toxicity as a cause of indeterminate acute liver failure. Hepatology 2011;53:565–76.

80. Roberts DW, Lee WM, Hinson JA, et al. An immunoassay to rapidly measure acetaminophen protein adducts accurately identifies patients with acute liver injury or failure. Clin Gastroenterol Hepatol 2017;15:555–62.

81. Martin P, DiMartini A, Feng S, et al. Evaluation for liver transplantation in adults: 2013 practice guideline by the American Association for the Study of Liver Diseases and the American Society of Transplantation. Hepatology 2014;59: 1144–65.

82. Karkhanis J, Verna EC, Chang MS, et al, Acute Liver Failure Study Group. Steroid use in acute liver failure. Hepatology 2014;59:612–21.

83. Zhao B, Zhang HY, Xie GJ, et al. Evaluation of the efficacy of steroid therapy on acute liver failure. Exp Ther Med 2016;12:3121–9.

84. Darweesh SK, Ibrahim MF, El-Tahawy MA. Effect of N-acetylcysteine on mortality and liver transplantation rate in non-acetaminophen-induced acute liver failure: a multicenter study. Clin Drug Investig 2017;37:473–82.

85. Kortsalioudaki C, Taylor RM, Cheeseman P, et al. Safety and efficacy of N-acetylcysteine in children with non-acetaminophen-induced acute liver failure. Liver Transpl 2008;14:25–30.

86. Reuben A, Tillman H, Fontana RJ, et al. Outcomes in adults with acute liver failure between 1998 and 2013: an observational cohort study. Ann Intern Med 2016;164:724–32.

87. Lee WM, Hynan LS, Rossaro L, et al, Acute Liver Failure Study Group. Intravenous N-acetylcysteine improves transplant-free survival in early stage non-acetaminophen acute liver failure. Gastroenterology 2009;137:856–64.

88. Singh S, Hynan LS, Lee WM, Acute Liver Failure Study Group. Improvements in hepatic serological biomarkers are associated with clinical benefit of intravenous N-acetylcysteine in early stage non-acetaminophen acute liver failure. Dig Dis Sci 2013;58:1397–402.

89. Nabi T, Nabi S, Rafiq N, et al. Role of N-acetylcysteine treatment in non-acetaminophen-induced acute liver failure: a prospective study. Saudi J Gastro-enterol 2017;23:169–75.

90. Stravitz RT, Sanyal AJ, Reisch J, et al, Acute Liver Failure Study Group. Effects of N-acetylcysteine on cytokines in non-acetaminophen acute liver failure: potential mechanism of improvement in transplant-free survival. Liver Int 2013; 33:1324–31.

91. Squires RH, Dhawan A, Alonso E, et al, Pediatric Acute Liver Failure Study Group. Intravenous N-acetylcysteine in pediatric patients with nonacetaminophen acute liver failure: a placebo-controlled clinical trial. Hepatology 2013; 57:1542–9.

92. Koch DG, Tillman H, Durkalski V, et al. Development of a model to predict transplant-free survival of patients with acute liver failure. Clin Gastroenterol Hepatol 2016;14:1199–206.

93. Fontana RJ, Ellerbe C, Durkalski VE, et al, US Acute Liver Failure Study Group. Two-year outcomes in initial survivors with acute liver failure: results from a prospective, multicentre study. Liver Int 2015;35:370–80.

94. Reddy KR, Ellerbe C, Schilsky M, et al, Acute Liver Failure Study Group. Determinants of outcome among patients with acute liver failure listed for liver transplantation in the United States. Liver Transpl 2016;22:505–15.

95. Robles-Diaz M, Lucena MI, Kaplowitz N, et al. Use of Hy's law and a new composite algorithm to predict acute liver failure in patients with drug-induced liver injury. Gastroenterology 2014;147:109–18.e5.

96. Rathi C, Pipaliya N, Patel R, et al. Drug induced liver injury at a tertiary hospital in India: etiology, clinical features and predictors of mortality. Ann Hepatol 2017; 16:442–50.

97. Devarbhavi H, Singh R, Patil M, et al. Outcome and determinants of mortality in 269 patients with combination anti-tuberculosis drug-induced liver injury. J Gastroenterol Hepatol 2013;28:161–7.

98. Mindikoglu AL, Magder LS, Regev A. Outcome of liver transplantation for drug-induced acute liver failure in the United States: analysis of the United Network for Organ Sharing database. Liver Transpl 2009;15:719–29.

99. Fontana RJ, Hayashi PH, Barnhart H, et al, DILIN Investigators. Persistent liver biochemistry abnormalities are more common in older patients and those with cholestatic drug induced liver injury. Am J Gastroenterol 2015;110:1450–9.

100. Levy C, Lindor KD. Drug-induced cholestasis. Clin Liver Dis 2003;7:311–30.

101. Moradpour D, Altorfer J, Flury R, et al. Chlorpromazine-induced vanishing bile duct syndrome leading to biliary cirrhosis. Hepatology 1994;20:1437–41.

102. Davies MH, Harrison RF, Elias E, et al. Antibiotic-associated acute vanishing bile duct syndrome: a pattern associated with severe, prolonged, intrahepatic cholestasis. J Hepatol 1994;20:112–6.

103. Medina-Caliz I, Robles-Diaz M, Garcia-Muñoz B, et al, Spanish DILI registry. Definition and risk factors for chronicity following acute idiosyncratic drug-induced liver injury. J Hepatol 2016;65:532–42.

104. Mosedale M, Watkins PB. Drug-induced liver injury: advances in mechanistic understanding that will inform risk management. Clin Pharmacol Ther 2017; 101:469–80.

105. Antoine DJ, Jenkins RE, Dear JW, et al. Molecular forms of HMGB1 and keratin-18 as mechanistic biomarkers for mode of cell death and prognosis during clinical acetaminophen hepatotoxicity. J Hepatol 2012;56:1070–9.

106. Antoine DJ, Williams DP, Kipar A, et al. High-mobility group box-1 protein and keratin-18, circulating serum proteins informative of acetaminophen-induced necrosis and apoptosis in vivo. Toxicol Sci 2009;112:521–31.
107. Yamamoto T, Tajima Y. HMGB1 is a promising therapeutic target for acute liver failure. Expert Rev Gastroenterol Hepatol 2017;11:673–82.
108. Starkey Lewis PJ, Dear J, Platt V, et al. Circulating microRNAs as potential markers of human drug-induced liver injury. Hepatology 2011;54:1767–76.
109. Ward J, Kanchagar C, Veksler-Lublinsky I, et al. Circulating microRNA profiles in human patients with acetaminophen hepatotoxicity or ischemic hepatitis. Proc Natl Acad Sci U S A 2014;111:12169–74.
110. Rosen HR, Biggins SW, Niki T, et al. Association between plasma level of galectin-9 and survival of patients with drug-induced acute liver failure. Clin Gastroenterol Hepatol 2016;14:606–12.
111. Srungaram P, Rule JA, Yuan HF, et al, Acute Liver Failure Study Group. Plasma osteopontin in acute liver failure. Cytokine 2015;73:270–6.
112. Tsipotis E, Shuja A, Jaber BL. Albumin dialysis for liver failure: a systematic review. Adv Chronic Kidney Dis 2015;22:382–90.
113. Wittebole X, Hantson P. Use of the molecular adsorbent recirculating system (MARS™) for the management of acute poisoning with or without liver failure. Clin Toxicol (Phila) 2011;49:782–93.
114. de Geus H, Mathôt R, van der Hoven B, et al. Enhanced paracetamol clearance with molecular adsorbents recirculating system (MARS®) in severe autointoxication. Blood Purif 2010;30:118–9.
115. Kantola T, Koivusalo AM, Höckerstedt K, et al. The effect of molecular adsorbent recirculating system treatment on survival, native liver recovery, and need for liver transplantation in acute liver failure patients. Transpl Int 2008;21:857–66.
116. Saliba F, Camus C, Durand F, et al. Albumin dialysis with a noncell artificial liver support device in patients with acute liver failure: a randomized, controlled trial. Ann Intern Med 2013;159:522–31.
117. Gerth HU, Pohlen M, Thölking G, et al. Molecular adsorbent recirculating system (MARS) in acute liver injury and graft dysfunction: results from a case-control study. PLoS One 2017;12:e0175529.
118. Hanish SI, Stein DM, Scalea JR, et al. Molecular adsorbent recirculating system effectively replaces hepatic function in severe acute liver failure. Ann Surg 2017;266:677–84.
119. Diaz FC, Saez-Gonzalez E, Beniloch S, et al. Albumin dialysis with MARS for the treatment of anabolic steroid-induced cholestasis. Ann Hepatol 2016;15:939–43.
120. Gonzalez HC, Jafri SM, Gordon SC. Management of acute hepatotoxicity including medical agents and liver support systems. Clin Liver Dis 2017;21:163–80.
121. Huber W, Henschel B, Schmid R, et al. First clinical experience in 14 patients treated with ADVOS: a study on feasibility, safety and efficacy of a new type of albumin dialysis. BMC Gastroenterol 2017;17:32.
122. Larsen FS, Schmidt LE, Bernsmeier C, et al. High-volume plasma exchange in patients with acute liver failure: an open randomised controlled trial. J Hepatol 2016;64:69–78.
123. Lee KC, Baker LA, Stanzani G, et al. Extracorporeal liver assist device to exchange albumin and remove endotoxin in acute liver failure: results of a pivotal pre-clinical study. J Hepatol 2015;63:634–42.

124. Stravitz RT, Gottfried M, Durkalski V, et al, Acute Liver Failure Study Group. Safety, tolerability and pharmacokinetics of L-ornithine phenylacetate in patients with acute liver injury/failure and hyperammonemia. Hepatology 2017. [Epub ahead of print].

Acetaminophen (APAP or N-Acetyl-p-Aminophenol) and Acute Liver Failure

Chalermrat Bunchorntavakul, MD[a,b], K. Rajender Reddy, MD[a,*]

KEYWORDS

- Acetaminophen • Hepatotoxicity • Overdose • Drug-induced liver injury
- Acute liver failure • N-acetylcysteine • Liver transplantation

KEY POINTS

- Acetaminophen (APAP) is the leading cause of acute liver failure (ALF) worldwide, either following intentional overdose or unintentional ingestion (therapeutic misadventure).
- Spontaneous survival is more common in APAP-induced ALF compared to non-APAP etiologies.
- N-acetylcysteine is recommended for all patients with APAP-induced ALF and liver transplantation should be offered early to those who are unlikely to survive based on described prognostic criteria.

INTRODUCTION

A safe and effective antipyretic and analgesic, acetaminophen (APAP or N-acetyl-p-aminophenol), has had global and common use since 1955. Various formulations, both as a single-ingredient medication (eg, immediate-release and extended-release tablets/capsules, suspensions, rectal suppositories, and for intravenous use) and also as a component of numerous combination over-the-counter and prescription products, have been in wide use.[1,2] More than 28 billion doses of APAP were distributed in the United States in 2003, and the most commonly dispensed medication among 89 million outpatient prescriptions in 2005 was hydrocodone/APAP.[3,4]

Conflict of Interest: The authors have nothing to disclose.
[a] Division of Gastroenterology and Hepatology, Department of Medicine, University of Pennsylvania, Hospital of the University of Pennsylvania, 2 Dulles, 3400 Spruce Street, Philadelphia, PA 19104, USA; [b] Division of Gastroenterology and Hepatology, Department of Medicine, Rajavithi Hospital, College of Medicine, Rangsit University, Rajavithi Road, Ratchathewi, Bangkok 10400, Thailand
* Corresponding author.
E-mail address: rajender.reddy@uphs.upenn.edu

Although APAP is generally considered to be safe at the usual therapeutic doses (1–4 g/d), there have been concerns over the past few decades because APAP-induced acute liver failure (ALF) is being commonly encountered in adults in the United States and many other countries worldwide.[5–10] Single overdose ingestion typically follows suicidal attempt and doses exceeding 15 to 25 g may cause severe liver injury and can be lethal in up to 25% of the cases.[1,5,10–12] More often though nowadays, 30% to 50% of cases of hospitalized APAP hepatotoxicity result from an "unintentional overdose," a "therapeutic misadventure," or an "alcohol/Tylenol syndrome" wherein the daily dose may not have greatly exceeded the recommended safe limits but certain risk factors, such as concomitant alcohol use, obesity, nutritionally depleted state, and drugs that stimulate the cytochrome P450 (CYP) system are present.[1,5,10–12]

EPIDEMIOLOGY OF ACETAMINOPHEN OVERDOSE AND ACETAMINOPHEN-INDUCED ACUTE LIVER FAILURE

APAP has been a major cause of overdose-related ALF and death in the United States (40%–50% of cases) and in the United Kingdom (40%–70% of cases).[5–8,13–16] In the United States, APAP overdose is the leading reason for calls to the Poison Control Centers (>100,000 per year) and accounts yearly for more than 56,000 emergency room visits, 2600 hospitalizations, and ~450 deaths due to ALF.[5] In the US ALF Study Group, APAP overdose accounted for 42% (275/662) of ALF cases; with rising rates during the study from 28% in 1998 to 51% in 2003.[11] Unintentional overdoses accounted for 48%, intentional (suicide attempts) 44%, and 8% were of unknown intent.[11] Most unintentional patients reported taking APAP for acute or chronic pain syndromes; 38% took 2 or more APAP preparations simultaneously, and 63% used narcotic-containing compounds.[11] In contrast, unintentional overdose appears to be less recognized in Europe (based on published experience), accounting for 10% to 17% of ALF cases.[10,17,18] It appears that the prevalence of APAP overdose among ALF cases has been relatively stable over the past decade, with APAP still being the most important etiology of ALF in the United States as per the recent data from the US ALF Study Group as of January 2017 (n = 2436); APAP accounted for 46% of all ALF cases, which was several fold more than all prescription drugs combined.[10] Notably, APAP combination products (14% with APAP/diphenhydramine and 57% with APAP/opioids) accounted for ~70% of APAP-induced ALF cases in the United States.[19] It is known that the incidence of APAP-related ALF also varies among developed countries. Unlike in the United States and United Kingdom, APAP overdose accounts for only 3% to 9% of ALF in Spain and Germany, reflecting the differences in population behavior and oversight through the national regulatory system with regard to access to large doses of APAP.[18,20,21] By contrast, Asia-Pacific countries have a higher incidence of ALF due to hepatitis viruses with fewer cases of APAP overdose being observed (**Table 1**).[6,10,15,16,18,21–30]

PHARMACOLOGY AND MECHANISM OF ACETAMINOPHEN-INDUCED HEPATOTOXICITY AND LIVER FAILURE

The therapeutic dose of APAP is 325 to 1000 mg/dose (10–15 mg/kg/dose in children), given every 4 to 6 hours, with a maximum recommended daily dose of 3250 mg.[1,31] Peak concentrations of APAP are achieved within 90 minutes of oral ingestion, and the therapeutic serum concentrations range from 10 to 20 μg/mL.[1,3,32] Peak serum concentration, however, after an overdose is generally noted within 4 hours, but may be delayed beyond 4 hours in cases of overdose of extended-release

Table 1
Epidemiology of acetaminophen overdose–related acute liver failure in various countries

Countries	No. of Subjects/ Years	APAP-Induced ALF, %	Non-APAP Etiologies
US[10]	2436/1998–2017	46	Non-APAP DILI 11%; hepatotropic viruses 18%; indeterminate 12%; other causes 13%
Canada[23]	81/1991–1999	15	Non-APAP DILI 12%; hepatotropic viruses 30%; indeterminate 27%; other causes 16%
UK[15]	310/1994–2004	43	Non-APAP DILI 8%; hepatotropic viruses 7%; indeterminate 30%; other causes 13%
Scotland[16]	669/1992–2014	70	Non-APAP DILI 5%; hepatotropic viruses 11%; indeterminate 3%; other causes 11%
Scandinavia[24]	315/1990–2001	17	Non-APAP DILI 10%; hepatotropic viruses 12%; indeterminate 43%; other causes 17%
France[22]	808/1997–2010	22	Non-APAP DILI 14%; hepatotropic viruses 17%; indeterminate 28%; other causes 19%
Germany[21]	109/2008–2009	9	Non-APAP DILI 32%; hepatotropic viruses 21%; indeterminate 24%; other causes 14%
Spain[25]	267/1992–2000	2	Non-APAP DILI 14%; hepatotropic viruses 37%; indeterminate 32%; other causes 15%
Australia[26]	80/1988–2001	36	Non-APAP DILI 6%; hepatotropic viruses 14%; indeterminate 34%; other causes 10%
India[27]	180/1989–1996	0	Non-APAP DILI <1%; hepatotropic viruses 68%; indeterminate 31%; other causes 0%
Japan[28]	460/2004–2009	0	Non-APAP DILI 15%; hepatotropic viruses 45%; indeterminate 30%; other causes 10%
Sudan[29]	37/2003–2004	0	Non-APAP DILI 8%; hepatotropic viruses 27%; indeterminate 38%; other causes 27%
Chile[30]	27/1995–2003	0	Non-APAP DILI 7%; hepatotropic viruses 37%; indeterminate 44%; other causes 11%

Abbreviations: ALF, acute liver failure; APAP, acetaminophen; DILI, drug-induced liver injury.

preparations or when there is concomitant use of drugs that delay gastric emptying time (eg, anticholinergics, opioids).[33,34] Protein binding is minimal at therapeutic doses with a volume of distribution of ~0.9 L/kg.[32] The serum half-life of APAP is 2 to 3 hours; however, it is prolonged to more than 4 hours in patients with significant liver injury and chronic liver disease, and in those who ingest extended-release preparations.[1,3,10,32,35]

Approximately 85% to 90% of APAP, at therapeutic doses, undergoes phase II conjugation to sulfated and glucuronidated metabolites, which are then excreted in the urine.[1,3,32,36] A relatively minor amount (~2%) of APAP is excreted in the urine unchanged. Up to 10% of APAP undergoes phase I oxidation via the hepatic CYP pathway (primarily responsible by cytochrome P450 2E1 [CYP2E1]) to a toxic, highly reactive intermediate, N-acetyl-para-benzoquinoneimine (NAPQI).[3,32,36] The small amount of NAPQI produced from normal doses of APAP is rapidly conjugated by hepatic glutathione (GSH), forming nontoxic mercaptate and cysteine compounds that are then excreted in the urine.[32,36,37] Minor proportions of APAP are oxidized by myeloperoxidase and cyclooxygenase-1 (COX-1), but the clinical significance of this pathway is unclear[1,36,37] (**Fig. 1**).

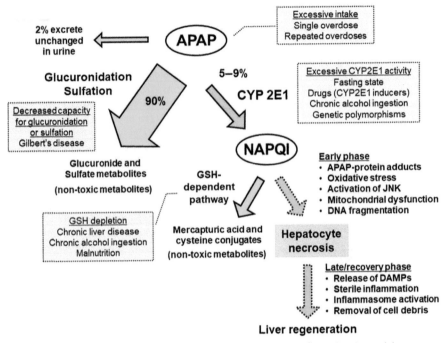

Fig. 1. Metabolism of acetaminophen and potential factors influencing its toxicity.

APAP is a unique drug in that it causes hepatotoxicity in a dose-dependent manner. At toxic doses of APAP, sulfation and glucuronidation pathways become readily saturated and most APAP is metabolized through CYP2E1 to NAPQI.[3,36] Thus, NAPQI is increasingly produced saturating and depleting GSH stores. When such depletion occurs by approximately 70% to 80%, NAPQI binds to hepatocytes, causing cellular injury.[3,36,38] In the absence of GSH, NAPQI covalently binds to cysteine groups on hepatocyte molecules forming NAPQI-protein adducts (so-called APAP-protein adducts). This process is an irreversible step that leads to oxidative injury and hepatocellular necrosis.[3,36] Other mechanisms that are likely to play an important role in the early-phase APAP-induced hepatotoxicity include mitochondrial damage, nuclear DNA fragmentation, and lipid peroxidation.[36,39–41] Additionally, depletion of GSH contributes to oxidative stress, activation of stress proteins, particularly c-jun N-terminal kinase (JNK), and gene transcription mediators, and alterations in the liver's innate immune system.[2,3,41,42] Eventually, mitochondrial oxidative stress triggers the mitochondrial permeability transition pore opening, resulting in mitochondrial damage and release of intermembrane proteins, such as endonuclease G and apoptosis-inducing factor, which then further triggers DNA fragmentation and cell necrosis.[41,42] It has been suggested that the abundance of CYP2E1 in Zone 3 hepatocytes makes that area most vulnerable to injury, and thus the characteristic histologic feature of centrilobular hepatocellular necrosis is observed in APAP hepatotoxicity.[3] Passive congestion and scattered infiltration of lymphocytes and neutrophils also may be observed.[36]

Accumulating evidence suggests a critical role of innate immunity, sterile inflammation, and inflammasome activation in the progression and repair of liver injury during the late/recovery phase of APAP hepatotoxicity.[42–44] The release of damage-associated molecular patterns (DAMPs), which subsequently activate pattern recognition receptors on macrophages, transcriptionally induce cytokine, chemokine formation, and the inflammasome, occurs following extensive necrotic cell death in cases of APAP overdose. Critical to this potential inflammatory process is the activation of caspase-1 and interleukin-1b by a molecular complex known as the inflammasome. In addition, in late-stage APAP hepatotoxicity, factors such formation of the NACHT, leucine-rich repeat, and pyrin domain-containing protein 3 (Nalp3) inflammasome in particular, could be mechanistically involved in liver injury.[42] Neutrophils and monocyte-derived macrophages are then recruited into the liver to remove necrotic cell debris, making room for liver cell regeneration.[42,43]

INGESTED DOSE AND OTHER FACTORS INFLUENCING ACETAMINOPHEN-INDUCED HEPATOTOXICITY

The total ingested dose of APAP is the most important factor determining the development and severity of APAP hepatotoxicity. In addition, the pattern of use and various factors (eg, chronic alcohol consumption, age, concurrent use of certain medications, genetic factors, preexisting liver disease, and nutritional status) also can influence the susceptibility to APAP hepatotoxicity through several mechanisms, including reduced capacity for glucuronidation or sulfation, excessive CYP activity, and depletion of glutathione stores[1,2] (**Table 2**).

An acute ingestion of $\geq$7.5 to 10 g in adults or 150 to 200 mg/kg in children older than 6 years (all APAP consumed within 8 hours) is likely to cause hepatotoxicity.[1,3] Repeated overdoses of $\geq$10 g in a 24-hour period or $\geq$6 g per 24-hour period for $\geq$48 hours may be associated with subsequent hepatotoxicity, and thus such patients should undergo a longer period of evaluation.[45] A lower threshold (4–10 g) for evaluation may be considered in a high-risk population, such as those with excess alcohol intake. Although most studies have reported safety of short-term and long-term use of APAP at the maximum recommended dose of 4 g,[46,47] a well-designed, randomized placebo-controlled study of 145 healthy volunteers reported that the daily intake of APAP of 4 g for 14 days was associated with asymptomatic elevations of alanine aminotransferase (ALT) (>3 times the upper limits of normal) in up to 40% of subjects.[48] These elevations of ALT occurred despite APAP concentrations being within therapeutic limits, and resolved after APAP discontinuation without any clinical consequences.[48] Although the US Food and Drug Administration (FDA) Advisory Committee proposed a decrease in the maximum daily dose from 4000 to 3250 mg, and the maximum individual dose from 1000 to 650 mg, and relegating 500-mg tablets to prescription status, these recommendations have not been fully implemented worldwide.[31]

Among several factors influencing APAP hepatotoxicity, chronic alcohol consumption seems to be the most important factor encountered in clinical practice. Those with alcoholic and nonalcoholic chronic liver disease and malnutrition are at risk for APAP hepatotoxicity. The interaction between ethanol, a competitive substrate or CYP2E1, and APAP is complex. Acute alcohol ingestion is not a risk factor for APAP hepatotoxicity and actually may be protective by competing with APAP for CYP2E1.[49–51] In a prospective observational study of 362 patients presenting within 24 hours after acute APAP overdose, concurrent acute alcohol intake was reported by 49% of patients. The prevalence of hepatotoxicity was 5.1% (95% confidence interval [CI] 2.6%–9.5%) in those who ingested ethanol, compared with 15.2% (95% CI 10.7%–21.2%) in those who did not ($P = .0027$).[51] In contrast, chronic alcohol ingestion may potentiate APAP hepatotoxicity by upregulating CYP2E1 (increased synthesis and half-life), and reducing GSH synthesis and storage.[1,12,36,49] Most available

Table 2
Factors influencing acetaminophen hepatotoxicity

Factors	Mechanisms	Potential Clinical Consequences
Chronic alcohol ingestion	• ↑ CYP2E1 activity • ↓ GSH synthesis and storage	↑ APAP hepatotoxicity, particularly with repeated overdoses
Acute alcohol ingestion	• Competing with APAP for CYP2E1	Possibly ↓ APAP hepatotoxicity
Medications and herbs	• ↑ CYP2E1 activity (eg, INH, rifampicin, St. John wort, garlic, grapefruit juice, and germander) • Competing hepatic glucuronidation (eg, zidovudine and TMP/SMX)	Possibly ↑ APAP hepatotoxicity
Gilbert disease	• ↓ capacity for hepatic glucuronidation	Possibly ↑ APAP hepatotoxicity
Genetic susceptibility	• Polymorphisms in enzymes involved in APAP metabolism (eg, UGT, SULT, CYP2E1, GST, N-deacetylase, NAT2, and fatty acid amide hydrolase)	Possibly ↑ or ↓ APAP hepatotoxicity
Malnutrition	• ↓ Capacity for hepatic glucuronidation • ↓ GSH storage	↑ APAP hepatotoxicity, in individuals with alcoholism
Fasting state	• ↓ GSH storage	↑ APAP hepatotoxicity, in individuals with alcoholism
Chronic liver disease	• ↓ Capacity for hepatic glucuronidation • ↓ GSH storage • ↓ Hepatic reserve	↑ APAP hepatotoxicity, particularly in individuals with alcoholism
Advanced age	• Age-dependent APAP metabolism	Possibly ↑ APAP hepatotoxicity after acute overdose (compared with younger age)
Pregnancy	• ↑ Activity of glucuronidation • ↑ Oxidative pathways	Inconclusive (APAP can cross the placenta, so there is a potential for APAP hepatotoxicity in the fetus)
Obesity and fatty liver disease	• ↓ APAP plasma levels (↓ GI absorption, ↑ volume of distribution) • ↑ Activity of glucuronidation • ↑ CYP2E1 activity • ↓ GSH storage • ↑ Oxidative stress	Inconclusive

Abbreviations: APAP, acetaminophen; CYP2E1, cytochrome P450 2E1; GI, gastrointestinal; GSH, glutathione; GST, glutathione S-transferases; INH, isoniazid; NAT2, N-acetyltransferase 2; SULT, sulfotransferase; TMP/SMX, trimethoprim-sulfamethoxazole; UGT, UDP-glucuronosyltransferase. ↑, increased; ↓, decreased.

data have concluded that chronic alcohol consumption is associated with an increased risk of APAP hepatotoxicity in patients with repeated overdoses or chronic ingestion in doses considered "acceptable" (therapeutic misadventure).[3,12,36,52] However, whether chronic alcohol consumption increases APAP hepatotoxicity at a therapeutic dose or in a single overdose setting is less clear.[1,53–55]

CLINICAL MANIFESTATIONS OF ACETAMINOPHEN-INDUCED HEPATOTOXICITY AND LIVER FAILURE
The 4 Classic Stages of Acetaminophen Hepatotoxicity

Timely recognition of APAP overdose is likely to prevent subsequent morbidity and mortality. The early manifestations of APAP overdose are frequent, mild, and nonspecific, and include nausea, vomiting, malaise, and abdominal pain. At large, these symptoms do not reliably predict subsequent hepatotoxicity. Nevertheless, a study of 291 patients suggested that an increase in episodes of vomiting at first presentation appears to be a risk indicator of subsequent hepatotoxicity.[56] The clinical course of APAP hepatotoxicity in patients with a single overdose can be classically divided into 4 consecutive stages (**Table 3**), although it should be noted that the course is variable and influenced by several factors, such as dose and formulation of APAP, coingested drug, and preexisting liver disease.[1]

APAP hepatotoxicity is characterized by marked acute elevation of serum aminotransferase (often >3000 IU/L), which typically is noted within 24 to 36 hours, and peaks approximately 72 hours after overdose.[57] The aspartate aminotransferase (AST) can be >10,000 IU/L, and typically more elevated than the ALT.[36] The degree of aminotransferase elevation correlates roughly with the degree of hepatocellular damage.[36] Maximal hepatotoxicity often peaks between 3 and 5 days after ingestion, and may be associated with jaundice, coagulopathy, and encephalopathy.[3] Prothrombin time (PT) that continues to increase beyond 4 seconds after overdose, and with a peak PT $\geq$180 seconds, has been reported to be associated with approximately 90% mortality without LT.[58] Patients may develop progressive central nervous system

Table 3
Clinical manifestations of acetaminophen hepatotoxicity

Stage I (first 24 h)	• Nausea, vomiting, malaise, lethargy, diaphoresis (some patients remain asymptomatic) • AST/ALT are typically normal (AST/ALT may begin to rise at 8–12 h after massive overdose)
Stage II (24–72 h)	• Stage I symptoms usually improve or resolve (so-called latent period) • Subclinical AST/ALT elevation • In severe cases, RUQ pain, tender hepatomegaly, jaundice, and prolonged PT may be seen • Nephrotoxicity (elevated creatinine and oliguria) may become evident
Stage III (72–96 h)	• Systemic symptoms of stage I reappear • AST/ALT elevation, typically peak at 72–96 h after ingestion (often >3000 IU/L) • Jaundice, encephalopathy, prolonged PT, and lactic acidosis may develop • AKI (10%–25%; >50% if ALF) and acute pancreatitis (0.3%–5%) may develop • Death often in this stage, usually from multiorgan system failure
Stage IV (96 h–2 wk)	• Survivors of stage III will enter recovery phase, which often lasts 1–2 wk, but may take several wk in severe cases • Histologic recovery occurs slower than clinical recovery and may take up to 3 mo • When recovery occurs, it is complete; chronic hepatitis has not been reported

Abbreviations: AKI, acute kidney injury; ALT, alanine aminotransferase; AST, aspartate aminotransferase; PT, prothrombin time; RUQ, right upper quadrant.
From Bunchorntavakul C, Reddy KR. Acetaminophen-related hepatotoxicity. Clin Liver Dis 2013;17(4):593; with permission.

symptoms of lethargy, confusion, and coma, requiring intubation. Lactic acidosis is a poor prognostic marker in APAP hepatotoxicity that can manifest as 2 scenarios: (1) early onset following massive overdose and before the onset of hepatotoxicity in which a large amount of NAPQI critically inhibits mitochondrial function; and (2) later in course, usually after day 2, resulting from tissue hypoxia together with decreased hepatic clearance of lactate in those with ALF.[1,59] Central nervous system symptoms and metabolic acidosis early in the course of disease (stage I) are not common features of APAP toxicity, and other possible causes should be excluded, particularly coingestion of other substances.[1] Further, the pharmacologic mechanism of APAP as a cannabinoid system modulator has recently been alluded to as causing "in situ" toxicity by high APAP doses in brain tissue.[60]

Acute kidney injury (AKI) develops in 10% to 25% of patients with significant APAP hepatotoxicity and in more than 50% of those with ALF.[61–64] It often becomes evident approximately 1 to 3 days after ingestion, peaking over 7 to 10 days, and often manifests as acute tubular necrosis with oliguria, either alone or in combination with hepatic necrosis.[61–63] The mechanism of nephrotoxicity is thought to be related to the toxic metabolites of APAP in the kidney.[62] APAP-related AKI is typically reversible, but approximately one-third of patients may require renal replacement therapy (RRT) before the recovery occurs.[61–63] On the other hand, almost all fatal cases of APAP-induced ALF are accompanied by severe AKI (stage 3).[64] When compared with other etiologies of ALF, AKI associated with APAP-induced ALF has tended to be more frequent and more severe.[63] Although the development of AKI reduced the overall survival in ALF, more than 50% of patients with APAP-induced ALF survived without LT (even with RRT), compared with 19% of those with ALF from other causes.[63] Interestingly, the development of AKI in APAP-induced ALF was not associated with the dose and pattern of ingestion or the use or nonuse of N-acetylcysteine (NAC), but rather was associated with alcohol use, vasopressor requirement, mechanical ventilation, higher serum phosphate and lactate, and lower serum sodium and hematocrit.[63,64]

An elevated serum amylase is frequently seen in patients with APAP poisoning (13%–36%), particularly in patients with ALF (~80%), and serum amylase level of greater than 150 U/L was associated with an approximate fivefold increase in mortality.[65] However, clinical acute pancreatitis, including severe acute pancreatitis, occurs infrequently (0.3%–5%).[65,66]

Patterns of Ingestion: Intentional Versus Unintentional Overdoses

Despite the apparently different clinical scenarios with suicidal and unintentional APAP ingestions, patients who progress to ALF owing to either phenotype somewhat resemble each other in many ways.[10] Patients who unintentionally ingest more than the therapeutic APAP doses are more likely to present late (when hepatotoxicity is clinically apparent), often with a background of ingesting APAP combination products, and/or coingesting other medications, and/or have alcohol/substance abuse and/or known risk factors for hepatotoxicity.[10,11,52,67] In addition, this group tends to have lower peak AST/ALT levels, have advanced encephalopathy on presentation, and have higher rates of morbidity and mortality than those who attempted suicide, even though the latter group had taken a higher total amount of APAP.[10,11,17,52,67,68]

Acetaminophen Combination Products

A significant proportion of patients with APAP-induced ALF have been reported to have ingested APAP combination products, either with or without opioids.[19] Patients taking APAP/opioids were more likely to be unintentional overdose, older age, have more comorbidities, and have advanced encephalopathy on presentation, whereas patients taking APAP/diphenhydramine tended to have higher peak serum AST/ALT levels.[19] There were no differences noted in delayed hepatotoxicity or clinical outcomes based on types of APAP product ingested.[19]

EVALUATIONS FOR PATIENTS WITH ACETAMINOPHEN-INDUCED HEPATOTOXICITY AND LIVER FAILURE

General approach promptly begins with careful history taking and physical examination. If encephalopathy is present, the history may be unavailable or can be provided only by the family. The precise time and amount of APAP intake, as well as serum APAP level, should be obtained. The Rumack-Matthew nomogram is a valuable tool for predicting the risk of hepatotoxicity in patients with single acute overdose ingestion who present to a health care facility within 24 hours; however, it is not applicable in cases with established hepatotoxicity and ALF.[1,69,70] Given the consequences of missed APAP poisoning, a screening for APAP seems reasonable in patients with unknown or possible APAP overdose, or in those with indeterminate hepatitis/ALF.[3,71] Supratherapeutic APAP levels of greater than 20 µg/mL (or >10 µg/mL with risk factors for APAP hepatotoxicity) are predictors of APAP hepatotoxicity; however, serum APAP concentration already may be negative at the time of established hepatotoxicity, thus not eliminating the possibility of APAP etiology for liver injury. Regardless, prompt empiric therapy with NAC should be considered in any patient with acute elevations of AST/ALT and a significant history of APAP ingestion (>4 g), irrespective of serum APAP level.[1,2] Dramatic elevations in the serum total bilirubin level (>10 µg/mL), although uncommon early on following APAP overdose, can cause a false-positive serum assay for APAP (APAP level can be falsely reported in up to 10–30 µg/mL depending on the bilirubin levels) in patients with other causes of acute hepatitis, which then may delay recognition of the underlying problem.[1,72,73]

In patients with established APAP hepatotoxicity, cautious monitoring of clinical and laboratory parameters is vital, as more than 90% of cases can be expected to resolve spontaneously.[36,74] Levels of ALT may not correlate well with the severity of liver injury, but PT and bilirubin are the key indicators of clinical progress.[75,76] Careful monitoring of PT and neurologic sings are vital, and early transfer to an intensive care unit and a facility where LT is available, should be considered if the patient has an international normalized ratio (INR) greater than 1.5, onset of encephalopathy, or other poor prognostic features.[75] Based on the data from the US ALF Study Group (n = 386), patients with severe and acute liver injury (ALI) from APAP (defined as an acute increase in ALT ≥10 times upper limit of normal and INR ≥2.0, without encephalopathy irrespective of bilirubin level) are more likely to have poor outcomes (progress to ALF, LT, or death) when compared with ALI from other etiologies (7.2% vs 40%, respectively).[77] Of note, the significance of specific biochemical markers of liver injury also may vary by etiology. For example, an INR of 2.5 would be of immediate concern in subacute ALF but not, or to a lesser extent, in APAP hepatotoxicity.[76] Bilirubin level, relatively, is not of prominent prognostic value in patients with APAP hepatotoxicity, but is a key predictor of outcome in many cases with non-APAP causes.[76] When ALF develops, APAP-induced ALF represents a unique form of ALF that differs from most other etiologies, with an expected good overall outcome in which spontaneous survivors are more than twice as likely than in the non-APAP etiologies.[6,11]

Role of Acetaminophen Adducts and Other Serum Biomarkers

APAP-protein adducts are released into blood during hepatocyte lysis, and the concentration of adducts in serum of overdose patients has correlated with toxicity.[78] The median elimination half-life of APAP-protein adducts in adults with ALF has been noted to be 42.0 (22.6–61.2) hours exceeded that of the parent drug APAP: median 5.4 (0.8–119.7) hours.[35,78] The detection of serum APAP-protein adducts has reliably identified APAP hepatotoxicity, particularly in patients who may present more than 12 to 24 hours after ingestion, and thus may be a useful diagnostic test for ALF of unknown etiology or unclear history.[1,71,78,79] Patients with ALF often have impaired mental status and/or may not be forthcoming about their ingestion of APAP. Thus, serum APAP concentrations typically are low or undetectable in patients with unintentional APAP hepatotoxicity due to the delay in presentation after ingestion.[80] Interestingly, up to 19% of indeterminate cases in the US ALF Study demonstrated adducts in serum suggesting that unrecognized APAP toxicity caused or contributed to ALF in these patients.[71,79] In addition to the application for diagnosis, the role of APAP-protein adducts for determining prognosis and for justifying intervention requires further study.[1,76] Quantitation of APAP-protein adducts in serum through high-pressure liquid chromatography with electrochemical detection (HPLC-EC) has been shown in both experimental models and clinical studies.[71,79] However, this assay is sophisticated, requiring complex analytical equipment and highly trained laboratory personnel. Recently, a more rapid and simple quantitative APAP-protein adducts immunoassay has been introduced and has shown a high degree of concordance with HPLC-EC, with 100% sensitivity and 100% negative predictive value, thus likely to increase early detection of APAP hepatotoxicity and aid in clinical management.[80]

Serum markers of mitochondrial damage and DAMPs, including glutamate dehydrogenase, nuclear DNA, and mitochondrial DNA have been investigated as clinically useful surrogate markers capable of indicating mitochondrial lysis following hepatocyte necrosis in APAP hepatotoxicity.[40,81] In addition, intranuclear product high mobility group B1, a chromatin protein involved in nuclear DNA organization and transcription regulation, and circulating kidney injury molecule 1 also are detectable in serum, and are associated with poor prognosis in the setting of APAP hepatotoxicity.[82,83] A panel of these serum biomarkers, if validated and readily available, may help in decision making of therapeutic strategies, including LT, as well as to identify future potential targets of medical therapy.[2,40,81]

MANAGEMENT OF ACETAMINOPHEN-INDUCED LIVER FAILURE

ALF is considered a "hepatology emergency," in that early discussion with a transplant team or rapid transfer to an experienced center that has LT availability is advisable once stabilized (even if the patient has not deteriorated).[75] As ALF often leads to infections and multiple organ failure, intensive care unit admission should be considered as early as possible. The general principles of the management of APAP-induced ALF do not differ from those for other causes of ALF. Careful monitoring and general management to prevent/treat infections and the use of organ support systems, where applicable and available, are very important and should follow the principles as in generally critically-ill patients, but with some specific etiology and organ failure–directed attention.[75,76,84]

N-ACETYLCYSTEINE
Mechanism of Actions and Clinical Efficacy

NAC, a GSH precursor, is an established antidote for APAP overdose and should be given in all patients with APAP hepatotoxicity, as well as in patients at significant risk for developing hepatotoxicity. The key to effective treatment is to initiate therapy before the onset of liver injury, as indicated by ALT elevation. When given early after acute APAP overdose, NAC provides cysteine for the replenishment and maintenance of hepatic GSH stores and thus presenting more substrate for the detoxification of the reactive metabolites. Further, it also may enhance the sulfation pathway and directly reduce NAPQI.[3,85,86] Based on mechanism of APAP hepatotoxicity, administration of NAC is an effective antidote when given before the onset of liver injury, although it is less effective in the early phase of liver injury (mainly driven by oxidative injury); whether NAC can alleviate late-stage APAP hepatotoxicity (mainly drives by sterile inflammation) is less certain. Several case series have observed that severe hepatotoxicity was uncommon (<5%–10%) when NAC was administered within 8 hours following acute APAP overdose, whereas delays beyond 10 hours were associated with an increased risk of hepatotoxicity (20%–30%).[3,87–89]

Patients with established liver injury also may benefit from NAC, as it has been shown to improve LT-free survival among patients with APAP-induced ALF (~20%–30% reduction in mortality).[90,91] Instead of detoxifying NAPQI, the potential mechanisms of NAC in this state are of increasing nitric oxide production, improving hepatic perfusion and oxygen delivery, scavenging reactive oxygen and nitrogen species, and refining mitochondrial energy production.[3,36] In the only randomized placebo-controlled study that assessed NAC in APAP-induced ALF (n = 50), overall survival was increased in the NAC group compared with the control group (48% vs 20%, respectively; $P = .037$).[91] Thus, NAC-treated patients had a lower incidence of cerebral edema (40% vs 68%; $P = .047$) and hypotension requiring inotropic support (48% vs 80%; $P = .018$).[91] Subsequently, there has been no randomized placebo-controlled trial evaluating the efficacy of NAC for APAP overdose, as such trials were considered unethical. As a result, 2 systematic reviews performed by the Cochrane Group in 2006[92] and by the American Gastroenterological Association in 2017[93] concluded that NAC may reduce mortality in APAP-induced ALF, but had low-quality evidence of investigations done thus far. Given the seriousness of the disease and the potential benefits with minor side effects of NAC, immediate NAC therapy has long been a standard of care for patients with APAP-induced ALF in most centers, and is recommended by the international guidelines.[76,84,93] In addition, the benefits of NAC also have been observed in patients with early-grade encephalopathy and with non-APAP ALF.[93,94]

Dosage Regimen and Side Effects

NAC is available in both oral and intravenous (IV) form; however, the IV regimen is generally preferred in the setting of ALF because the patients often have nausea, vomiting, ileus, and/or alteration in consciousness. The recommended dose of NAC (standard 24-hour regimen) is IV loading dose of 150 mg/kg in 200 mL diluent in 15 to 60 minutes, followed by 50 mg/kg in 500 mL diluent over 4 hours, and then 100 mg/kg in 1000 mL diluent over 16 hours (IV NAC solution is hyperosmolar and is compatible with 5% dextrose in water, 0.45% NSS (normal saline), and sterile water).[1,84] The doses of NAC are calculated using patient body weight with a ceiling weight of 100 kg for IV therapy.[95] An observational study of APAP poisoning in patients weighing more than 100 kg found that both maximum weight cutoff and actual weight-based NAC dose were safe, but clinicians preferred the latter, and hepatotoxicity was similar (up to 33%) with both strategies.[96] Anaphylactoid reactions (eg, rash, itching, angioedema, bronchospasm, tachycardia, and hypotension) develop in 10% to 20% of patients treated with IV NAC.[97,98] Patients with flushing alone or mild symptoms do not require intervention and the infusion can be continued with careful monitoring. Patients who develop urticaria, angioedema, hypotension, and bronchospasm should be treated with 1 or more medications of diphenhydramine, corticosteroids, and bronchodilators. The infusion should be stopped and can be restarted at a slower rate and with close monitoring.[95,99] In a randomized trial, slowing the loading infusion time from 15 minutes to 60 minutes had not compromised efficacy but also did not lower the incidence of anaphylactoid reactions.[98]

A 12-hour modified regimen has been evaluated in a randomized-controlled study and found to be associated with less vomiting, fewer anaphylactoid reactions, and reduced need for treatment interruption, compared with a standard 24-hour protocol; however, this study was not powered to detect noninferiority of the shorter treatment duration protocol.[100] After the initial NAC protocol, the recommendation for continuation and monitoring in patients with established severe APAP hepatotoxicity or ALF is not well defined. Controversy exists over when to stop the use of NAC; whether a 72-hour period is sufficient or continuation until liver biochemical tests have improved is necessary.[84] Based on limited evidence, most experts have advised a standard IV regimen with continuation of infusion at a rate of 6.25 mg/kg per hour until LT or reversal of hepatotoxicity (ALT and/or AST have peaked and are decreasing, encephalopathy resolves, and INR is <1.5) and with undetectable serum APAP concentration.[1–3,91,95,101] However, some experts have suggested to limit the use of NAC to a maximum of 5 days, given its antiinflammatory effects that may increase risk of sepsis in the later phase.[76] NAC (FDA Pregnancy Category B) is not contraindicated in pregnant women with APAP overdose and is the most important intervention to prevent pregnancy loss. In a prospective observational study of 60 pregnant women with acetaminophen overdose, increasing time to NAC administration was associated with an increased risk of miscarriage and fetal death.[102]

LIVER TRANSPLANTATION
Selection of Patient and Prognostic Systems

Although APAP-induced ALF is associated with more favorable outcomes compared with all other causes of ALF, it still has a high mortality (~30%) without LT.[8,11,36,74] LT is life-saving in patients with APAP overdose who progress to severe ALF. The decision to proceed with LT in APAP-induced ALF is challenging and involves balancing the inherent risks associated with delay in listing and LT against the potential for spontaneous recovery from medical therapy alone, the risk of major surgery in the context of severe and critical illness, shortage of organ pool, and the necessity for long-term immunosuppression.[103] In addition, the psychosocial issues in patients with APAP overdose need to be considered, as more than 30% of patients who fulfill transplant criteria have challenges of major psychiatric illnesses or alcohol and/or substance abuse.[104]

To identify patients with APAP-induced ALF who are unlikely to survive without LT, several clinical features and laboratory parameters have been evaluated and prognostic models have been developed (**Table 4**). In 1989, O'Grady and colleagues[105,106] introduced the King's College Criteria (KCC) to determine which patients with APAP-induced and non-APAP ALF had a poor prognosis, and thus are likely to benefit most from LT. Without LT, patients with APAP-induced ALF who met the criteria had very high mortality (80%–90%),[36,105,106] and, as such, these patients deserve consideration of LT. KCC has good specificity (82%–94%) but has limited sensitivity (68%–82%). The positive predictive values (PPV) are reasonable (70%–95%) but negative predictive values (NPV) are variable (25%–90%).[11,35,82,100,102–106] Therefore, a significant number of patients who do not fulfill the KCC will eventually die without LT. Of note, the performance of KCC is slightly different for the 2 categories of ALF, as the pooled meta-analyses revealed specificity to be high for APAP-induced ALF at 89% to 95% and less for the non-APAP category at 74% to 81%. Sensitivity was

Table 4
Prognostic criteria serving as guidance for liver transplantation in acetaminophen-induced acute liver failure

Prognostic Variable	Etiology	Predictors of Poor Outcome Providing Guidance for Liver Transplantation	Sensitivity, %	Specificity, %
King's College criteria[76,103]	APAP	Arterial pH <7.3 after fluid resuscitation OR all 3 of the following: (I) Grade III or IV HE; (II) Prothrombin time >100 s (or INR >6.5); (III) Serum creatinine >3.4 mg/dL (or >300 μmol/L)	58–69	92–95
Lactate[109]	APAP	Admission arterial lactate >3.5 mmol/L or >3.0 mmol/L after fluid resuscitation	81	95
Clichy criteria[22]	All	Grade III-IV HE + Factor V <20% (age <30 y) or <30% (age >30 y)	81[a] 75[a] (LT patients excluded)	56[a] 56[a] (LT patients excluded)
Factor V; factor VIII/V ratio[134]	APAP	Factor V <10% Factor VIII/V ratio >30	91 91	100 91
Phosphate[110]	APAP	Phosphate >1.2 mmol/L on day 2 or 3 after overdose	89	100
Gc-globulin[112]	APAP	Gc-globulin <100 mg/L	73	68
Alfa-feto protein[111]	APAP	Alfa-feto protein <3.9 μg/L 24 h after peak ALT	100	74
FABP1[117]	APAP	FABP1 >350 ng/mL on day 1 FABP1 >350 ng/mL on day 3–5	64 71	62 84
APACHE II[11,123]	All	APACHE II >19 APACHE II >15 on admission	68[a] 82[a]	87[a] 98[a]
SOFA[121]	APAP	SOFA score >6 by 72 h after overdose SOFA score >7 by 96 h after overdose	91 96	70 73
SOFA[122]	Staggered APAP overdose[b]	SOFA score >5 on admission SOFA score >10 at 24 h after admission SOFA score >13 at 48 h after admission	100 92 100	58 83 97
MELD[108,119,121]	APAP	MELD >33 at onset of HE MELD >37 by 72 h after overdose MELD >42 by 96 h after overdose	60–80 100 86	53–69 50 71
ALFSG Prognostic Index[117]	All	ALFSG Index on day 1 ALFSG Index on day 3–5	52[a] 54[a]	85[a] 89[a]

Abbreviations: ALFSG, the Acute Liver Failure Study Group; APACHE, the Acute Physiology and Chronic Health Evaluation; APAP, acetaminophen; FABP1, serum liver-type fatty acid binding protein; HE, hepatic encephalopathy; INR, international normalized ratio; LT, liver transplantation; MELD, the Model of End-stage Liver Disease; SOFA, the sequential organ failure assessment.
[a] Numbers taken from the cohorts of patients with APAP-induced ALF.
[b] Multiple supratherapeutic doses over more than 8 h, resulting in cumulative dose of greater than 4 g/d.

relatively poor for both groups: 58% for APAP and 58% to 68% for non-APAP.[103,107,108] In addition, KCC perform best in groups with high-grade encephalopathy in historically earlier studies, suggesting that modern medical management of ALF may modify performance of KCC; sensitivity was noted to be reduced in studies published after 2005 (46%–71%) compared with studies before 1995 (76%–82%).[107]

Modifications of KCC and several alternative prognostic variables or scoring systems have been proposed in an attempt to improve or replace the KCC in the setting of APAP-induced ALF. Arterial blood lactate greater than 3.5 mmol/L is an early predictor of mortality in APAP-ALF (sensitivity 67%, specificity 95%, PPV 79%, NPV 91%) and may increase the predictive accuracy of the KCC.[109] In addition, several other laboratory parameters and serum biomarkers for predicting outcomes in APAP-induced ALF, such as phosphate,[110] alfa-feto protein,[111] Gc-globulin,[112] interleukin-6,[113] galectin-9,[114] procoagulant microparticles,[115] neutrophil-lymphocyte ratio,[116] liver-type fatty acid binding protein (FABP1),[117] and brain-type fatty acid binding protein (FABP7),[118] also have been proposed. The Model of End-stage Liver Disease (MELD) is also useful in APAP-induced ALF, but has not proved to be a better discriminator than the KCC.[108,119] The Sequential Organ Failure Assessment score, originally designed for grading dysfunction of multiple organ systems, has been shown to be prognostically superior to the KCC and MELD criteria for APAP-induced ALF due to both single and repeated overdoses.[120–122] The Acute Physiology and Chronic Health Evaluation (APACHE) II score of greater than 15 on admission has been noted to be a sensitive tool to predict progression to ALF and was more sensitive than the KCC on the day of admission.[11,123] An APACHE II score of greater than 19 was associated with a lower LT-free survival.[11,76] The US ALF Study Group has introduced a highly specific (but low sensitivity) logistic regression model, so-called ALFSG Prognostic Index, to predict LT-free survival in ALF using admission variables including hepatic encephalopathy (HE) grade, ALF etiology, vasopressor use, bilirubin, and INR.[124] More recently, a novel Classification and Regression Tree model to predict LT-free survival in APAP-induced ALF has been proposed by the US ALF Study Group.[125] This model offered improved sensitivity and model performance over traditional KCC, while maintaining similar accuracy and negligibly worse specificity.[125] Last, a new high-performance statistical model to support decision making for LT in patients with APAP-induced ALF also has been proposed using the dataset from the United Kingdom and Denmark.[126]

It should be kept in mind that although these proposed prognostic markers and mathematical scoring systems for APAP-induced ALF demonstrated encouraging performance, they were evaluated only in a single or limited number of studies with variable quality; thus, more external validation is required. As it stands, KCC remains the most validated and widely used prognostic model for APAP-induced ALF, and one that has been adopted by most international guidelines and transplant centers.[1,76,84,127] Apart from medical issues, psychiatric illnesses and family support also should be carefully evaluated before offering LT, especially in patients with intentional APAP overdose, as there remains a concern of the risk of reattempting suicide after LT.[1]

Clinical Outcomes

There has been some controversy concerning the outcomes of LT for APAP-induced ALF. A large experience of 1144 ALF cases (54% were APAP-related) from the US ALF Study Group observed that APAP patients, compared with non-APAP patients, had better 2-year survival in those not transplanted but lower survival in those transplanted, indicating a good discriminatory ability of the physicians in observing versus transplanting those with APAP-induced ALF.[9] In this analysis, patients were classified into 3 groups: (A) not listed for LT (n = 697); (B) listed, not transplanted (n = 177); and (C) listed, transplanted (n = 270), and the 2-year survival among APAP and non-APAP etiology in groups A, B, and C was 31% and 34%, 59% and 83%, and 72% and 53%, respectively.[9] A significant number of patients did not receive LT for a variety of reasons, including milder disease and psychosocial disqualifiers.[9] More recent data from the US ALF Study Group focusing on 617 patients with ALF listed for LT (36% of overall ALF group) reported on the 3-week outcomes and noted that 117 (19%) spontaneously survived, 108 (17.5%) died without LT, and 392 (63.5%) underwent LT.[128] When compared with other slowly evolving etiologies of ALF, such as autoimmune hepatitis, drug-induced, and hepatitis B virus, patients with APAP-induced ALF were less likely to be listed (22% vs 57%), less likely to receive an LT (36% vs 74%), more likely to die (24% vs 17%), and the median time to death was sooner (2.0 vs 4.5 days). Despite greater severity of illness, the listed APAP group still had a higher spontaneous survival rate than the non-APAP group (40% vs 11%, P<.001).[128]

Over the long run, it is relevant that survival benefit, the long-term adherence to immunosuppression, and quality of life following LT are important considerations. In a UK experience of 858 patients with APAP hepatotoxicity, 63% (60/95) of listed patients eventually underwent the procedure.[8] Of 60 patients transplanted, 73% survived to discharge and 58% survived to an average of 9 years post-LT. When compared with non-APAP etiologies, the incidence of psychiatric disease (principally depression) and 30-day mortality were greatest in the APAP group, but for those who survived beyond 30 days, there was no difference in long-term survival rates between APAP and non-APAP groups.[8] Adherence to follow-up appointments and compliance with immunosuppressive regimens were lower in the APAP overdose group, and was not predicted by any identifiable premorbid psychiatric conditions.[8] In addition, another experience from the United Kingdom reported that despite a high prevalence of psychiatric disturbance (56% had formal psychiatric diagnosis and 22% previously attempted suicide), the 5-year outcomes for patients transplanted emergently for APAP-induced ALF were comparable to those transplanted for non-APAP ALF and electively for cirrhosis.[129] On the other hand, the European Liver Transplant Registry database observed that social problems post-LT were a cause of death or graft failure; suicide and nonadherence to immunosuppression were nearly 10% higher in the APAP group than for other etiologies.[130] In a similar vein, spontaneous survivors from APAP-induced ALF in the US ALF Study Group had a significant decrease in quality of life, with high rates of psychiatric disease and substance abuse during the long-term follow-up, raising further questions as to the appropriateness of emergency LT for APAP-induced ALF.[131,132] Therefore, decisions to list and proceed with LT must be made early in APAP-induced ALF, with additional considerations for psychiatric/social problems. Multidisciplinary approaches with long-term psychiatric follow-up may help lower posttransplant suicide rates and enhance compliance with medication use and follow-up, thus lowering risk of graft loss.[133]

REFERENCES

1. Bunchorntavakul C, Reddy KR. Acetaminophen-related hepatotoxicity. Clin Liver Dis 2013;17(4):587–607, viii.

2. Yoon E, Babar A, Choudhary M, et al. Acetaminophen-induced hepatotoxicity: a comprehensive update. J Clin Transl Hepatol 2016;4(2):131–42.

3. Hodgman MJ, Garrard AR. A review of acetaminophen poisoning. Crit Care Clin 2012;28(4):499–516.

4. Wysowski DK, Governale LA, Swann J. Trends in outpatient prescription drug use and related costs in the US: 1998-2003. Pharmacoeconomics 2006;24(3): 233–6.

5. Lee WM. Acetaminophen and the U.S. Acute Liver Failure Study Group: lowering the risks of hepatic failure. Hepatology 2004;40(1):6–9.

6. Ostapowicz G, Fontana RJ, Schiodt FV, et al. Results of a prospective study of acute liver failure at 17 tertiary care centers in the United States. Ann Intern Med 2002;137(12):947–54.

7. Ayonrinde OT, Phelps GJ, Hurley JC, et al. Paracetamol overdose and hepato-toxicity at a regional Australian hospital: a 4-year experience. Intern Med J 2005; 35(11):655–60.

8. Cooper SC, Aldridge RC, Shah T, et al. Outcomes of liver transplantation for paracetamol (acetaminophen)-induced hepatic failure. Liver Transpl 2009; 15(10):1351–7.

9. Reddy KR, Schilsky ML, Stravitz R, et al. Liver transplantation for acute liver failure: results from the NIH Acute Liver Failure Study Group. Hepatology 2012;56(4 Suppl):246A–7A.

10. Lee WM. Acetaminophen (APAP) hepatotoxicity-Isn't it time for APAP to go away? J Hepatol 2017;67(6):1324–31.

11. Larson AM, Polson J, Fontana RJ, et al. Acetaminophen-induced acute liver failure: results of a United States multicenter, prospective study. Hepatology 2005; 42(6):1364–72.

12. Zimmerman HJ, Maddrey WC. Acetaminophen (paracetamol) hepatotoxicity with regular intake of alcohol: analysis of instances of therapeutic misadventure. Hepatology 1995;22(3):767–73.

13. Ichai P, Samuel D. Etiology and prognosis of fulminant hepatitis in adults. Liver Transpl 2008;14(Suppl 2):S67–79.

14. Lee WM. Etiologies of acute liver failure. Semin Liver Dis 2008;28(2):142–52.

15. Bernal W, Cross TJ, Auzinger G, et al. Outcome after wait-listing for emergency liver transplantation in acute liver failure: a single centre experience. J Hepatol 2009;50(2):306–13.

16. Donnelly MC, Davidson JS, Martin K, et al. Acute liver failure in Scotland: changes in aetiology and outcomes over time (the Scottish Look-Back Study). Aliment Pharmacol Ther 2017;45(6):833–43.

17. Craig DG, Bates CM, Davidson JS, et al. Overdose pattern and outcome in paracetamol-induced acute severe hepatotoxicity. Br J Clin Pharmacol 2011; 71(2):273–82.

18. Gulmez SE, Larrey D, Pageaux GP, et al. Liver transplant associated with para-cetamol overdose: results from the seven-country SALT study. Br J Clin Pharma-col 2015;80(3):599–606.

19. Serper M, Wolf MS, Parikh NA, et al. Risk factors, clinical presentation, and out-comes in overdose with acetaminophen alone or with combination products: re-sults from the Acute Liver Failure Study Group. J Clin Gastroenterol 2016;50(1): 85–91.

20. Mas A, Escorsell A, Fernandez J. Liver transplantation for acute liver failure: a Spanish perspective. Transplant Proc 2010;42(2):619–21.

21. Hadem J, Tacke F, Bruns T, et al. Etiologies and outcomes of acute liver failure in Germany. Clin Gastroenterol Hepatol 2012;10(6):664–9.e2.

22. Ichai P, Legeai C, Francoz C, et al. Patients with acute liver failure listed for superurgent liver transplantation in France: reevaluation of the Clichy-Villejuif criteria. Liver Transpl 2015;21(4):512–23.

23. Tessier G, Villeneuve E, Villeneuve JP. Etiology and outcome of acute liver failure: experience from a liver transplantation centre in Montreal. Can J Gastroenterol 2002;16(10):672–6.

24. Brandsaeter B, Hockerstedt K, Friman S, et al. Fulminant hepatic failure: outcome after listing for highly urgent liver transplantation-12 years experience in the Nordic countries. Liver Transpl 2002;8(11):1055–62.

25. Escorsell A, Mas A, de la Mata M. Acute liver failure in Spain: analysis of 267 cases. Liver Transpl 2007;13(10):1389–95.

26. Gow PJ, Jones RM, Dobson JL, et al. Etiology and outcome of fulminant hepatic failure managed at an Australian liver transplant unit. J Gastroenterol Hepatol 2004;19(2):154–9.

27. Khuroo MS, Kamili S. Aetiology and prognostic factors in acute liver failure in India. J Viral Hepat 2003;10(3):224–31.

28. Oketani M, Ido A, Nakayama N, et al. Etiology and prognosis of fulminant hepatitis and late-onset hepatic failure in Japan: summary of the annual nationwide survey between 2004 and 2009. Hepatol Res 2013;43(2):97–105.

29. Mudawi HM, Yousif BA. Fulminant hepatic failure in an African setting: etiology, clinical course, and predictors of mortality. Dig Dis Sci 2007;52(11):3266–9.

30. Uribe M, Buckel E, Ferrario M, et al. Epidemiology and results of liver transplantation for acute liver failure in Chile. Transplant Proc 2003;35(7):2511–2.

31. Krenzelok EP. The FDA Acetaminophen Advisory Committee meeting - what is the future of acetaminophen in the United States? The perspective of a committee member. Clin Toxicol (Phila) 2009;47(8):784–9.

32. Forrest JA, Clements JA, Prescott LF. Clinical pharmacokinetics of paracetamol. Clin Pharmacokinet 1982;7(2):93–107.

33. Bizovi KE, Aks SE, Paloucek F, et al. Late increase in acetaminophen concentration after overdose of Tylenol extended relief. Ann Emerg Med 1996;28(5):549–51.

34. Douglas DR, Sholar JB, Smilkstein MJ. A pharmacokinetic comparison of acetaminophen products (Tylenol Extended Relief vs regular Tylenol). Acad Emerg Med 1996;3(8):740–4.

35. Schiodt FV, Ott P, Christensen E, et al. The value of plasma acetaminophen half-life in antidote-treated acetaminophen overdosage. Clin Pharmacol Ther 2002;71(4):221–5.

36. Larson AM. Acetaminophen hepatotoxicity. Clin Liver Dis 2007;11(3):525–48, vi.

37. Graham GG, Scott KF, Day RO. Tolerability of paracetamol. Drug Saf 2005;28(3):227–40.

38. Mitchell JR, Jollow DJ, Potter WZ, et al. Acetaminophen-induced hepatic necrosis. IV. Protective role of glutathione. J Pharmacol Exp Ther 1973;187(1):211–7.

39. Knight TR, Fariss MW, Farhood A, et al. Role of lipid peroxidation as a mechanism of liver injury after acetaminophen overdose in mice. Toxicol Sci 2003;76(1):229–36.

40. McGill MR, Sharpe MR, Williams CD, et al. The mechanism underlying acetaminophen-induced hepatotoxicity in humans and mice involves mitochondrial damage and nuclear DNA fragmentation. J Clin Invest 2012;122(4):1574–83.

41. Jaeschke H. Acetaminophen: dose-dependent drug hepatotoxicity and acute liver failure in patients. Dig Dis 2015;33(4):464–71.

42. Woolbright BL, Jaeschke H. Role of the inflammasome in acetaminophen-induced liver injury and acute liver failure. J Hepatol 2017;66(4):836–48.

43. Jaeschke H, Williams CD, Ramachandran A, et al. Acetaminophen hepatotoxicity and repair: the role of sterile inflammation and innate immunity. Liver Int 2012; 32(1):8–20.

44. Liu ZX, Govindarajan S, Kaplowitz N. Innate immune system plays a critical role in determining the progression and severity of acetaminophen hepatotoxicity. Gastroenterology 2004;127(6):1760–74.

45. Dart RC, Erdman AR, Olson KR, et al. Acetaminophen poisoning: an evidence-based consensus guideline for out-of-hospital management. Clin Toxicol (Phila) 2006;44(1):1–18.

46. Temple AR, Benson GD, Zinsenheim JR, et al. Multicenter, randomized, double-blind, active-controlled, parallel-group trial of the long-term (6-12 months) safety of acetaminophen in adult patients with osteoarthritis. Clin Ther 2006;28(2): 222–35.

47. Temple AR, Lynch JM, Vena J, et al. Aminotransferase activities in healthy subjects receiving three-day dosing of 4, 6, or 8 grams per day of acetaminophen. Clin Toxicol (Phila) 2007;45(1):36–44.

48. Watkins PB, Kaplowitz N, Slattery JT, et al. Aminotransferase elevations in healthy adults receiving 4 grams of acetaminophen daily: a randomized controlled trial. JAMA 2006;296(1):87–93.

49. Lee WM. Drug-induced hepatotoxicity. N Engl J Med 2003;349(5):474–85.

50. Schmidt LE, Dalhoff K, Poulsen HE. Acute versus chronic alcohol consumption in acetaminophen-induced hepatotoxicity. Hepatology 2002;35(4):876–82.

51. Waring WS, Stephen AF, Malkowska AM, et al. Acute ethanol coingestion confers a lower risk of hepatotoxicity after deliberate acetaminophen overdose. Acad Emerg Med 2008;15(1):54–8.

52. Schiodt FV, Rochling FA, Casey DL, et al. Acetaminophen toxicity in an urban county hospital. N Engl J Med 1997;337(16):1112–7.

53. Dart RC, Kuffner EK, Rumack BH. Treatment of pain or fever with paracetamol (acetaminophen) in the alcoholic patient: a systematic review. Am J Ther 2000;7(2):123–34.

54. Kuffner EK, Dart RC, Bogdan GM, et al. Effect of maximal daily doses of acetaminophen on the liver of alcoholic patients: a randomized, double-blind, placebo-controlled trial. Arch Intern Med 2001;161(18):2247–52.

55. Rumack BH. Acetaminophen misconceptions. Hepatology 2004;40(1):10–5.

56. Zyoud SH, Awang R, Sulaiman SA, et al. Assessing the impact of vomiting episodes on outcome after acetaminophen poisoning. Basic Clin Pharmacol Toxicol 2010;107(5):887–92.

57. Singer AJ, Carracio TR, Mofenson HC. The temporal profile of increased transaminase levels in patients with acetaminophen-induced liver dysfunction. Ann Emerg Med 1995;26(1):49–53.

58. Harrison PM, O'Grady JG, Keays RT, et al. Serial prothrombin time as prognostic indicator in paracetamol induced fulminant hepatic failure. BMJ 1990; 301(6758):964–6.

59. Shah AD, Wood DM, Dargan PI. Understanding lactic acidosis in paracetamol (acetaminophen) poisoning. Br J Clin Pharmacol 2011;71(1):20–8.

60. Ghanem CI, Perez MJ, Manautou JE, et al. Acetaminophen from liver to brain: new insights into drug pharmacological action and toxicity. Pharmacol Res 2016;109:119–31.

61. Blakely P, McDonald BR. Acute renal failure due to acetaminophen ingestion: a case report and review of the literature. J Am Soc Nephrol 1995;6(1):48–53.

62. Mazer M, Perrone J. Acetaminophen-induced nephrotoxicity: pathophysiology, clinical manifestations, and management. J Med Toxicol 2008;4(1):2–6.

63. Tujios SR, Hynan LS, Vazquez MA, et al. Risk factors and outcomes of acute kidney injury in patients with acute liver failure. Clin Gastroenterol Hepatol 2015; 13(2):352–9.

64. O'Riordan A, Brummell Z, Sizer E, et al. Acute kidney injury in patients admitted to a liver intensive therapy unit with paracetamol-induced hepatotoxicity. Nephrol Dial Transplant 2011;26(11):3501–8.

65. Schmidt LE, Dalhoff K. Hyperamylasaemia and acute pancreatitis in paracetamol poisoning. Aliment Pharmacol Ther 2004;20(2):173–9.

66. Caldarola V, Hassett JM, Hall AH, et al. Hemorrhagic pancreatitis associated with acetaminophen overdose. Am J Gastroenterol 1986;81(7):579–82.

67. Gyamlani GG, Parikh CR. Acetaminophen toxicity: suicidal vs. accidental. Crit Care 2002;6(2):155–9.

68. Craig DG, Bates CM, Davidson JS, et al. Staggered overdose pattern and delay to hospital presentation are associated with adverse outcomes following paracetamol-induced hepatotoxicity. Br J Clin Pharmacol 2012;73(2):285–94.

69. Prescott LF, Illingworth RN, Critchley JA, et al. Intravenous N-acetylcysteine: the treatment of choice for paracetamol poisoning. Br Med J 1979;2(6198): 1097–100.

70. Rumack BH, Peterson RC, Koch GG, et al. Acetaminophen overdose. 662 cases with evaluation of oral acetylcysteine treatment. Arch Intern Med 1981;141(3 Spec No):380–5.

71. Khandelwal N, James LP, Sanders C, et al. Unrecognized acetaminophen toxicity as a cause of indeterminate acute liver failure. Hepatology 2011;53(2): 567–76.

72. Beuhler MC, Curry SC. False positive acetaminophen levels associated with hyperbilirubinemia. Clin Toxicol (Phila) 2005;43(3):167–70.

73. Polson J, Wians FH Jr, Orsulak P, et al. False positive acetaminophen concentrations in patients with liver injury. Clin Chim Acta 2008;391(1–2):24–30.

74. Bernal W, Wendon J, Rela M, et al. Use and outcome of liver transplantation in acetaminophen-induced acute liver failure. Hepatology 1998;27(4):1050–5.

75. Bunchorntavakul C, Reddy KR. Acute liver failure. Clin Liver Dis 2017;21(4): 769–92.

76. Wendon J, Cordoba J, Dhawan A, et al. EASL clinical practical guidelines on the management of acute (fulminant) liver failure. J Hepatol 2017;66(5):1047–81.

77. Koch DG, Speiser JL, Durkalski V, et al. The natural history of severe acute liver injury. Am J Gastroenterol 2017;112(9):1389–96.

78. James LP, Letzig L, Simpson PM, et al. Pharmacokinetics of acetaminophen-protein adducts in adults with acetaminophen overdose and acute liver failure. Drug Metab Dispos 2009;37(8):1779–84.

79. Davern TJ 2nd, James LP, Hinson JA, et al. Measurement of serum acetaminophen-protein adducts in patients with acute liver failure. Gastroenterology 2006;130(3):687–94.

80. Roberts DW, Lee WM, Hinson JA, et al. An immunoassay to rapidly measure acetaminophen protein adducts accurately identifies patients with acute liver injury or failure. Clin Gastroenterol Hepatol 2017;15(4):555–62.e3.

81. McGill MR, Staggs VS, Sharpe MR, et al. Serum mitochondrial biomarkers and damage-associated molecular patterns are higher in acetaminophen overdose patients with poor outcome. Hepatology 2014;60(4):1336–45.

82. Antoine DJ, Sabbisetti VS, Francis B, et al. Circulating kidney injury molecule 1 predicts prognosis and poor outcome in patients with acetaminophen-induced liver injury. Hepatology 2015;62(2):591–9.

83. Woolbright BL, McGill MR, Staggs VS, et al. Glycodeoxycholic acid levels as prognostic biomarker in acetaminophen-induced acute liver failure patients. Toxicol Sci 2014;142(2):436–44.

84. Lee WM, Stravitz RT, Larson AM. Introduction to the revised American Association for the Study of Liver Diseases position paper on acute liver failure 2011. Hepatology 2012;55(3):965–7.

85. Lin JH, Levy G. Sulfate depletion after acetaminophen administration and replenishment by infusion of sodium sulfate or N-acetylcysteine in rats. Biochem Pharmacol 1981;30(19):2723–5.

86. Lauterburg BH, Corcoran GB, Mitchell JR. Mechanism of action of N-acetylcysteine in the protection against the hepatotoxicity of acetaminophen in rats in vivo. J Clin Invest 1983;71(4):980–91.

87. Prescott LF. Treatment of severe acetaminophen poisoning with intravenous acetylcysteine. Arch Intern Med 1981;141(3 Spec No):386–9.

88. Smilkstein MJ, Knapp GL, Kulig KW, et al. Efficacy of oral N-acetylcysteine in the treatment of acetaminophen overdose. Analysis of the national multicenter study (1976 to 1985). N Engl J Med 1988;319(24):1557–62.

89. Prescott LF, Park J, Ballantyne A, et al. Treatment of paracetamol (acetaminophen) poisoning with N-acetylcysteine. Lancet 1977;2(8035):432–4.

90. Harrison PM, Keays R, Bray GP, et al. Improved outcome of paracetamol-induced fulminant hepatic failure by late administration of acetylcysteine. Lancet 1990;335(8705):1572–3.

91. Keays R, Harrison PM, Wendon JA, et al. Intravenous acetylcysteine in paracetamol induced fulminant hepatic failure: a prospective controlled trial. BMJ 1991;303(6809):1026–9.

92. Brok J, Buckley N, Gluud C. Interventions for paracetamol (acetaminophen) overdose. Cochrane Database Syst Rev 2006;(2):CD003328.

93. Herrine SK, Moayyedi P, Brown RS Jr, et al. American Gastroenterological Association Institute technical review on initial testing and management of acute liver disease. Gastroenterology 2017;152(3):648–64.e5.

94. Lee WM, Hynan LS, Rossaro L, et al. Intravenous N-acetylcysteine improves transplant-free survival in early stage non-acetaminophen acute liver failure. Gastroenterology 2009;137(3):856–64, 864.e1.

95. Heard KJ. Acetylcysteine for acetaminophen poisoning. N Engl J Med 2008;359(3):285–92.

96. Varney SM, Buchanan JA, Kokko J, et al. Acetylcysteine for acetaminophen overdose in patients who weigh >100 Kg. Am J Ther 2014;21(3):159–63.

97. Dawson AH, Henry DA, McEwen J. Adverse reactions to N-acetylcysteine during treatment for paracetamol poisoning. Med J Aust 1989;150(6):329–31.

98. Kerr F, Dawson A, Whyte IM, et al. The Australasian Clinical Toxicology Investigators Collaboration randomized trial of different loading infusion rates of N-acetylcysteine. Ann Emerg Med 2005;45(4):402–8.

99. Bailey B, McGuigan MA. Management of anaphylactoid reactions to intravenous N-acetylcysteine. Ann Emerg Med 1998;31(6):710–5.

100. Bateman DN, Dear JW, Thanacoody HK, et al. Reduction of adverse effects from intravenous acetylcysteine treatment for paracetamol poisoning: a randomised controlled trial. Lancet 2014;383(9918):697–704.

101. Fontana RJ. Acute liver failure including acetaminophen overdose. Med Clin North Am 2008;92(4):761–94, viii.

102. Riggs BS, Bronstein AC, Kulig K, et al. Acute acetaminophen overdose during pregnancy. Obstet Gynecol 1989;74(2):247–53.

103. Craig DG, Ford AC, Hayes PC, et al. Systematic review: prognostic tests of paracetamol-induced acute liver failure. Aliment Pharmacol Ther 2010;31(10): 1064–76.

104. Simpson KJ, Bates CM, Henderson NC, et al. The utilization of liver transplantation in the management of acute liver failure: comparison between acetaminophen and non-acetaminophen etiologies. Liver Transpl 2009;15(6):600–9.

105. O'Grady JG, Alexander GJ, Hayllar KM, et al. Early indicators of prognosis in fulminant hepatic failure. Gastroenterology 1989;97(2):439–45.

106. O'Grady JG, Langley PG, Isola LM, et al. Coagulopathy of fulminant hepatic failure. Semin Liver Dis 1986;6(2):159–63.

107. McPhail MJ, Wendon JA, Bernal W. Meta-analysis of performance of Kings's College Hospital criteria in prediction of outcome in non-paracetamol-induced acute liver failure. J Hepatol 2010;53(3):492–9.

108. McPhail MJ, Farne H, Senvar N, et al. Ability of King's College criteria and model for end-stage liver disease scores to predict mortality of patients with acute liver failure: a meta-analysis. Clin Gastroenterol Hepatol 2016;14(4):516–25.e5 [quiz: e43–5].

109. Bernal W, Donaldson N, Wyncoll D, et al. Blood lactate as an early predictor of outcome in paracetamol-induced acute liver failure: a cohort study. Lancet 2002;359(9306):558–63.

110. Schmidt LE, Dalhoff K. Serum phosphate is an early predictor of outcome in severe acetaminophen-induced hepatotoxicity. Hepatology 2002;36(3):659–65.

111. Schmidt LE, Dalhoff K. Alpha-fetoprotein is a predictor of outcome in acetaminophen-induced liver injury. Hepatology 2005;41(1):26–31.

112. Schiodt FV, Bondesen S, Petersen I, et al. Admission levels of serum Gc-globulin: predictive value in fulminant hepatic failure. Hepatology 1996;23(4): 713–8.

113. Bernal W, Auzinger G, Sizer E, et al. Early prediction of outcome of acute liver failure using bedside measurement of interleukin-6. Hepatology 2007;46(S1): 617A.

114. Rosen HR, Biggins SW, Niki T, et al. Association between plasma level of galectin-9 and survival of patients with drug-induced acute liver failure. Clin Gastroenterol Hepatol 2016;14(4):606–12.e3.

115. Stravitz RT, Bowling R, Bradford RL, et al. Role of procoagulant microparticles in mediating complications and outcome of acute liver injury/acute liver failure. Hepatology 2013;58(1):304–13.

116. Craig DG, Kitto L, Zafar S, et al. An elevated neutrophil-lymphocyte ratio is associated with adverse outcomes following single time-point paracetamol (acetaminophen) overdose: a time-course analysis. Eur J Gastroenterol Hepatol 2014;26(9):1022–9.

117. Karvellas CJ, Speiser JL, Tremblay M, et al. Elevated FABP1 serum levels are associated with poorer survival in acetaminophen-induced acute liver failure. Hepatology 2017;65(3):938–49.

118. Karvellas CJ, Speiser JL, Tremblay M, et al. The association between FABP7 serum levels with survival and neurological complications in acetaminophen-induced acute liver failure: a nested case-control study. Ann Intensive Care 2017;7(1):99.

119. Schmidt LE, Larsen FS. MELD score as a predictor of liver failure and death in patients with acetaminophen-induced liver injury. Hepatology 2007;45(3): 789–96.

120. Cholongitas E, Theocharidou E, Vasianopoulou P, et al. Comparison of the sequential organ failure assessment score with the King's College Hospital criteria and the model for end-stage liver disease score for the prognosis of acetaminophen-induced acute liver failure. Liver Transpl 2012;18(4):405–12.

121. Craig DG, Reid TW, Wright EC, et al. The sequential organ failure assessment (SOFA) score is prognostically superior to the model for end-stage liver disease (MELD) and MELD variants following paracetamol (acetaminophen) overdose. Aliment Pharmacol Ther 2012;35(6):705–13.

122. Craig DG, Zafar S, Reid TW, et al. The sequential organ failure assessment (SOFA) score is an effective triage marker following staggered paracetamol (acetaminophen) overdose. Aliment Pharmacol Ther 2012;35(12):1408–15.

123. Mitchell I, Bihari D, Chang R, et al. Earlier identification of patients at risk from acetaminophen-induced acute liver failure. Crit Care Med 1998;26(2):279–84.

124. Koch DG, Tillman H, Durkalski V, et al. Development of a model to predict transplant-free survival of patients with acute liver failure. Clin Gastroenterol Hepatol 2016;14(8):1199–206.e2.

125. Speiser JL, Lee WM, Karvellas CJ. Predicting outcome on admission and post-admission for acetaminophen-induced acute liver failure using classification and regression tree models. PLoS One 2015;10(4):e0122929.

126. Bernal W, Wang Y, Maggs J, et al. Development and validation of a dynamic outcome prediction model for paracetamol-induced acute liver failure: a cohort study. Lancet Gastroenterol Hepatol 2016;1(3):217–25.

127. Lee WM. Acute liver failure. Semin Respir Crit Care Med 2012;33(1):36–45.

128. Reddy KR, Ellerbe C, Schilsky M, et al. Determinants of outcome among patients with acute liver failure listed for liver transplantation in the United States. Liver Transpl 2016;22(4):505–15.

129. Karvellas CJ, Safinia N, Auzinger G, et al. Medical and psychiatric outcomes for patients transplanted for acetaminophen-induced acute liver failure: a case-control study. Liver Int 2010;30(6):826–33.

130. Germani G, Theocharidou E, Adam R, et al. Liver transplantation for acute liver failure in Europe: outcomes over 20 years from the ELTR database. J Hepatol 2012;57(2):288–96.

131. Fontana RJ, Ellerbe C, Durkalski VE, et al. Two-year outcomes in initial survivors with acute liver failure: results from a prospective, multicentre study. Liver Int 2015;35(2):370–80.

132. Rangnekar AS, Ellerbe C, Durkalski V, et al. Quality of life is significantly impaired in long-term survivors of acute liver failure and particularly in acetaminophen-overdose patients. Liver Transpl 2013;19(9):991–1000.

133. Crone C, DiMartini A. Liver transplant for intentional acetaminophen overdose: a survey of transplant clinicians experiences with recommendations. Psychosomatics 2014;55(6):602–12.

134. Pereira LM, Langley PG, Hayllar KM, et al. Coagulation factor V and VIII/V ratio as predictors of outcome in paracetamol induced fulminant hepatic failure: relation to other prognostic indicators. Gut 1992;33(1):98–102.

Nonviral or Drug-Induced Etiologies of Acute Liver Failure

Russell Rosenblatt, MD, Robert S. Brown Jr, MD, MPH*

KEYWORDS

- Acute liver failure • Autoimmune hepatitis • Budd-Chiari syndrome • Wilson disease
- Fulminant hepatic failure

KEY POINTS

- When viral hepatitis and drug-induced liver injury are ruled out as etiologies of acute liver failure, Budd-Chiari, autoimmune hepatitis, and Wilson disease need to be evaluated as possible underlying etiologies.
- If no infection is present in a patient with acute liver failure from autoimmune hepatitis, consider corticosteroid therapy if MELD-Na is less than 28 and reassess for improvement within 1 week.
- Following an algorithm in patients presenting with acute Budd-Chiari syndrome is associated with improved outcomes and can lead to reversal of acute liver failure.
- Acute liver failure in patients with Wilson disease requires urgent liver transplantation evaluation because spontaneous survival is unlikely.
- In patients with acute liver failure and pregnancy, prompt delivery is recommended.

INTRODUCTION

Acute liver failure (ALF) is a highly fatal but rare condition with approximately 2000 cases occurring annually in the United States.[1] ALF is diagnosed by the following criteria: absence of pre-existing liver disease, acute onset less than 26 weeks, coagulopathy defined as international normalized ratio greater than 1.5, and the presence of encephalopathy.[2] Patients can present with a wide range of symptoms including fatigue, jaundice, and confusion. In the pre–liver transplant era, outcomes were poor with survival of 15% but now are steadily improving to more than 65% and climbing with increased liver transplantation (LT) success rates.[3] Patients with ALF are listed as United Network for Organ Sharing status 1a and given top priority over all forms

Disclosure Statement: The authors have nothing to disclose.
Division of Gastroenterology and Hepatology, Weill Cornell Medical College, 1305 York Avenue, 4th Floor, New York, NY 10021, USA
* Corresponding author.
E-mail address: Rsb2005@med.cornell.edu

Clin Liver Dis 22 (2018) 347–360
https://doi.org/10.1016/j.cld.2018.01.008
1089-3261/18/© 2018 Elsevier Inc. All rights reserved.

liver.theclinics.com

of chronic liver disease in adults because their expected survival is thought to be less than 7 days, requiring urgent prioritization.[4]

There are a wide range of causes of ALF and regional differences that affect health behaviors, exposures, and genetics.[5] Drug-induced liver injury, more specifically acetaminophen, is the most common cause of ALF and has a high likelihood of spontaneous survival.[6] Although the most common causes of ALF are drug-induced liver injury and viral hepatitis, other causes of ALF can account for up to 48% of cases, with indeterminate causes making up 17% to 38% (**Fig. 1**).[3,5] Diagnosis is complicated because biopsy is often not possible given the presence of severe coagulopathy. Identification of the cause as early as possible in the clinical course is essential because certain disease processes are potentially reversible and prognosis can help drive transplant decision-making. This article reviews nonviral and nondrug-induced causes of ALF.

AUTOIMMUNE HEPATITIS

Autoimmune hepatitis (AIH) is an inflammatory disorder of the liver with a prevalence of 11 to 17 per 100,000 persons[7] and accounts for up to 6% of patients presenting with ALF.[8] Classically, patients present in the third to sixth decade of life and are female.[7] The severity of presenting symptoms can range from asymptomatic to acute, which accounts for approximately 25% to 40% of patients with AIH.[7,9] AIH is frequently associated with other autoimmune diseases including thyroiditis, synovitis, ulcerative colitis, and celiac disease.[7]

Diagnosis revolves around laboratory testing and biopsy results.[10] Along with a hepatocellular injury pattern, patients frequently have elevated serum globulin levels. AIH type 1 is associated with positive antinuclear antibody (ANA) and anti–smooth muscle antibody, whereas anti-liver cytosol type 1 and antiliver/kidney microsome type 1 are present in AIH type 2.[11] The International Autoimmune Hepatitis Group created criteria for diagnosis for AIH in 1999[10] and a simplified version in 2008.[12] Classic biopsy findings for AIH are the presence of interface hepatitis along with plasma cell infiltrate.[13] The diagnosis of AIH in ALF is more complicated because the histology is similar to that of a drug-induced liver injury.[9] Additionally, serum immunoglobulin G levels are normal in 25% to 39% of patients with acute presentation of AIH, whereas ANA is weakly positive or absent in 39% of patients.[14] Furthermore, in patients with ALF, only 50% and 60% of those clinically diagnosed to have AIH were diagnosed by the simplified 2008 and 1999 criteria, respectively.[15] Therefore, AIH is likely a frequent cause of indeterminate ALF, and in a study of 72 patients

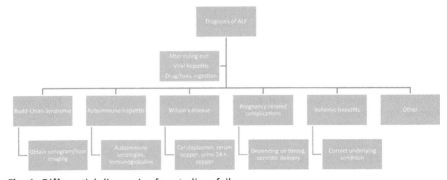

Fig. 1. Differential diagnosis of acute liver failure.

with ALF and indeterminate pathology, 58% had probable AIH. These patients had higher serum globulin levels, and were more likely to have elevated ANA or anti–smooth muscle antibody.[8]

In patients with acute presentations of AIH, corticosteroids are first-line therapy. Prednisone and azathioprine can improve laboratory findings in up to 68% to 75% of patients presenting acutely.[16] However, those with ALF from AIH have more variable outcomes because 20% to 80% of patients improve with corticosteroids.[17–20] A study of five retrospective studies assessing outcomes in patients with AIH and ALF noted that 89% were treated with corticosteroids and between 8.3% and 50% of those patients went into remission. All patients who did not respond to corticosteroids and who were not rescued by LT died, and no patients with a model for end stage liver disease (MELD) higher than 28 responded to corticosteroid therapy.[21] Another study noted that simply presenting acutely conferred a higher risk of not responding to steroids.[22] Yeoman and colleagues[17] found that patients who responded to corticosteroids had a decrease in MELD-Na score by Day 7. Czaja and colleagues[23] noted that a hyperbilirubinemia that does not resolve with corticosteroid use is highly predictive of treatment failure and need for rescue with LT. However, corticosteroids are not without risks, and chief among them is infection. In a study by the ALF study group assessing patients who received corticosteroids for various indications of ALF, there was no difference in spontaneous or overall survival for those who received corticosteroids. In fact, corticosteroid use was associated with decreased survival in the entire cohort.[24] Therefore, given the risk factors of corticosteroid treatment, it is recommended to have clearly defined end points.[25] Our recommendation is, if no infection is present, to attempt corticosteroid therapy in patients with MELD-Na less than 28 with a reassessment of improvement within 1 week (**Box 1**).

LT is the treatment of last resort for patients who have fulminant hepatic failure from AIH. In a review of eight patients with fulminant ALF from AIH, three patients underwent LT, four patients responded to treatment, two died, and one patient was still listed for LT.[26] Although the 5-year outcomes for LT for AIH are 73% to 78%[27] and comparable with outcomes for other liver disease etiologies, higher rates of rejection[28] and rarely recurrence[29] are noted in this cohort.

BUDD-CHIARI SYNDROME

Budd Chiari syndrome (BCS) is a rare syndrome with an annual incidence of 2.3 per 1,000,000 persons.[30] It presents as ALF in 7.3% to 49% of cases[31–33] and accounts for 0.9% to 1.5% of ALF cases.[34,35] BCS is a result of hepatic venous outflow obstruction caused by either a thrombotic or, less frequently, nonthrombotic condition at the level of the hepatic veins, inferior vena cava, or even right atrium.[36] In response, caudate lobe is enlarged in up to 75% of cases because of its direct venous drainage into the inferior vena cava.[37]

Box 1
Parameters for corticosteroid use in patients with autoimmune hepatitis and acute liver failure

No presence of infection

MELD-Na less than 28

Monitor for improvement of MELD-Na within 1 week

Monitor for improvement of bilirubin within 1 week

The underlying cause of BCS is identified in up to 87% to 90% of patients.[33,38] The most common causes include myeloproliferative disorders related to Janus tyrosine kinase 2 mutations (39%–50%), factor V Leiden (12%–25%), protein C deficiency (3%–12.5%), antiphospholipid syndrome (up to 25%), and rarely paroxysmal nocturnal hemoglobinuria (up to 10%).[39,40] Oral contraceptive pills, although a common risk factor for BCS in Western countries (up to 33% of women), is rarely if at all implicated in BCS cases in Asia, and pregnancy (6% of women) can also be implicated in BCS.[39,40] Additionally, there is a higher prevalence of pure hepatic vein obstruction in Western countries compared with Asian countries. Other rarer causes include obstruction of venous outflow from masses, such as hepatocellular carcinoma, renal cell carcinoma, hemangiosarcomas, focal nodular hyperplasia, polycystic liver disease, or parasitic cysts.[37,41]

Patients with BCS can present with right upper quadrant pain, ascites, edema, jaundice, and encephalopathy.[41] Depending on the severity and timing of venous outflow obstruction, portal hypertension and other manifestations of liver disease can present acutely or more chronically. In the subacute setting, transaminase elevation tends to be less marked than in acute venous obstruction but ascites can be more severe. Similar to patients with cardiac disease, the serum-ascitic fluid albumin gradient is elevated along with an ascitic protein greater than 2.5 g/dL.[37] Diagnosis is typically made by either contrast-enhanced imaging (computed tomography or MRI) with attention to a venogram, Doppler sonogram, or, if needed for confirmation, invasive hepatic venography.[37]

Treatment of BCS is based on expert opinion because it is a rare condition, and most data are presented in case series. Guidelines recommend starting anticoagulation immediately, followed by investigation for a lesion that is amenable to stenting or angioplasty (**Fig. 2**).[37,39,42] If these interventions fail, transjugular intrahepatic portosystemic shunt (TIPS), and ultimately, as a last resort, LT, should be considered.[39] Outcomes using this algorithm have been excellent, ranging from 77% to

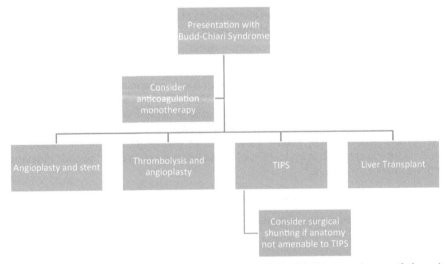

Fig. 2. Treatment options for patients presenting with Budd-Chiari syndrome. If there is technical failure or failure to respond to angioplasty or thrombolysis, can proceed to TIPS. If no improvement with TIPS or TIPS cannot be performed, can proceed to LT. TIPS, transjugular intrahepatic portosystemic shunt.

89% 5-year survival.[37,41,42] In a study of 157 patients following this algorithm, 69 received only anticoagulation and 40% of those patients died. Of the 88 patients who underwent invasive treatments, most (70%) underwent TIPS, whereas 23% ultimately required LT. The overall survival in this cohort was 77%.[42] Another case series of 163 patients had 56 patients undergo TIPS, and only three required LT.[39] However, the application and outcomes of this algorithm to patients with ALF is less clear because the subjects included in these studies have a wide variety of presentations ranging from chronic to subacute to acute.

More commonly, patients who present in ALF tended to undergo TIPS as first-line therapy[43] and had survival ranging from 50% to 80%.[32,44,45] Those with ALF who were not rescued with LT after a failed TIPS tended to die within days of the procedure from progressive liver failure or procedure-related complications.[32,44] Thrombolysis, typically by catheter or less commonly systemic administration, carries risk of hemorrhage but, when combined with angioplasty, can relieve obstruction in up to 87.5% cases.[42] Outcomes for LT for BCS have drastically improved since the dawn of the MELD era and are no different than for other causes.[31,46] Given that the previously mentioned algorithm is associated with excellent outcomes but has not been validated in patients with ALF, we recommend pursuing an approach favoring early intervention to relieve the obstruction if it can be performed safely. If there is no improvement with this intervention, we recommend pursuing LT evaluation.

WILSON DISEASE

Wilson disease (WD) is an autosomal-recessive disease characterized by a mutation at the ATP7B gene that encodes a metal-transporting P-type adenosine triphosphatase, mainly expressed in hepatocytes. The disease is characterized by hepatic copper retention and accumulation that can also be released into the bloodstream and deposited into other organs, such as the brain.[47] It is a rare disease that occurs in approximately 1 in 30,000 to 100,000 live births.[48]

WD can present at any age with a wide variety of manifestations ranging from ALF to chronic liver disease to psychosis. Most patients present between ages 5 and 35 but can present as late as 70.[47] Patients with classic WD are between 5 and 40 years old with low serum ceruloplasmin and detectable Kayser-Fleischer rings. Patients with earlier onset, before 10 years old, of WD tend to present with hepatic manifestations, whereas later onset presents with more neuropsychiatric manifestations.[49] Most patients presenting with ALF from WD have a Coombs-negative hemolytic anemia, coagulopathy, renal failure, transaminase elevation (usually <2000 IU/L), normal or low alkaline phosphatase, and are more likely female.[47] However, it is rare for all of these findings to be evident, especially on presentation, and diagnosis is challenging (**Fig. 3**). In a study of 55 patients diagnosed but not yet treated for WD, 17 patients presented with chronic liver disease, five patients with ALF, three patients with hemolysis, 20 patients with neurologic disease, and 10 patients by genetic testing from family history.[50] Neurologic symptoms are subtle, ranging from changes in handwriting to personality changes, to spasticity and dystonia.[47] A study by the ALF study group compared laboratory parameters in 140 patients, 16 of whom had ALF from WD, with 29 patients with other chronic liver disease and 17 with treated chronic WD. The authors found that a decreased alkaline phosphatase to total bilirubin ratio less than four has a sensitivity of 94% and specificity 96% along with a likelihood ratio of 23 for ALF from WD. When combined with an aspartate transaminase to alanine transaminase ratio greater than 2.2, the sensitivity and specificity of diagnosis of ALF from WD rose to 100% for both tests. This study also noted

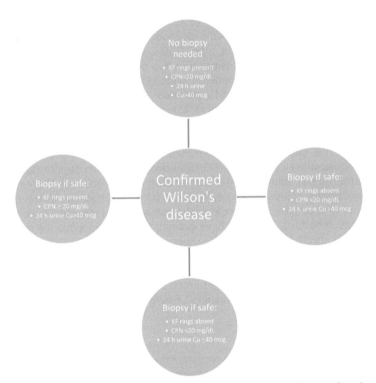

Fig. 3. Diagnosis of Wilson disease in patients presenting with liver disease of unclear cause. CPN, ceruloplasmin; Cu, copper; KF, Kayser-Fleischer. *Adapted from* Roberts EA, Schilsky ML. Diagnosis and treatment of Wilson disease: an update. Hepatology 2008;47(6):2090; with permission.

that the median hemoglobin was 7.1 in ALF from WD compared with 11.6 in all other patients, demonstrating the likely effect of Coombs-negative hemolytic anemia.[51] An older study by Sallie and coworkers[52] found the alkaline phosphatase to bilirubin ratio to be less specific, however. In this cohort of patients with WD and ALF, more than 10% of patients had normal ceruloplasmin, whereas all had abnormal urinary copper levels.[52]

The prognosis of WD presenting with ALF is poor, typically requiring LT for survival. Multiple studies have been performed attempting to stabilize patients until LT can be performed. Case reports have demonstrated the potential for success of plasmapheresis and albumin dialysis and Molecular Absorbents Recirculating System (MARS) as a bridge to LT.[53,54] There are little data that chelation therapy can improve WD in the setting of ALF and it generally is not used.

LT is an effective treatment for children and adults with ALF from WD. Patients who presented only with hepatic manifestations had significantly improved post-LT survival compared with those who had with both hepatic and neuropsychiatric symptoms. Additionally, patients who presented with ALF had similar outcomes to those who did not.[55] In a study of 75 adults and 46 children who underwent LT for WD from 1985 to 2009 in France, there was an 87% survival at 5, 10, and 15 years.[56] Another cohort of 37 patients who underwent LT for WD, accounting for 1.2% of all LTs, had eight patients present with ALF. Our recommendation is to evaluate patients presenting with ALF from WD for LT. If the patient requires bridging to LT, plasmapheresis, which is much more widely available than molecular absorbents recirculating system, can be used.

CONDITIONS DURING PREGNANCY

Liver test abnormalities in pregnancy are not uncommon, whereas ALF is rare. ALF in pregnant women can certainly be caused by viral hepatitis, notably hepatitis E,[57] but can also be caused by three pregnancy-specific conditions: (1) preeclampsia; (2) hemolysis, elevated liver tests, low platelets (HELLP) syndrome; and (3) acute fatty liver of pregnancy (AFLP) (Table 1). All three syndromes present with major risks to the mother (placental abruption, disseminated intravascular coagulopathy, death) and infant (preterm delivery, fetal growth restriction, hypoxic-induced neurologic injury, and perinatal death).[58]

Preeclampsia is present in approximately 3.4% of pregnancies and has an unclear pathophysiology but is related to the presence of the placenta itself or a maternal reaction to the placenta.[59] Risk factors include nulliparity, multifetal gestation, advanced maternal age, obesity, and a history of preeclampsia, because it recurs in about 20% of pregnancies.[59] It is characterized by the presence of edema, hypertension, and proteinuria detected after 20 weeks gestation.[58] HELLP syndrome is present in up to 20% of cases of severe preeclampsia[60,61] and is thought to have a similar pathophysiology to preeclampsia but with a more severe hepatic inflammation and activation of the coagulation cascade.[62] Presentation in HELLP syndrome is notable for elevated transaminases, hemolysis markers, thrombocytopenia, along with right upper quadrant or epigastric pain, nausea, and headache.[58,63] The pattern of liver injury is typically hepatocellular in nature and caused by vasoconstriction and fibrin precipitation.[61] A feared hepatic complication of both preeclampsia and HELLP syndrome, are hepatic rupture and hematoma beneath Glisson capsule. Embolization is successful in treating rupture and hematoma[64] but surgery is sometimes required

Table 1			
Description of pregnancy-specific causes of acute liver failure			
Disease	Presentation Timing	Presentation	Management[68]
Preeclampsia	After 20 wk	Range from asymptomatic to hepatic rupture, hypertension, proteinuria, transaminitis, RUQ pain[61]	Supportive management Deliver after 36 wk
HELLP	After 22 wk	Hemolysis, transaminitis RUQ pain, thrombocytopenia, hypertension, proteinuria[66]	Deliver after 34 wk Consider platelet transfusion to 40,000–50,000 cells/μL before delivery, especially if C-section is planned
Acute fatty liver of pregnancy	Late third trimester	Abdominal pain, jaundice, nausea, vomiting, confusion, transaminitis, hyperbilirubinemia, coagulopathy, hypoglycemia, preeclampsia/HELLP symptoms	Prompt delivery Monitor infant for signs of LCHAD deficiency

Abbreviations: LCHAD, long-chain 3-hydroxyacyl-coenzyme A dehydrogenase; RUQ, right upper quadrant.

to control bleeding.[57] A randomized trial showed the benefit of treatment based on the Mississippi Protocol, consisting of corticosteroids, magnesium sulfate, and systolic blood pressure control, in improving maternal outcomes.[65] A Cochrane review analyzed 11 studies in which corticosteroids were given to patients with HELLP and found no difference in maternal mortality, severe morbidity, or perinatal or infant death. The only objective improvement of steroid use was a statistically significant increase in platelet count.[66] Therefore, the only indication for steroid administration in HELLP should be limited to promote fetal lung maturity. Rarely, LT is required, but outcomes are comparable with outcomes for other causes.[67]

AFLP is a rapidly progressive and potentially fatal liver disease with an incidence of 5 to 15 cases per 100,000 births.[68–70] AFLP typically presents in the third trimester and is more common in twin pregnancies.[68] The underlying pathophysiology of AFLP resides in a mutation in long-chain 3-hydroxyacyl-coenzyme A dehydrogenase (LCHAD), an enzyme instrumental in B-oxidation of mitochondrial fatty acids.[71] However, not all women with LCHAD deficiency have liver disease because it typically manifests when the fetus has deficient LCHAD enzymatic activity.[72] Offspring should be monitored for signs and symptoms of LCHAD deficiency including hypoketotic hypoglycemia and fatty liver. ALF is present in up to 10.7% to 37.5% of patients with AFLP, and liver function frequently recovers soon after delivery.[69,70,73] Renal failure is also prevalent in up to 72% in patients with AFLP.[74] AFLP is diagnosed clinically or by the Swansea criteria (**Box 2**).[73,75] The Swansea criteria had an 85% and 100% positive predictive value and negative predictive value, respectively, in 20 patients who were biopsied postmortem, before, or just after delivery. In that study 40% of patients met criteria for HELLP, 20% for partial HELLP, and 10% for preeclampsia with liver

---

Box 2
Swansea criteria for diagnosis of acute fatty liver disease of pregnancy

Six or more criteria required in the absence of another cause

Vomiting

Abdominal pain

Polydipsia/polyuria

Encephalopathy

Elevated bilirubin greater than 14 μmol/L

Hypoglycemia less than 4 mmol/L

Elevated urate greater than 340 μmol/L

Leukocytosis greater than 11×10^6 cells/L

Ascites or bright liver on ultrasound

Elevated transaminases (AST or ALT) >42 IU/L

Elevated ammonia greater than 47 μmol/L

Renal impairment; creatinine greater than 150 μmol/L

Coagulopathy; prothrombin time greater than 14 s or aPPT greater than 34 s

Microvesicular steatosis on liver biopsy

Abbreviations: ALT, alanine transaminase; aPPT, activated partial thromboplastin time; AST, aspartate transaminase.
Adapted from Tran TT, Ahn J, Reau NS. ACG clinical guideline: liver disease and pregnancy. Am J Gastroenterol 2016;111(2):183; with permission.

involvement.[73] In the pretransplant era, mortality reached 85% but now ranges from 0% to 7.1% in case series.[68,69]

ISCHEMIC HEPATITIS

Ischemic hepatitis, often referred to as "shock liver," is characterized by a rapid rise in transaminases in the setting of significant cardiovascular, respiratory, or circulatory insult.[76,77] Ischemic hepatitis is present in 0.02% of hospital admissions, 2.5% of intensive care unit admissions, and in up to 40% of patients with transaminase elevation greater than 10 times the upper limit of normal.[76] The transaminases typically downtrend within 48 hours.[78] The most common precipitating events are cardiac or sepsis-related, with a prevalence of 66% to 78% and 23% of cases, respectively.[2,76] These events are frequently associated with episodes of hypotension, hypoxemia, or decreased hepatic blood flow, but are subclinical in up to 52.9%.[76] The underlying pathophysiology is thought to involve a two-hit hypothesis: a low flow state in addition to an acute insult.[77] When poor substrate is combined with a hypoxemic or hypotensive episode, the patient often suffers hepatic ischemia and necrosis. Biopsy, although not usually performed, demonstrates centrilobular (zone 3) necrosis.[79] Statins have been noted to be a protective factor against developing ischemic hepatitis, whereas active alcohol consumption is a risk factor.[80]

Ischemic hepatitis accounts for 0.3% to 6% of ALF cases.[81,82] Prognosis is poor with an early 29% to 45% mortality typically from multiorgan failure,[81,83] and patients are rarely transplanted given other existing comorbidities. However, a study of the ALF study group cohort noted that ischemic hepatitis accounted for 4.4% of 1147 cases of ALF, with only 2 of 51 patients undergoing LT. One patient survived more than 5 years, whereas the other died within 13 days of LT. Grade 3 or 4 encephalopathy and lack of normalization of liver tests were powerful predictors of short-term and long-term mortality, respectively.[81] However, it should be noted that the diagnosis of ALF is especially difficult to make in these patients given the high incidence of multiorgan failure, sepsis, and other conditions that can affect mental status and make it challenging to identify hepatic encephalopathy.[77] According to American Association for the Study of Liver Diseases guidelines, recommendations for treatment of ischemic hepatitis with ALF are to provide cardiovascular support.[2]

MUSHROOM POISONING

Mushroom poisoning leading to liver failure is typically caused by *Amanita phalloides*.[84–87] Toxicity occurs through amatoxin binding to DNA-dependent RNA polymerase II and inhibiting the chain elongation that is necessary for transcription.[88] Typically, there are three phases of poisoning after a 6- to 12-hour asymptomatic period. The first phase is marked by gastrointestinal distress with diarrhea, vomiting, and abdominal pain and is followed 24 to 48 hours after by a phase of hepatotoxicity and coagulopathy. The third and final phase, occurring 4 to 7 days after ingestion is characterized by fulminant hepatic failure with convulsions and hemorrhage.[86]

Mushroom poisoning causing acute liver injury or ALF is quite morbid with a spontaneous survival rate between 33.8% and 55.6%.[84,87] Predictors of poor outcome include diarrhea within 8 hours of ingestion, meeting King's College Criteria,[85] and prothrombin index.[84] In a study by the ALF study group of 2224 patients, 5 and 13 patients had amatoxin-induced acute liver injury or ALF, respectively, and 10 of the 18 spontaneously survived. Of the patients with only acute liver injury, one was transplanted and four spontaneously survived.[87] Because of the rarity of the condition, validated treatment trials have not been performed. *N*-Acetylcysteine and penicillin are common therapies given. Penicillin is thought to be effective through a variety of mechanisms including reducing γ-aminobutyric acid–producing bacteria and even displacing α-amatoxicin.[86] Silibinin, an extract of milk thistle, is another therapy that can help increase excretion of amatoxin in the bile and inhibit amatoxin uptake by competing for the same transporter.[89] In a pooled analysis of 452 patients, the use of silibinin was shown to significantly reduce mortality. Overall, penicillin and silibinin, if available, are administered to attempt to avoid LT, but if these treatments fail, LT should be used as a rescue therapy.

SUMMARY

ALF is a rare but highly morbid disease with improving outcomes because of the increased use of LT, and likely improvements in critical care. When viral and drug-induced causes of liver injury have been ruled out, other common causes including AIH, BCS, and WD need to be worked up and ruled out. AIH and BCS are treated in some cases with corticosteroids and interventional procedures to relieve hepatic vein obstruction, respectively, and even reverse the course of ALF. However, in all of these nonviral and nondrug etiologies of ALF, if rapid improvement is not seen, patients should proceed to LT.

REFERENCES

1. Lee WM, Squires RH, Nyberg SL, et al. Acute liver failure: summary of a workshop. Hepatology 2008;47(4):1401–15.
2. Lee WM, Stravitz RT, Larson AM. Introduction to the revised American Association for the Study of Liver Diseases position paper on acute liver failure 2011. Hepatology 2012;55(3):965–7.
3. Ostapowicz G, Fontana RJ, Schiødt FV, et al. Results of a prospective study of acute liver failure at 17 tertiary care centers in the United States. Ann Intern Med 2002;137(12):947–54.
4. Organ procurement and transplantation network policies. 2017. Available at: https://optn.transplant.hrsa.gov/media/1200/optn_policies.pdf. Accessed November 10, 2017.
5. Bernal W, Auzinger G, Dhawan A, et al. Acute liver failure. Lancet 2010;376: 190–201.
6. Larson AM, Polson J, Fontana RJ, et al. Acetaminophen-induced acute liver failure: results of a United States multicenter, prospective study. Hepatology 2005; 42(6):1364–72.
7. Manns MP, Czaja AJ, Gorham J, et al. Diagnosis and management of autoimmune hepatitis. Hepatology 2010;51:2193–213.
8. Stravitz RT, Lefkowitch JH, Fontana RJ, et al. Autoimmune acute liver failure: proposed clinical and histological criteria. Hepatology 2011;53(2):517–26.
9. Manns MP, Lohse AW, Vergani D. Autoimmune hepatitis: update 2015. J Hepatol 2015;62(S1):S100–11.
10. Alvarez F, Berg P, Bianchi FB, et al. International autoimmune hepatitis group report: review of criteria for diagnosis of autoimmune hepatitis. J Hepatol 1999; 31(5):929–38.
11. Bogdanos DP, Mieli-Vergani G, Vergani D. Autoantibodies and their antigens in autoimmune hepatitis. Semin Liver Dis 2009;29(3):241–53.
12. Hennes EM, Zeniya M, Czaja AJ, et al. Simplified criteria for the diagnosis of autoimmune hepatitis. Hepatology 2008;48(1):169–76.
13. Krawitt EL. Autoimmune hepatitis. N Engl J Med 2006;354(1):54–66.

14. Yasui S, Fujiwara K, Yonemitsu Y, et al. Clinicopathological features of severe and fulminant forms of autoimmune hepatitis. J Gastroenterol 2011;46(3):378–90.

15. Yeoman AD, Westbrook RH, Al-Chalabi T, et al. Diagnostic value and utility of the simplified International Autoimmune Hepatitis Group (IAIHG) criteria in acute and chronic liver disease. Hepatology 2009;50(2):538–45.

16. Czaja AJ. Acute and acute severe (fulminant) autoimmune hepatitis. Dig Dis Sci 2013;58(4):897–914.

17. Yeoman AD, Westbrook RH, Zen Y, et al. Early predictors of corticosteroid treatment failure in icteric presentations of autoimmune hepatitis. Hepatology 2011; 53(3):926–34.

18. Ichai P, Duclos-Vallée JC, Guettier C, et al. Usefulness of corticosteroids for the treatment of severe and fulminant forms of autoimmune hepatitis. Liver Transpl 2007;13(7):996–1003.

19. Sugawara K, Nakayama N, Mochida S. Acute liver failure in Japan: definition, classification, and prediction of the outcome. J Gastroenterol 2012;47(8):849–61.

20. Takikawa Y, Suzuki K. Clinical epidemiology of fulminant hepatitis in Japan. Hepatol Res 2008;38(Suppl 1):S14–8.

21. Potts JR, Verma S. Optimizing management in autoimmune hepatitis with liver failure at initial presentation. World J Gastroenterol 2011;17(16):2070–5.

22. Montano-Loza AJ, Carpenter HA, Czaja AJ. Features associated with treatment failure in type 1 autoimmune hepatitis and predictive value of the model of end-stage liver disease. Hepatology 2007;46(4):1138–45.

23. Czaja AJ, Rakela J, Ludwig J. Features reflective of early prognosis in corticosteroid-treated severe autoimmune chronic active hepatitis. Gastroenterology 1988;95(2):448–53.

24. Karkhanis J, Verna EC, Chang MS, et al. Steroid use in acute liver failure. Hepatology 2014;59(2):612–21.

25. Czaja AJ. Corticosteroids or not in severe acute or fulminant autoimmune hepatitis: therapeutic brinksmanship and the point beyond salvation. Liver Transpl 2007;13(7):953–5.

26. Kessler WR, Cummings OW, Eckert G, et al. Fulminant hepatic failure as the initial presentation of acute autoimmune hepatitis. Clin Gastroenterol Hepatol 2004; 2(7):625–31.

27. Schramm C, Bubenheim M, Adam R, et al. Primary liver transplantation for autoimmune hepatitis: a comparative analysis of the European liver transplant registry. Liver Transpl 2010;16(4):461–9.

28. Vogel A, Heinrich E, Bahr MJ, et al. Long-term outcome of liver transplantation for autoimmune hepatitis. Clin Transplant 2004;18(1):62–9.

29. Duclos-Vallée JC, Sebagh M, Rifai K, et al. A 10 year follow up study of patients transplanted for autoimmune hepatitis: histological recurrence precedes clinical and biochemical recurrence. Gut 2003;52(6):893–7.

30. Ki M, Choi HY, Kim KA, et al. Incidence, prevalence and complications of Budd-Chiari syndrome in South Korea: a nationwide, population-based study. Liver Int 2016;36(7):1067–73.

31. Segev DL, Nguyen GC, Locke JE, et al. Twenty years of liver transplantation for Budd-Chiari syndrome: a national registry analysis. Liver Transpl 2007;13(9): 1285–94.

32. Garcia-Pagán JC, Heydtmann M, Raffa S, et al. TIPS for Budd-Chiari syndrome: long-term results and prognostics factors in 124 patients. Gastroenterology 2008; 135(3):808–15.

33. Harmanci O, Kav T, Peynircioglu B, et al. Long-term follow-up study in Budd-Chiari syndrome: single-center experience in 22 years. J Clin Gastroenterol 2013;47(8):706–12.
34. Marudanayagam R, Shanmugam V, Gunson B, et al. Aetiology and outcome of acute liver failure. HPB (Oxford) 2009;11(5):429–34.
35. Parekh J, Matei VM, Canas-Coto A, et al. Budd-Chiari syndrome causing acute liver failure: a multicenter case series. Liver Transpl 2017;23(2):135–42.
36. Ludwig J, Hashimoto E, McGill D, et al. Classification of hepatic venous outflow obstruction: ambiguous terminology of the Budd-Chiari syndrome. Mayo Clin Proc 1990;65(1):51–5.
37. DeLeve L, Valla D-C, Garcia-Tsao G. Vascular disorders of the liver. Hepatology 2009;49(5):1729–64.
38. Denninger MH, Chaït Y, Casadevall N, et al. Cause of portal or hepatic venous thrombosis in adults: the role of multiple concurrent factors. Hepatology 2000; 31(3):587–91.
39. Murad SD, Plessier A, Hernandez-Guerra M, et al. Etiology, management, and outcome of the Budd-Chiari syndrome. Ann Intern Med 2009;151(3):167–75.
40. Valla D, Paris U, Diderot D, et al. Hepatic venous outflow tract obstruction etiopathogenesis: Asia versus the West. J Gastroenterol Hepatol 2004;19:204–11.
41. Plessier A, Valla DC. Budd-Chiari syndrome. Semin Liver Dis 2008;28(3):259–69.
42. Seijo S, Plessier A, Hoekstra J, et al. Good long-term outcome of Budd-Chiari syndrome with a step-wise management. Hepatology 2013;57(5):1962–8.
43. Eapen CE, Velissaris D, Heydtmann M, et al. Favourable medium term outcome following hepatic vein recanalisation and/or transjugular intrahepatic portosystemic shunt for Budd Chiari syndrome. Gut 2006;55(6):878–84.
44. Kavanagh PM, Roberts J, Gibney R, et al. Acute Budd-Chiari syndrome with liver failure: the experience of a policy of initial interventional radiological treatment using transjugular intrahepatic portosystemic shunt. J Gastroenterol Hepatol 2004; 19(10):1135–9.
45. Mancuso A, Fung K, Mela M, et al. TIPS for acute and chronic Budd-Chiari syndrome: a single-centre experience. J Hepatol 2003;38(6):751–4.
46. Ulrich F, Pratschke J, Neumann U, et al. Eighteen years of liver transplantation experience in patients with advanced Budd-Chiari syndrome. Liver Transpl 2008;14(2):144–50.
47. Roberts EA, Schilsky ML. Diagnosis and treatment of Wilson disease: an update. Hepatology 2008;47(6):2089–111.
48. Frydman M. Genetic aspects of Wilson's disease. J Gastroenterol Hepatol 1990; 5(4):483–90.
49. Catana AM, Medici V. Liver transplantation for Wilson disease. World J Hepatol 2012;4(1):5–10.
50. Steindl P, Ferenci P, Dienes H, et al. Wilson's disease in patients presenting with liver disease: a diagnostic challenge. Gastroenterology 1997;113(1):212–8.
51. Korman JD, Volenberg I, Balko J, et al. Screening for Wilson disease in acute liver failure: a comparison of currently available diagnostic tests. Hepatology 2008; 48(4):1167–74.
52. Sallie R, Katsiyiannakis L, Baldwin D, et al. Failure of simple biochemical indexes to reliably differentiate fulminant Wilson's disease from other causes of fulminant liver failure. Hepatology 1992;16(5):1206–11.
53. Jhang JS, Schilsky ML, Lefkowitch JH, et al. Therapeutic plasmapheresis as a bridge to liver transplantation in fulminant Wilson disease. J Clin Apher 2007; 22(1):10–4.

54. Sen S, Felldin M, Steiner C, et al. Albumin dialysis and molecular adsorbents re-circulating system (MARS) for acute Wilson's disease. Liver Transpl 2002;8(10): 962–7.

55. Medici V, Mirante VG, Fassati LR, et al. Liver transplantation for Wilson's disease: the burden of neurological and psychiatric disorders. Liver Transpl 2005;11(9): 1056–63.

56. Guillaud O, Dumortier J, Sobesky R, et al. Long term results of liver transplantation for Wilson's disease: experience in France. J Hepatol 2014;60(3):579–89.

57. Tran TT, Ahn J, Reau NS. ACG clinical guideline: liver disease and pregnancy. Am J Gastroenterol 2016;111(2):176–94.

58. Sibai B, Dekker G, Kupferminc M. Pre-eclampsia. Lancet 2005;365(9461): 785–99.

59. Ananth CV, Keyes KM, Wapner RJ. Pre-eclampsia rates in the United States, 1980-2010: age-period-cohort analysis. BMJ 2013;347:f6564.

60. Haram K, Svendsen E, Abildgaard U. The HELLP syndrome: clinical issues and management. A review. BMC Pregnancy Childbirth 2009;9:8.

61. Vigil-De Gracia P, Ortega-Paz L. Pre-eclampsia/eclampsia and hepatic rupture. Int J Gynecol Obstet 2012;118(3):186–9.

62. Benedetto C, Marozio L, Tancredi A, et al. Biochemistry of HELLP syndrome. Adv Clin Chem 2011;53:85–104.

63. Sibai BM. Diagnosis, controversies, and management of the syndrome of hemo-lysis, elevated liver enzymes, and low platelet count. Obstet Gynecol 2004;103(5, Part 1):981–91.

64. Grand'maison S, Sauve N, Weber F, et al. Hepatic rupture in hemolysis, elevated liver enzymes, low platelets syndrome. Obstet Gynecol 2012;119(3):617–25.

65. Martin JN, Owens MY, Keiser SD, et al. Standardized Mississippi protocol treatment of 190 patients with HELLP syndrome: slowing disease progression and preventing new major maternal morbidity. Hypertens Pregnancy 2012;31:79–90.

66. Woudstra DM, Chandra S, Hofmeyr GJ. Corticosteroids for HELLP (hemolysis, elevated liver enzymes, low platelets) syndrome in pregnancy. Cochrane Database Syst Rev 2010;(9):CD008148.

67. Zarrinpar A, Farmer DG, Ghobrial RM, et al. Liver transplantation for HELLP syndrome. Am Surg 2007;73(10):1013–6.

68. Knight M, Nelson-Piercy C, Kurinczuk JJ, et al. A prospective national study of acute fatty liver of pregnancy in the UK. Gut 2008;57(7):951–6.

69. Castro MA, Fassett MJ, Reynolds TB, et al. Reversible peripartum liver failure: a new perspective on the diagnosis, treatment, and cause of acute fatty liver of pregnancy, based on 28 consecutive cases. Am J Obstet Gynecol 1999; 181(2):389–95.

70. Nelson DB, Yost NP, Cunningham FG. Acute fatty liver of pregnancy: clinical outcomes and expected duration of recovery. Am J Obstetrics Gynecol 2013;209(5): 456.e1–7.

71. Ibdah JA, Bennett MJ, Rinaldo P, et al. A fetal fatty-acid oxidation disorder as a cause of liver disease in pregnant women. N Engl J Med 1999;340(22):1723–31.

72. Treem WR, Shoup ME, Hale DE, et al. Acute fatty liver of pregnancy, hemolysis, elevated liver enzymes, and low platelets syndrome, and long chain 3-hydrox-yacyl-coenzyme A dehydrogenase deficiency. Am J Gastroenterol 1996;91(11): 2293–300.

73. Goel A, Ramakrishna B, Zachariah U, et al. How accurate are the Swansea criteria to diagnose acute fatty liver of pregnancy in predicting hepatic microve-sicular steatosis? Gut 2011;60(1):138–9.

74. Xiong HF, Liu JY, Guo LM, et al. Acute fatty liver of pregnancy: over six months follow-up study of twenty-five patients. World J Gastroenterol 2015;21(6): 1927–31.

75. Ch'ng CL. Prospective study of liver dysfunction in pregnancy in Southwest Wales. Gut 2002;51(6):876–80.

76. Tapper EB, Sengupta N, Bonder A. The incidence and outcomes of ischemic hepatitis: a systematic review with meta-analysis. Am J Med 2015;128(12): 1314–21.

77. Lightsey JM, Rockey DC. Current concepts in ischemic hepatitis. Curr Opin Gastroenterol 2017;33(3):158–63.

78. Giannini EG, Testa R, Savarino V. Liver enzyme alteration: a guide for clinicians. CMAJ 2005;172(3):367–79.

79. Hofer H, Oesterreicher C, Wrba F, et al. Centrilobular necrosis in autoimmune hepatitis: a histological feature associated with acute clinical presentation. J Clin Pathol 2006;59(3):246–9.

80. Drolz A, Horvatits T, Michl B, et al. Statin therapy is associated with reduced incidence of hypoxic hepatitis in critically ill patients. J Hepatol 2014;60(6):1187–93.

81. Taylor RM, Tujios S, Jinjuvadia K, et al. Short and long-term outcomes in patients with acute liver failure due to ischemic hepatitis. Dig Dis Sci 2012;57(3):777–85.

82. Brandsœter B, Höckerstedt K, Friman S, et al. Fulminant hepatic failure: outcome after listing for highly urgent liver transplantation - 12 years' experience in the Nordic countries. Liver Transpl 2002;8(11):1055–62.

83. Birrer R, Takuda Y, Takara T. Hypoxic hepatopathy: pathophysiology and prognosis. Intern Med 2007;46(14):1063–70.

84. Ganzert M, Felgenhauer N, Zilker T. Indication of liver transplantation following amatoxin intoxication. J Hepatol 2005;42(2):202–9.

85. Escudié L, Francoz C, Vinel JP, et al. *Amanita phalloides* poisoning: reassessment of prognostic factors and indications for emergency liver transplantation. J Hepatol 2007;46(3):466–73.

86. Enjalbert F, Rapior S, Nouguier-Soulé J, et al. Treatment of amatoxin poisoning: 20-year retrospective analysis. J Toxicol Clin Toxicol 2002;40(6):715–57.

87. Karvellas CJ, Tillman H, Leung AA, et al. Acute liver injury and acute liver failure from mushroom poisoning in North America. Liver Int 2016;36(7):1043–50.

88. Wienland T, Faulstich H. Fifty years of amanitin. Experientia 1991;47(11–12): 1186–93.

89. Saller R, Meier R, Brignoli R. The use of silymarin in the treatment of liver diseases. Drugs 2001;61(14):2035–63.

The Clinical Spectrum and Manifestations of Acute Liver Failure

Sarah Zahra Maher, MD[a],*, Ian Roy Schreibman, MD[b]

KEYWORDS

- Acute liver failure • Acetaminophen toxicity • Cerebral edema
- Hepatic encephalopathy

KEY POINTS

- Acute liver failure is a rare condition defined by the onset of hepatic encephalopathy and coagulopathy in patients without preexisting cirrhosis or liver disease.
- Management includes early recognition and administration of cause-specific therapy preferably in an intensive care unit setting as well as transfer to a liver transplantation center.
- Complications can be life threatening and include metabolic and acid-base disturbances, renal failure, cardiopulmonary complications, bleeding, and coagulopathy.
- Cerebral edema and intracranial hypertension are complications of acute liver failure that result in high morbidity and mortality.

INTRODUCTION

Acute liver failure (ALF) is a rare, life-threatening condition that is defined by the onset of hepatic encephalopathy (HE) and coagulopathy (international normalized ratio [INR] ≥ 1.5) in patients without cirrhosis or preexisting liver disease of less than 26 weeks.[1,2] In addition, patients can develop acute on chronic liver disease with autoimmune hepatitis, Wilson disease, and alcohol-induced liver injury (ie, severe alcoholic hepatitis). The time frame of ALF is classified as hyperacute (<7 days), acute (7–21 days), or subacute (22 days to <26 weeks) based on the onset of encephalopathy and jaundice.[3,4] The most common causes of ALF in the United States include acetaminophen (acetyl-p-aminophenol) toxicity, idiosyncratic drug-induced liver failure, viral hepatitis, and indeterminate causes. Early recognition of ALF and initiation of cause-specific therapy and immediate contact with a liver transplant center have led to improved outcomes

Disclosure: The authors have nothing to disclose.
[a] Internal Medicine, Penn State Health Milton S. Hershey Medical Center, 500 University Drive, Hershey, PA 17033, USA; [b] Division of Gastroenterology and Hepatology, Penn State Health Milton S. Hershey Medical Center, 500 University Drive, Hershey, PA 17033, USA
* Corresponding author.
E-mail address: smaher@pennstatehealth.psu.edu

Clin Liver Dis 22 (2018) 361–374
https://doi.org/10.1016/j.cld.2018.01.012
1089-3261/18/© 2018 Elsevier Inc. All rights reserved.

liver.theclinics.com

over the past few decades.[5,6] In this article the authors discuss the clinical spectrum and manifestations of ALF.

PATHOPHYSIOLOGY

ALF occurs when the rate of hepatocyte death, characterized by apoptosis or necrosis, exceeds the rate of hepatocyte regeneration. The cellular damage that occurs varies by disease process. For example, acetaminophen toxicity results in apoptosis, whereas ischemia results in necrosis. The end result, however, is the same, in that hepatocyte death leads to multi-organ failure.[7]

CAUSE

ALF results from a wide variety of causes and varies by country. The causes of ALF have also changed over the past few decades. In the United States and Western Europe, there has been a decline in viral hepatitis and an increase in acetaminophen-induced ALF, which, along with idiosyncratic drug-induced liver failure, accounts for 60% of cases of ALF. In contrast, Asian countries have a higher incidence of hepatitis viruses leading to ALF with hepatitis E virus in India and Pakistan and hepatitis B virus (HBV) in Japan, China, and Thailand.[8–10] Determining the specific cause of ALF can help practitioners manage the condition and predict its prognosis. Knowing the cause also helps predict how certain manifestations will present. For example, acetaminophen-induced ALF and mushroom poisoning both have a rapid presentation, whereas other forms of drug-induced liver failure tend to have a more insidious onset. Causes of ALF are listed in **Table 1** and briefly discussed later.

DIAGNOSIS AND INITIAL EVALUATION

A thorough history and physical examination helps aid in the diagnosis. Specifically, it is important to illicit potential exposures, including drugs, herbs, toxins, and viruses, to help determine the cause of ALF and to initiate cause-specific treatment.

The most widely accepted definition of ALF includes the onset of encephalopathy as well as evidence of coagulation abnormalities (prolonged prothrombin time, INR $\geq$1.5) in patients without preexisting cirrhosis and with an illness of less than 26 weeks of duration. This definition includes patients with Wilson disease, autoimmune hepatitis, or a viral hepatitis, as long as the duration of illness has only been recognized for less than 26 weeks. Patients with severe alcoholic hepatitis, however, are considered to have acute-on-chronic liver failure as most patients have a long-standing history of heavy alcohol use.

Initial laboratory tests should include routine chemistries, complete blood count, coagulation panel, and an arterial blood gas. It is also important to evaluate for complications, including an arterial lactate, ammonia, amylase, and lipase, as well as monitoring urinary output. Depending on the cause of ALF, variations in laboratory testing can be seen, which is discussed in detail in the following section. The following laboratory abnormalities can be seen in most patients with ALF[4,11]:

- Prolonged prothrombin time, INR greater than 1.5
- Elevated aminotransferase levels
- Elevated bilirubin
- Anemia and thrombocytopenia
- Elevated serum creatinine and blood urea nitrogen

Table 1
Causes of acute liver failure

Cause	Examples	Comments
Drugs and toxins	• Acetaminophen • Idiosyncratic drug reactions[a] • Herbal supplements[b] • Mushroom poisoning • Other toxins[c]	• ALF due to acetaminophen toxicity is dose related • Idiosyncratic drug reactions are dose independent
Infectious	• Hepatitis A, B, D, E • Herpes simplex virus • Varicella zoster virus • CMV • EBV • Parasites (dengue, leptospirosis, malaria)	—
Ischemia	• Ischemic hepatitis • Shock: cardiogenic, septic, hypovolemic • Heat stroke	—
Vascular	• Acute Budd-Chiari • Venoocclusive disease	—
Metabolic/ miscellaneous	• Wilson disease • Acute fatty liver of pregnancy, eclampsia, HELLP syndrome • Alpha-1 antitrypsin deficiency • Autoimmune hepatitis • Malignant infiltration	—
Indeterminate	Unknown	15%–20% of ALF in adults and 50% of ALF in children cannot be attributed to a specific cause

Abbreviations: CMV, cytomegalovirus; EBV, Epstein-Barr virus; HELLP, hemolysis, elevated liver enzymes, low platelet count.

[a] Examples include, but are not limited to, abacavir, allopurinol, amiodarone, amoxicillin, aspirin, carbamazepine, ciprofloxacin, dapsone, didanosine, doxycycline, efavirenz, gemtuzumab, isoniazid, itraconazole, methamphetamine, methyldopa, nitrofurantoin, nonsteroidal antiinflammatory drugs, phenytoin, rifampin, statins, sulfonamides, tetracycline, tricyclic antidepressants, trimethoprim-sulfamethoxazole, valproic acid.

[b] Examples include, but are not limited to, comfrey, greater celandine, He Shon, Wu, Herbalife, Hydroxycut, kava kava, ma huang.

[c] Examples include, but are not limited to, alcohol, carbon tetrachloride, cocaine, MDMA (ecstasy).

- Electrolytes abnormalities: hypoglycemia, hypomagnesemia, hypokalemia, hypophosphatemia
- Acidosis or alkalosis
- Elevated ammonia level
- Elevated lactate dehydrogenase level

Liver biopsy has an uncertain role in ALF, as it could add diagnostic information, however, carries the risks of bleeding and death. Only 2 studies assessed the diagnostic accuracy of liver biopsy, with the diagnosis changing in only 18% of cases. The studies did not report on whether or not the diagnosis changed the management plan or outcome. The American Gastroenterological Association (AGA) suggests against routine use of liver biopsy for diagnosis in ALF.[4,5]

DETERMINING CAUSES AND SPECIFIC THERAPIES

Regardless of the cause of ALF, there is high morbidity and mortality associated with ALF. Without a transplant, spontaneous survival has been reported at 15% or less. Accordingly, the single most important step is transferring patients to a tertiary care center where liver transplant may be offered.

Acetaminophen hepatotoxicity: This cause is rapidly deduced with evidence of excessive ingestion of acetaminophen and acetaminophen-containing pain medications. It is a dose-related toxin, and ingestions of greater than 10 g/d or sometimes as low as 3 to 4 g/d can result in hepatotoxicity.[12]

Very high aminotransferase levels are typically seen, with levels exceeding 3500 IU/L. As acetaminophen-induced ALF is the leading cause of ALF in the United States and the United Kingdom, it is recommended that levels should be drawn in all patients presenting with ALF. Because the time of ingestion may be unknown, low or absent levels of acetaminophen do not rule out acetaminophen-induced hepatotoxicity and should not stall management.[4,12–14] Early administration of N-acetylcysteine (NAC) has been shown to be both safe and effective for acetaminophen-induced ALF. Even following 48 hours of ingestion, intravenous (IV) NAC (loading dose with 150 mg/kg over 15 minutes; maintenance dose if 50 mg/kg given over 4 hours followed by 100 mg/kg administered over 16 hours) has been shown to improve outcomes.[15,16] The mechanism of action of NAC is well established. Acetaminophen in therapeutic doses is converted to nontoxic metabolites via sulfidation and glucuronidation pathways. A small component of acetaminophen is metabolized by cytochrome P450 into the hepatotoxic metabolite N-acetyl-p-benzoquinone imine (NAPQI). NAPQI is then excreted via conjugation to glutathione. When a toxic threshold is reached, the sulfidation and glucuronidation pathways are saturated, leading to toxic accumulation of NAPQI. NAC acts by replenishing glutathione levels helping to excrete the toxic NAPQI. If acetaminophen ingestion has occurred within a few hours of presentation, activated charcoal (dose 1 g/kg orally) is useful for gastrointestinal decontamination.[17]

As mentioned earlier, doses less than the toxic threshold, as low as 3 to 4 g/d, can result in hepatotoxicity. This circumstance is the so-called therapeutic misadventure and can be seen in the following conditions[15,18]:

- Chronic alcoholics: Chronic alcohol use induces cytochrome p450 2E1 (CYP2E1), shunting acetaminophen through the cytochrome p450 pathway, leading to increased concentrations of NAPQI. As these patients are often malnourished, they have diminished capacity to excrete NAPQI due to depleted glutathione reserves.
- Malnutrition and fasting states: Glucuronidation stores are reduced, resulting in increased NAPQI levels.
- Drugs that induce CYP2E1 include anticonvulsants (phenytoin, carbamazepine, phenobarbital), isoniazid, and rifampin.
- Drugs that increase the metabolism of CYP2E1 by competing with glucuronidation pathways include sulfamethoxazole and trimethoprim (Bactrim) and zidovudine.
- Advanced age: The elderly have less glutathione and decreased activity of glucuronidation enzymes.
- Genetic predisposition

Ischemic injury: This condition, also known as shock liver, occurs following any insult that results in significant hypoperfusion of the liver, including cardiac arrest/cardiogenic shock, septic shock, hypovolemic shock, and hemorrhagic shock. There is a marked elevation in aminotransferase levels as well as elevated lactate dehydrogenase, indicating cell necrosis. Management consists of optimizing hemodynamics and results in early recovery of hepatic function.[19]

Viral hepatitis: As previously mentioned, the incidence of viral hepatitis has declined in the United States and is more frequently seen in endemic regions.[20]

- *Hepatitis A virus (HAV)*: Acute HAV is associated with travel to or living in endemic regions and can be evaluated by measuring serum anti-HAV immunoglobulin M (IgM). Management consists of supportive care.
- *HBV*: ALF can occur in acute hepatitis B or in patients with chronic hepatitis B with reactivation in the setting of chemotherapy or immunosuppression. Serologies, including hepatitis B surface antigen and anti–hepatitis B core antigen IgM, should be measured. In patients with active infection, treatment with nucleos(t)ide analogues is recommended and supported by case reports.[21,22]
- *Hepatitis C virus (HCV)*: HCV does not seem to cause ALF and is more so associated with chronic liver disease and cirrhosis.
- *Hepatitis D*: It may occasionally be diagnosed in HBV-positive individuals.
- *Hepatitis E virus (HEV)*: Acute HEV in endemic parts of the world has been observed as a cause of ALF, and is more severe in pregnant women, with mortality rates ranging from 33% to 71%.The AGA suggests testing for HEV in pregnant women presenting with ALF by measuring anti-hepatitis E virus. Management consists of supportive measures. It is also recommended that HEV serologic testing be obtained before any patient is labeled with ALF from drug-induced or idiopathic causes.
- *Herpes simplex virus (HSV)*: HSV itself is a rare cause of ALF and is caused by both HSV-1 and HSV-2. The AGA suggests testing for HSV in patients with ALF by checking HSV serologies and HSV DNA. HSV in patients with ALF carries a poor prognosis, even with acyclovir therapy (5–10 mg/kg IV every 8 hours). However, there are case reports that demonstrate that patients with acute hepatitis secondary to HSV do better with treatment compared with those who are left untreated.
- *Varicella zoster virus (VZV)*: It is rarely implicated as a cause of ALF; however, the AGA recommends routine testing for VZV in immunocompetent patients with ALF.[5]

Drug-induced liver injury (DILI): Drugs, including both nutritional and herbal supplements other than acetaminophen, listed in **Table 2**, typically do not cause dose-related ALF. ALF is seen within the first 6 months of drug initiation and is traditionally a diagnosis of exclusion. There are no specific therapies for DILI apart from supportive management and removing the offending agent.[4,22]

Wilson disease: This disease is an uncommon cause of ALF that is more commonly seen in young patients. Patients may have preexisting, undetected liver disease, however, are considered to be in ALF when a rapid deterioration occurs. Because of the fulminant presentation of this condition, early detection and referral to a transplant-capable center is critical. Laboratory abnormalities include marked elevation of indirect bilirubin, due to the presence of hemolysis. A high bilirubin to alkaline phosphatase ratio (>2.0) is an indirect indicator of Wilson disease. Testing for Wilson disease includes serum ceruloplasmin, serum and hepatic copper assessment, and 24-hour urine collection for copper. These tests have high false-positive and false-negative rates, and no large studies have been performed to assess the diagnostic accuracy of testing specifically for Wilson disease in ALF. Treatment to acutely lower serum copper includes albumin dialysis, hemofiltration, plasmapheresis, or plasma

Table 2
Causes, clinical characteristics, diagnostic testing, and guidelines for specific causes of acute liver failure

Causes	Clinical Characteristics	Diagnostic Tests	Guidelines	Specific Therapy
Acetaminophen	• Dose-related overdose with ingestions >10 g/d; can be seen with doses as low as 3–4 g/d • Marked elevated of aminotransferase levels (>3500 IU/L)	• Serum acetaminophen levels	—	• Activated charcoal within 4 h of ingestion • IV NAC
Ischemia	• Marked elevated aminotransferase levels	• Clinical history	—	• Optimizing hemodynamics, cardiovascular support
Viral hepatitis (A, B, C, E)	• HAV, HBV, HEV associated with living in or traveling to endemic areas • HEV incidence increased in pregnant women and has a more severe presentation • Aminotransferase levels of 1000–2000 IU/L	• Viral hepatitis serologies[a]	• The AGA suggests testing for HEV in pregnant women presenting with ALF.	• HAV and HEV managed with supportive measures • Should consider nucleos(t)ide analogues for HBV-associated liver failure
Autoimmune	• Often subacute presentation • Young or middle-aged women	• Autoimmune markers[b]	• The AGA recommends autoantibody testing in patients presenting with ALF.	• Prednisone 40–60 mg/d • Consider liver transplant
HSV	• Often seen in immunocompromised and pregnant hosts	• HSV-1 IgM	• The AGA suggests testing for and treating patients with ALF and HSV.	• Acyclovir (5–10 mg/kg IV q8h)
VZV	—	• VZV serology	• The AGA recommends routine testing for VZV in immunocompetent patients with ALF.	• Acyclovir (5–10 mg/kg IV q8h)
Wilson disease	• Rare cause of ALF • Typically occurs in young patients • Associated with Coombs negative hemolytic anemia	• Serum ceruloplasmin, serum and hepatic copper assessment, and 24-h urine collection for copper	• The AGA suggests against routinely testing patients with ALF for Wilson disease.	• Must consider liver transplant early in course because of fulminant presentation

[a] Viral hepatitis serologies: anti–hepatitis A virus IgM, hepatitis B surface antigen, anti–hepatitis B core antigen IgM, anti-HEV, anti-HCV, HCV RNA.
[b] Autoimmune markers: anti–nuclear antibody, anti–smooth muscle antibody, anti-soluble liver antigen, anti-neutrophil cytoplasmic antibody, immunoglobulin levels.

exchange. As a diagnosis of Wilson disease is unlikely to alter the management of ALF, the AGA suggests against routinely testing patients with ALF for Wilson disease.[5,23,24]

Autoimmune hepatitis (AIH): AIH is an uncommon cause of ALF that, similar to Wilson disease, may be a chronic preexisting condition with an acute fulminant presentation of ALF. Diagnosis of AIH includes serum testing for antinuclear antibody, anti–smooth muscle antibody, anti–soluble liver antigen, anti–neutrophil cytoplasmic antibody, and immunoglobulin levels. Steroid therapy (prednisone dosed at 40–60 mg/d) may be considered in early stage ALF; however, there are little data suggesting a response to corticosteroid therapy. Patients are often considered for liver transplant. One study showed 93% of patients with AIH reportedly had positive AIH autoantibodies. The AGA recommends autoantibody testing in patients presenting with ALF.[25]

Table 2 demonstrates causes, diagnostic testing, guidelines for testing, and management for specific causes of ALF.[4,5]

CLINICAL MANIFESTATIONS AND COMPLICATIONS OF ACUTE LIVER FAILURE

Initial symptoms in patients with ALF are nonspecific and include fatigue, lethargy, nausea/vomiting, anorexia, pruritus, right upper quadrant pain, and abdominal distension from ascites. As liver failure progresses, patients develop jaundice and mental status changes, known as HE, which is graded on severity on a scale from 0 to IV, as is described in **Table 3**. Physical examination findings include jaundice, right upper quadrant tenderness, hepatomegaly, ascites, and signs of intravascular volume depletion, including orthostatic hypotension.[11,26]

The following complications of ALF are now discussed in detail:

- Cerebral edema
- Infection
- Coagulopathy and bleeding
- Renal failure
- Cardiopulmonary complications
- Acid-base and metabolic disturbances.

Cerebral Edema

The most serious complication of ALF is cerebral edema (CE). CE is caused by an increase in intracranial pressure (ICP), which ultimately causes a decrease in cerebral perfusion pressure (CPP). CE accounts for 80% of the fatalities in ALF. CE should be suspected with findings of HE, systemic hypertension, bradycardia, and respiratory depression, known as the Cushing triad.[25,26] CE is observed in 65% to 70% of patients with grade IV encephalopathy. Development of grade III encephalopathy is associated with a very poor prognosis and requires rapid and early detection and management in a critical care unit, as patients have a precipitous rate of decline and high likelihood to develop CE.[26] In severe cases, increased ICP can lead to seizures, ischemic and hypoxic brain injury, as well as death from uncal herniation.[2]

The pathogenesis of CE and intracranial hypertension (ICH) is not well understood and beyond the scope of this article. However, it is thought to be multifactorial including the following[27]:

- Hyperammonia leading to osmotic disturbances from glutamine accumulation within astrocytes
- Loss of cerebrovascular autoregulation resulting in increased cerebral blood flow
- Inflammation

- Infection
- Metabolic disturbances
- Hypoxia

The use of ICP monitors to aid in the management of CE remains a controversial issue. ICP monitors provide early recognition of CE and are an accurate method of monitoring patients with grade III or IV encephalopathy, allowing for early intervention, as clinical signs of elevated ICP (Cushing triad, neurologic examination findings discussed earlier) are not uniformly present. By assessing CPP (calculated as mean arterial pressure [MAP] – ICP), ICP monitoring can aid in avoiding cerebral hypoperfusion by targeting CPP greater than 60 mm Hg and ICP less than 20 mm Hg. However, bleeding complications may occur and the use of ICP monitors has not been shown to change outcomes. The European Association for the Study of the Liver recommends invasive ICP monitoring in patients with grade III or IV coma that are mechanically ventilated with the presence of 1 or more of the following criteria, placing them at high risk for ICH:

- Young patients with hyperacute or acute ALF
- Ammonia level greater than 150 to 200 μmol/L that does not improve with initial interventions
- Renal impairment
- Vasopressor support

Other less invasive approaches for monitoring ICP include jugular bulb catheters, transcranial Doppler ultrasonography, ocular ultrasonography, and continuous electroencephalography; however, studies showing their use across various centers have not been performed.[1,3,28] The authors' own center favors the use of transcranial Doppler ultrasonography.

The management of CE and ICH is related to the grade of HE. Thus, a stepwise approach in management is advised, as highlighted in **Table 4**.[4,29–31]

It is unclear what method of reducing ICP is best and whether or not decreasing ICP decreases mortality. Five randomized controlled trials have assessed methods of reducing ICP, including moderate hypothermia, hypertonic saline, L-ornithine L-aspartate, IV mannitol, and hyperventilation. The results showed no statistically significant improvement in mortality with any of the individual treatments. The AGA suggests against the empirical use of treatments to reduce ICP.[5,32]

Table 3
Grading of hepatic encephalopathy

Grade	Intellectual Function	Neuromuscular Abnormality
0	Normal	Normal
Minimal	Subtle changes in driving/work	Minor abnormalities on psychometric tests
I	Personality changes, attention deficits, irritability, depressed state	Tremor and incoordination
II	Sleep-wake cycle alterations, behavioral changes, cognitive dysfunction, fatigue	Asterixis, ataxia, slow speech
III	Somnolence, confusion, disorientation	Muscle rigidity, nystagmus, sluggish pupillary response, clonus, plantar extensor response, hyporeflexia
IV	Stupor and coma	Unresponsive to noxious stimuli

Table 4
Summary of management of cerebral edema and intracranial hypertension in acute liver failure, based off of grade of encephalopathy

Grade	Management
I/II	• Transfer to ICU with decline in level of consciousness (grade II) and consider transfer to liver transplant facility and listing for transplant • Non-contrast CT to exclude other intracranial pathologies • Avoid sedation if possible; however, can give short-activing Benzodiazepines if needed for agitation • PO and PR lactulose as well as xifaxan[a]
III/IV	• Continue the aforementioned measures • Airway protection with intubation and mechanical ventilation • Propofol is agent of choice for sedation because of its short half-life and it may reduce cerebral blood flow • Position bed with head elevated at 30° • Hyperventilation *may* be useful for impending herniation with goal P_{CO_2} between 25 and 30 mm Hg • Minimize agitation, tactile stimuli, and suctioning • Close monitoring and correction of electrolytes and acid-base status • Consider induced hypothermia with external cooling blankets to maintain core temperature between 34°C and 35°C • Hypertonic saline to increase sodium to 145–155 mEq/L • Mannitol for severe elevation of ICP[b] • Immediate treatment of seizures with phenytoin and benzodiazepines with short half-lives

Abbreviations: CT, computed tomography; ICU, intensive care unit; PR, per rectum.
 [a] Combination lactulose and xifaxan is used to reduce ammonia levels. Caution must be taken to not give excessive lactulose, as this can cause gaseous bowel distention that may present technical difficulties during transplant.
 [b] Consider when ICP is greater than 20 mm Hg for more than 10 minutes. Given as 0.25 to 1.0 g/kg IV bolus every hour.

Infection

Patients with ALF are at an increased risk of both bacterial and fungal infections as a result of immune dysfunction, as the liver plays a key role in the function of leukocytes, macrophages, and complement systems. Risk of infection is further amplified in patients with ALF by the presence of multi-organ dysfunction, systemic inflammation, and the need for indwelling Foley catheters, central lines, and endotracheal intubation—all of which serve as a nidus for infection. Sepsis has been documented in more than 80% of ALF cases with infection sites including the chest (50%), urinary tract (22%), blood (16%), and IV catheters (12%). Common pathogens include staphylococcus, streptococcus, and gram-negative rods.[33,34] The following precautions may help prevent complications from infections in the setting of ALF:

- Examine wounds and venipuncture sites daily for any signs of infection.
- Proper hygiene, including handwashing, should be performed before patient contact.
- Change central lines and Foley catheters at appropriate intervals.
- Conduct regular surveillance for infection, including chest radiography and periodic blood, urine, and sputum cultures, to detect bacterial and fungal pathogens early.
- Monitor for signs of infection and have a low threshold to start empirical, broad-spectrum antibiotics with third-generation cephalosporins and vancomycin.

- Maintain a high index of suspicion for fungal infection if there is no improvement with broad-spectrum antibiotics.

The use of prophylactic antibiotics and antifungals remains controversial, as they have not been shown to improve overall outcomes in ALF. However, some centers advocate the use of broad-spectrum antimicrobial therapy in the setting of ALF.[35]

Coagulopathy and Bleeding

Coagulopathy and bleeding are common manifestations of ALF, as the synthesis of coagulation factors is decreased while consumption of clotting factors and platelets concurrently occurs. Although an elevated INR is a component of the definition of ALF, overall hemostasis is normal by several compensatory mechanisms. Furthermore, the synthesis of procoagulants (eg, protein C and protein S) is also reduced leading to balanced disequilibrium. Both a qualitative and quantitative platelet dysfunction occurs. A reduction in factors II, V, VII, IX, X, as well as circulating fibrinogen is observed. As there is increased levels of thrombin-antithrombin III complex, disseminated intravascular coagulation (DIC) may ensue. As the INR is an important marker of prognosis in ALF, correction of the INR with blood products is not advised, as this action will obscure both spontaneous improvement and worsening of the INR. Plasma transfusion also poses the risk of volume overload as well as transfusion-related acute lung injury. Similarly, the administration of platelets is discouraged in the absence of active bleeding. Only in the setting of clinically significant bleeding or in anticipation of a high-risk invasive procedure should the following measures be taken[36–38]:

- Transfuse the following with the goal INR less than 1.5
  - Transfuse vitamin K (5–10 mg subcutaneously), although its utility may be limited.
  - Fresh frozen plasma provides temporary correction.
  - Recombinant activated factor VIIa (40 μg/kg bolus) may be given as a last resort and also provides temporary correction.
- Transfuse platelets to maintain a platelet count greater than 50,000.
- Transfuse packed red blood cells to maintain hemoglobin greater than 7.
- In DIC, transfuse cryoprecipitate or desmopressin acetate for fibrinogen less than 100 mg/dL and active bleeding.

As patients with ALF are at high risk for gastrointestinal bleeding, it is recommended to empirically start acid suppression therapy with either proton pump inhibitors or histamine-2 blocking agents. Sucralfate may be used as a second-line agent.[36,37]

Renal Failure

Acute kidney injury (AKI) is a frequent complication of ALF that develops in 56% to 70% of patients and contributes to mortality as well as a poorer prognosis.[4] AKI is multifactorial, including prerenal azotemia (decreased oral intake, vomiting, diarrhea, sepsis, ischemia) as well as medication-induced renal toxicity (acetaminophen, diuretics, aminoglycosides, and so forth). Hepatorenal syndrome may occur in ALF, although it is more commonly seen in patients with long-standing cirrhosis. Most patients with AKI in the setting of ALF recover following proper management or liver transplant. Treatment of AKI in ALF entails maintaining adequate volume status, treatment of infections, and the avoidance of nephrotoxic agents. A third of cases require management with renal replacement therapy for the following indications:

- Volume overload
- Severe acidosis

- Metabolic derangements, including hyperkalemia and hyponatremia
- Toxic substance removal

Studies have shown that continuous renal replacement therapy has resulted in improved stability in both cardiovascular and intracranial parameters when compared with the intermittent mode and, thus, is the preferred method of dialysis.[39,40]

Cardiopulmonary Complications

Hemodynamic monitoring is critical, as patients with ALF demonstrate low systemic vascular resistance and systemic vasodilation, resulting in hypotension and multi-organ system failure. Hemodynamics, as discussed earlier, are imperative in the management of ICH and renal failure. Pulmonary complications include atelectasis, aspiration, pulmonary hemorrhage, and acute respiratory distress syndrome. The following are recommended for management[39,40]:

- Hemodynamic monitoring with target MAP 60 to 75 mm Hg or greater
  - Fluid resuscitation with normal saline is preferred.
  - Consider half-normal saline with 75 mEq/L sodium bicarbonate if patients are acidotic.
  - Consider dextrose in solution if patients are hypoglycemic.
  - Consider pressor support with if there is an inadequate hemodynamic response to IV fluids.
- Norepinephrine is the initial agent of choice.
- Vasopressin may be added to potentiate the effects of norepinephrine.
- Use a low threshold for intubation for airway protection.
  - Low positive end expiratory pressure (PEEP) is preferred, as high PEEP may compromise cardiac output, increase ICP, as well as worsen hepatic congestion.

Acid-Base and Metabolic Disturbances

Several metabolic derangements are commonly seen in ALF including alkalosis in the early stages and metabolic acidosis in the latter stages secondary to lactic acidosis, both of which are best managed by treating the underlying cause. Hyponatremia frequently occurs due to several factors including tissue hypoperfusion, antidiuretic hormone release, and impaired renal function. Hypoglycemia results from impaired gluconeogenesis as well as hepatic glycogen store depletion. Management involves frequent glucose checks and glucose infusions with target glucose ~140. Other electrolytes including calcium, potassium, phosphate, and magnesium should be frequently checked and replaced as these are often low in ALF.

In terms of nutrition, supplementation is recommended with early initiation of enteral feeds, which is preferred, or parenteral nutrition when enteral feeds are contraindicated. Early initiation of nutrition supplementation may reduce the risk of gastrointestinal bleeding from ulceration in these patients.[39–41]

SUMMARY

ALF is a life-threatening condition characterized by rapid progression and death associated with high morbidity and mortality. The causes have changed over the past few decades and vary according to geographic region, with acetaminophen and drug-induced ALF being the most common causes in the United States. Determining the cause aids in predicting the prognosis as well as the presentation of manifestations and guides providers to perform cause-specific management. At the initial presentation, nonspecific symptoms are present but may progress to more worrisome complications, including cerebral edema, infection, coagulopathy, renal failure, cardiopulmonary failure, and/or acid-base and metabolic disturbances. Although some cases of ALF have resolution with more conservative measures, liver transplantation is the ultimate treatment strategy in many cases. Transplantation, however, requires significant resources and a lifetime of immunosuppressive therapy.

REFERENCES

1. Wendon J, Cordoba J, Dhawan A, et al. EASL clinical practical guidelines on the management of acute (fulminant) liver failure. J Hepatol 2017;66(5):1047–81.
2. Lee WM, Stravitz RT, Larson AM. Introduction to the revised American Association for the Study of Liver Diseases position paper on acute liver failure 2011. Hepatology 2012;55:965–7.
3. Bunchorntavakul C, Reddy KR. Acute liver failure. Clin Liver Dis 2017;21(4):769–92.
4. Lee WM, Larson AM, Stravitz RT. AASLD position paper: the management of acute liver failure: update 2011. AASLD 2011.
5. Flamm SL, Yang YX, Singh S, et al. American Gastroenterological Association institute guidelines for the diagnosis and management of acute liver failure. Gastroenterology 2017;152(3):644–7.
6. Bernal W, Lee WM, Wendon J, et al. Acute liver failure: a curable disease by 2024? J Hepatol 2015;62:S112–20.
7. Riordan SM, Williams R. Mechanisms of hepatocyte injury, multi-organ failure, and prognostic criteria in acute liver failure. Semin Liver Dis 2003;23(3):203–15.
8. Lee WM. Etiologies of acute liver failure. Semin Liver Dis 2008;28:142–52.
9. Ichai P, Samuel D. Etiology and prognosis of fulminant hepatitis in adults. Liver Transpl 2008;14(Suppl 2):S67–79.
10. Khashab M, Tector AJ, Kwo PY. Epidemiology of acute liver failure. Curr Gastroenterol Rep 2007;9(1):66–73.
11. Gill RQ, Sterling RK. Acute liver failure. J Clin Gastroenterol 2001;33(3):191–8.
12. Schiødt FV, Rochling FA, Casey DL, et al. Acetaminophen toxicity in an urban county hospital. N Engl J Med 1997;337(16):1112–7.
13. Bunchorntavakul C, Reddy KR. Acetaminophen-related hepatotoxicity. Clin Liver Dis 2013;17(4):587–607, viii.
14. Roberts DW, Lee WM, Hinson JA, et al. An immunoassay to rapidly measure acetaminophen protein adducts accurately identifies patients with acute liver injury or failure. Clin Gastroenterol Hepatol 2017;15(4):555–62.e3.
15. Larson AM. Acetaminophen hepatotoxicity. Clin Liver Dis 2007;11:525–48.
16. Harrison PM, Keays R, Bray GP, et al. Improved outcome of paracetamol-induced fulminant hepatic failure by late administration of acetylcysteine. Lancet 1990;335(8705):1572–3.
17. Sato RL, Wong JJ, Sumida SM, et al. Efficacy of superactivated charcoal administered late (3 hours) after acetaminophen overdose. Am J Emerg Med 2003;21(3):189–91.
18. Larson AM, Polson J, Fontana RJ, et al. Acetaminophen-induced acute liver failure: results of a United States multicenter, prospective study. Hepatology 2005;42(6):1364–72.

19. Taylor RM, Tujios S, Jinjuvadia K, et al. Short and long-term outcomes in patients with acute liver failure due to ischemic hepatitis. Dig Dis Sci 2012; 57(3):777–85.

20. Schiodt FV, Davern TA, Shakil O, et al. Viral hepatitis-related acute liver failure. Am J Gastroenterol 2003;98:448–53.

21. Lok ASF, McMahon BJ. AASLD practice guideline, chronic hepatitis B: update of recommendation. Rom J Gastroenterol 2009;50:661–2.

22. Rockey DC, Seeff LB, Rochon J, et al. Causality assessment in drug-induced liver injury using a structured expert opinion process: comparison to the Roussel-Uclaf causality assessment method. Hepatology 2010;51(6):2117–26.

23. Korman JD, Volenberg I, Balko J, et al. Screening for Wilson disease in acute liver failure: a comparison of currently available diagnostic tests. Hepatology 2008; 48(4):1167–74.

24. Jhang JS, Schilsky ML, Lefkowitch JH, et al. Therapeutic plasmapheresis as a bridge to liver transplantation in fulminant Wilson disease. J Clin Apher 2007; 22(1):10–4.

25. Czaja AJ. Treatment of autoimmune hepatitis. Semin Liver Dis 2002;22:365–78.

26. Ellis AJ, Wendon JA, Williams R. Subclinical seizure activity and prophylactic phenytoin infusion in acute liver failure: a controlled clinical trial. Hepatology 2000;32(3):536–41.

27. Ware AJ, D'agostino AN, Combes B. Cerebral edema: a major complication of massive hepatic necrosis. Gastroenterology 1971;61(6):877–84.

28. Nielsen HB, Tofteng F, Wang LP, et al. Cerebral oxygenation determined by near-infrared spectrophotometry in patients with fulminant hepatic failure. J Hepatol 2003;38(2):188–92.

29. Bernal W, Hyyrylainen A, Gera A, et al. Lessons from look-back in acute liver failure? A single centre experience of 3300 patients. J Hepatol 2013;59(1):74–80.

30. Larsen FS, Wendon J. Brain edema in liver failure: basic physiologic principles and management. Liver Transpl 2002;8(11):983–9.

31. Mohsenin V. Assessment and management of cerebral edema and intracranial hypertension in acute liver failure. J Crit Care 2013;28(5):783–91.

32. Wijdicks EF, Nyberg SL. Propofol to control intracranial pressure in fulminant hepatic failure. Transplant Proc 2002;34(4):1220–2.

33. Daas M, Plevak DJ, Wijdicks EF, et al. Acute liver failure: results of a 5-year clinical protocol. Liver Transpl Surg 1995;1(4):210–9.

34. Dharel N, Bajaj JS. Antibiotic prophylaxis in acute liver failure: friend or foe? Clin Gastroenterol Hepatol 2014;12(11):1950–2.

35. Rolando N, Harvey F, Brahm J, et al. Prospective study of bacterial infection in acute liver failure: an analysis of fifty patients. Hepatology 1990;11(1): 49–53.

36. Stravitz RT, Lisman T, Luketic VA, et al. Minimal effects of acute liver injury/acute liver failure on hemostasis as assessed by thromboelastography. J Hepatol 2012; 56(1):129–36.

37. Pereira SP, Rowbotham D, Fitt S, et al. Pharmacokinetics and efficacy of oral versus intravenous mixed-micellar phylloquinone (vitamin K1) in severe acute liver disease. J Hepatol 2005;42(3):365–70.

38. Stravitz RT, Kramer DJ. Management of acute liver failure. Nat Rev Gastroenterol Hepatol 2009;6(9):542–53.

39. Tujios SR, Hynan LS, Vazquez MA, et al. Risk factors and outcomes of acute kidney injury in patients with acute liver failure. Clin Gastroenterol Hepatol 2015; 13(2):352–9.

40. Davenport A, Will EJ, Davidson AM. Improved cardiovascular stability during continuous modes of renal replacement therapy in critically ill patients with acute hepatic and renal failure. Crit Care Med 1993;21(3):328–38.
41. Raff T, Germann G, Hartmann B. The value of early enteral nutrition in the prophylaxis of stress ulceration in the severely burned patient. Burns 1997;23(4):313–8.

Prognostic Models in Acute Liver Failure

Avantika Mishra, MD[a],*, Vinod Rustgi, MD, MBA[b]

KEYWORDS

- Acute liver failure • Prognostic models • Model for End-Stage Liver Disease • MELD
- King's College Criteria

KEY POINTS

- There is a strong imperative to develop valid and accurate prognostic modeling for acute liver failure (ALF).
- Despite the numerous clinical models that have been proposed thus far and the use of some such models, that is, King's College Criteria and Model for End-Stage Liver Disease, in clinical practice to aid decision-making, there is a significant need for improvement for determining patients' clinical course, survival, and requirement for liver transplantation.
- Future prognostic models shall need a stronger statistical foundation and accountability for time and variability in the clinical course of ALF and be applied for pretransplant and posttransplant outcomes.

INTRODUCTION

Acute liver failure (ALF) is the rare and rapid clinical deterioration of liver function in the setting of coagulopathy and worsening mental status. This multisystem clinical syndrome was first reported in the literature by Trey and Davidson in the 1970s.[1] The definition of ALF is widely agreed to be a rapid-onset, severe hepatic dysfunction of less than 26 weeks' duration, coagulation abnormality (international normalized ratio [INR] ≥1.5), and encephalopathy in patients without preexisting cirrhosis.[1] Otherwise known as fulminant hepatitis,[2] fulminant hepatic failure,[1] fulminant liver failure,[3] and acute hepatic failure,[4] ALF is associated with high morbidity and mortality with most cases occurring de novo in patients without preexisting liver disease.[5,6]

The clinical presentation of liver failure can vary dramatically. Signs and symptoms include altered mental status or encephalopathy, cerebral edema, jaundice, right

Disclosure: The authors have nothing to disclose.
[a] Division of Gastroenterology and Hepatology, Rutgers Robert Wood Johnson University Hospital, Medical Education Building, Room 478, One Robert Wood Johnson Place, New Brunswick, NJ 08901, USA; [b] Division of Gastroenterology and Hepatology, Rutgers Robert Wood Johnson University Hospital, Medical Education Building, Room 466, 1 Robert Wood Johnson Place, New Brunswick, NJ 08901, USA
* Corresponding author.
E-mail address: Avantika23@gmail.com

Clin Liver Dis 22 (2018) 375–388
https://doi.org/10.1016/j.cld.2018.01.010
1089-3261/18/© 2018 Elsevier Inc. All rights reserved.

liver.theclinics.com

upper quadrant tenderness, ascites, along with numerous other clinical features that can be seen in any patient with acute-on-chronic liver disease. The most predominant causes of ALF worldwide include viral hepatitis (specifically acute infection with hepatitis A or B), followed by drug-induced liver injury (mostly acetaminophen [N-acetyl-p-aminophenol (APAP)] overdose), autoimmune-related liver disease, ischemic or shock liver, and hypoperfusion injury.[7] In the United States, APAP-related injury remains the most common cause of ALF.[8] Recent data suggest ALF results in approximately 2000 deaths annually in the United States, a number that has not improved in more than 20 years.[7,9] Given the various causes that contribute to ALF, the variable survival associated with its course, and the numerous clinical complications that occur concomitantly in this syndrome, prognostic models to determine outcomes would be highly useful, though currently have limited success.

It is critical to identify and risk stratify those patients with ALF to rapidly determine who is eligible for liver transplantation. Currently, liver transplantation is the only treatment that has proven survival benefit; however, given the often variable clinical course of ALF and its rapidly progressive nature, it is occasionally not a viable option.[10] Depending on the cause of liver injury, clinical outcomes can be favorable and transplant-free survival can be achieved as high as 70% of the time, whereas other causes of liver failure can lower the likelihood of clinical recovery to less than 30% without a transplantation.[7] Liver transplantation is the cornerstone of the treatment of irreversible fulminant hepatic failure and in the setting of rapid innovation can result in the survival of up to 88% of the patients who undergo it based on the most up-to-date data.[10,11] Currently, the diagnosis of ALF accounts for 8% of liver transplantation cases in both the United States and Europe.[12,13] Thus, to gauge the clinical status of patients and determine their eligibility for orthotopic transplantation, the use of prognostic models is crucial in stratifying the degree of liver failure. It is equally important to identify those patients who are not suitable candidates for transplantation to prevent morbidity associated with transplantation and the lifelong challenges of immunosuppression.

CAUSES OF ACUTE LIVER FAILURE

In order to characterize and determine the course and prognosis of patients with ALF, it is important to identify the cause of the underlying disorder first. Before 1999, the 3 largest studies investigating ALF deemed hepatitis B and non-A, non-B, or non-C hepatitis (ultimately, a largely cryptogenic cause) to be the most common causes for ALF.[6,14,15] In 1999, Schiødt and colleagues[16] conducted a large multicenter study gathering data on 295 patients in 13 hospitals between 1994 and 1996. The investigators of this study identified APAP to be the most frequent cause of ALF in the United States based on drug toxicity in 20% of their patient sample. These data were consistent with the patient data collected from the United Kingdom[17] and Denmark,[18] although there were considerable differences in frequency of APAP hepatotoxicity between the countries. Twenty percent of ALF cases in the United States were attributed to APAP toxicity versus 50% to 70% recorded in the United Kingdom and Denmark. This statistical underestimation of liver injury attributed to APAP toxicity in the United States was likely because data collected in the United States for this study were solely obtained from transplant databases; thus, by default, any patient who had APAP toxicity who was not listed for orthotopic transplantation was not included in the analysis.[19] Similar findings were confirmed in a study conducted by the US Acute Liver Failure Study Group in 2002, specifically that APAP toxicity and drug-induced liver injury were the predominant causes of ALF.[7] Several years later in 2008, another large multicenter prospective cohort study was conducted across 31 liver disease and transplant centers in the United States to determine clinical trends and outcomes in ALF. APAP-related hepatotoxicity, mostly from unintentional overdose, was confirmed as the principal cause of ALF, again surpassing viral hepatitis, which was previously the foremost underlying cause for liver failure.[8]

DEVELOPMENT OF PROGNOSTIC MODELS FOR ACUTE LIVER FAILURE

Eligibility for hepatic transplantation needs to be rapidly addressed in cases of decompensation from ALF. Since the 1960s, multiple models to identify early prognostic indicators and estimate prognosis for liver failure have been proposed and widely used as a resource; however, their accuracy and efficacy have been widely debated. Starting in 1964, Child and Turcotte[20] published an operative risk classification for cirrhotic patients recovering from variceal bleeding and undergoing portosystemic shunt surgery. Ascites, encephalopathy, serum bilirubin, serum albumin, and nutritional status were the 5 variables specifically selected based on clinical experience of the investigators. Each variable was graded 1 to 3, with the additive combined score used to classify the patients' cirrhosis status as the best (class A) or worst prognosis (class C).[20] The clinical implications of this risk stratification of A, B, or C are arbitrary and generally do not have consensus.[21] This scoring system was the first attempt at formal classification of the severity of liver disease.

Pugh and colleagues[22] conducted a study in 1973 for patients undergoing esophageal variceal surgical transection and used a modified version of the original classification by Child and Turcotte,[20] replacing nutritional status with prothrombin time (**Table 1**). This modified classification was the first to predict outcomes of surgery in cirrhotic patients based on the severity of their underlying liver disease. Neither the Child-Turcotte nor Pugh classifications have been validated over time, though medical

Table 1
Child-Turcotte-Pugh classification for severity of cirrhosis

	Points		
	1	2	3
Encephalopathy[a]	None	Grade 1–2	Grade 3–4
Ascites	None	Mild to moderate	Severe
Bilirubin (mg/dL)	<2	2–3	>3
Albumin (g/dL)	>3.5	2.8–3.5	<2.8
INR	<1.7	1.7–2.3	>2.3
CTP class obtained by adding above score for each parameter			
Class A = 5–6 points (least severe disease)			
Class B = 7–9 points (moderately severe disease)			
Class C = 10–15 points (most severe disease)			

The CTP classification system uses 2 clinical parameters (encephalopathy and ascites) and 3 laboratory values (bilirubin, albumin, and INR). Total points are used to classify patients as class A, B, or C.
   Pros: Multiorgan assessment of cirrhosis, simplicity of use.
   Cons: Arbitrary values, subjective scoring, oversimplification, variables not of equal prognostic importance.
   Abbreviation: CTP, Child-Turcotte-Pugh.
   [a] West Haven criteria for hepatic encephalopathy.
   From Pugh RN, Murray-Lyon IM, Dawson JL, et al. Transection of the esophagus for bleeding esophageal varices. Br J Surg 1973;60:646–9; with permission.

literature has shown prognostic value.[23] There are several weaknesses of the scoring system. First, cutoff points for each of the 5 variables reduce prognostic information and are thought to be arbitrary and suboptimal values. Each variable is not considered to be equally important and cannot be correlated linearly with mortality risk.[24] Moreover, the scoring classification is subjective, with physician characterization of hepatic encephalopathy and the presence of ascites as variable. This has improved in recent times given the use of ultrasound for ascites detection.[25] In addition, the Child-Turcotte-Pugh classification of liver disease does not account for other important prognostic indicators of ALF, including renal dysfunction, which is a well-established marker for organ dysfunction in liver failure.[26,27] It has also been shown before that prognostic variables and indicators that are based on statistical modeling may better predict prognosis than the methodology of the Child-Turcotte-Pugh classification.[24]

Another prognostic model was developed by O'Grady and colleagues[28] from the United Kingdom and coined the King's College Criteria for APAP-induced liver toxicity and non–APAP-induced liver toxicity (**Table 2**). After researching a prospective cohort of 588 patients in the liver unit of King's College Hospital between 1973 and 1975, the investigators determined that survival in APAP-induced ALF was correlated with arterial blood pH, prothrombin time, and serum creatinine. A pH less than 7.30, prothrombin time greater than 100 seconds, and creatinine greater than 300 μmol/L indicated a poor prognosis. For the subcohort of patients with viral hepatitis and drug-induced liver dysfunction, poor prognosis was determined to be associated with an age less than 11 years of age or greater than 40 years of age, duration of jaundice before onset of encephalopathy greater than 7 days, bilirubin greater than 300 μmol/L, and a prothrombin time greater than 50 seconds. The investigators of this study further attempted validation of these indicators after retrospectively researching a cohort of 175 patients from 1986 to 1987 to formally create the model known as the King's College Criteria. Studies surveying King's College Criteria have shown positive predictive

---

Table 2
The King's College Criteria for the assessment of acute liver failure

Acetaminophen-Induced ALF	Non–Acetaminophen-Induced ALF
1. Arterial pH <7.3	1. INR >6.5 (PT >100 s)
OR ALL 3 of the following	OR ANY 3 of the following
1. Encephalopathy grade 3 or 4[a]	1. Age between 10–40 y
2. INR >6.5 (PT >100 s)	2. Cause: non-A, non-B hepatitis or idiosyncratic drug reaction
3. Serum creatinine >3.4 (mg/dL)	3. Duration of jaundice before hepatic encephalopathy >7 d 4. INR >3.5 (PT >50) 5. Serum bilirubin >18 (mg/dL)

The King's College Criteria uses the cause of ALF (APAP induced or non–APAP induced), clinical information (encephalopathy, age, duration of jaundice), and laboratory values (INR, creatinine, bilirubin). This information is used to determine which patients should be referred for consideration of liver transplantation.

    Pros: high specificity, increased diagnostic accuracy in acetaminophen-induced ALF.

    Cons: low sensitivity and negative predictive value, subjective interpretation of encephalopathy.

    Abbreviation: PT, prothrombin time.

    [a] West Haven criteria for hepatic encephalopathy.

    From O'Grady JG, Alexander GJ, Hayllar KM, et al. Early indicators of prognosis in fulminant hepatic failure. Gastroenterology 1989;97(2):pp. 439-45; with permission.

values ranging from 70% to almost 100% and negative predictive values ranging from 25% to 94%.[29–31] In a large pooled meta-analysis, sensitivity was determined to be between 68% and 69% and specificity from 82% to 92%.[32,33] Data on the value of this predictive model have been mixed. In a further attempt to independently recreate and validate this prognostic model, another group of investigators[29] applied the aforementioned criteria to a population of 81 patients with ALF and determined that the King's College Criteria for predicting outcomes of ALF had slightly lower predictive accuracy than that originally suggested in the original O'Grady and colleagues'[28] study.

The Clichy criterion was developed by Bernuau and colleagues[34,35] in 1986 from a multivariate analysis of 115 patients with fulminant hepatitis B infection. The degree of coma and decreased factor V level less than 20% (age <30 years) or less than 30% (age >30 years) were determined to be valuable prognostic markers for determining needs for liver transplantation in patients with acute viral hepatitis (namely, patients with acute hepatitis B).[36] These criteria are predicted to have a positive predictive value of 82% and a negative predictive value of 98%.[32,37] Although the Clichy criteria were widely used in Northern Europe, its application has been stunted by the limited availability of factor V level measurement; moreover, the criteria were modeled from a cohort of patients with acute hepatic failure specifically from acute hepatitis B infection, thus, not immediately generalizable to all patients with ALF.[38] O'Grady and colleagues' criteria, colloquially deemed the London criteria, have been compared with the Clichy criteria to examine their predictive value and prognostic value in helping identify patients who would benefit from liver transplantation. In one study,[39] the London and Clichy criteria were both determined to have a low negative predictive value (<0.60) and would not have identified a subgroup of patients with a low risk of death. Any patient with grade 3 or 4 encephalopathy would have automatically been placed on an emergency waiting list for transplantation regardless based on the criteria, ultimately with a final decision to transplant when a donor organ was viable and available. The London Criteria had a positive predictive value of 1 for patients with grades 0 to 2 encephalopathy on admission to the hospital and, thus, may have allowed for a decision of liver transplantation at this earlier stage of ALF compared with the Clichy criteria.

Moving into the mid-1990s, another study of 61 patients with fulminant or subfulminant hepatic failure was conducted in the Veterans General Hospital in Taipei, Taiwan with the continued aim of identifying prognostic indicators for ALF.[40] Viral hepatitis accounted for 74% of the cause of ALF in this Taiwanese study population, whereas the most of the remaining patients developed drug-induced liver injury. The investigators collected data on 13 clinical parameters, of which 6 were considered significant on univariate analysis: prothrombin time prolongation, total bilirubin, creatinine, alpha-fetoprotein, age, and cholesterol. With stepwise logistic regression, age greater than 43 years, total bilirubin greater than 23, and prothrombin time prolongation of greater than 19 seconds were identified as independent predictors of nonsurvival with significant *P* values. These indicators had 100% sensitivity, 67% specificity, 95% positive predictive value, 100% negative predictive value, and 95% predictive accuracy; based on these data, they were identified as important and key prognostic factors for ALF. Similar findings were found in 1997 by Dhiman and colleagues[41] with notable factors adversely impacting the clinical course of liver failure, including presence of raised intracranial pressure at time of hospitalization, age greater than 50 years, prothrombin time greater than 100 seconds on admission, and onset of encephalopathy 7 days after onset of jaundice.

Less than a decade later, the Model for End-Stage Liver Disease (MELD) score was developed at the Mayo Clinic in Rochester, Minnesota by Kamath and colleagues[42] because of a health mandate to identify patients with ALF and appropriately allocate donor livers for hepatic transplantation. The MELD score was originally conceptualized to estimate the survival of patients undergoing a transjugular intrahepatic portosystemic shunt (TIPS) procedure using serum bilirubin, creatinine, and INR.[43]

Malinchoc and colleagues[43] used cox proportional hazard regression to identify serum concentration of creatinine and bilirubin, INR, and cause of cirrhosis as predictors of survival. The variables were used to calculate a risk score for patients undergoing elective TIPS: $R = 0.957 \times \log_e$ creatinine (mg/dL) + 0.378 × $\log_e$ bilirubin (mg/dL) + 1.120 × $\log_e$ INR + 0.643 × (cause of cirrhosis: 0 for alcohol-related and cholestatic liver disease; 1 for viral hepatitis and other cause liver disease). The MELD score was then modified from the original TIPS score: $R = 9.6 \times \log_e$ creatinine (mg/dL) + 3.8 × $\log_e$ bilirubin (mg/dL) + 11.20 × $\log_e$ INR + 0.64 × (cause of cirrhosis: 0 for alcohol-related or cholestatic liver disease; 1 for viral hepatitis and other cause of liver disease).[25] Kamath and colleagues[42] tested the MELD model's validity in 4 independent data sets, including patients hospitalized for hepatic decompensation, ambulatory patients with noncholestatic cirrhosis, patients with primary biliary cirrhosis, and a set of historical patients from the 1980s. This model was able to accurately determine the risk of mortality in patients with fulminant hepatic failure and ultimately was deemed a suitable prognostic model for disease severity in order to prioritize organ allocation for hepatic transplantation.[44] The United Network for Organ Sharing/Organ Procurement and Transplantation Network (UNOS/OPTN) adopted the MELD scoring system in 2002. In addition to its function of identifying disease severity for liver transplantation organ allocation, the MELD score has been extrapolated as an accurate predictor of 3-month mortality in liver disease,[45] with its concordance c-statistic (ie, the area under the receiver operating characteristic [AUROC] curve) being 0.78 to 0.87. The MELD score, now widely applicable and used, was recently updated in 2016 to incorporate hyponatremia to help improve prognostication of liver disease and renamed formally as the MELD-sodium (Na) score (**Table 3**).[46–49]

The aforementioned risk classifications and proposed prognostic model schemes for ALF have been widely debated about their true accuracy and value. Multiple

Table 3
Model for End-Stage Liver Disease Using Sodium

MELD-Na	Mortality Rate in Next 90 d (%)
MELD-Na Score	MELD − Na − [0.025 × MELD × (140 − Na)] + 140
≤9	1.9%
10–19	6.0%
20–29	19.6%
30–39	52.6%
≥40	71.3%

MELD-Na is calculated using 4 laboratory values (bilirubin, INR, creatinine, and sodium) and the aforementioned formula. The score represents the rate of mortality in the next 90 d.

Pros: extensively validated, statistical model currently used by UNOS for liver transplant graft allocation, mortality predictor.

Cons: absence of clear discriminant MELD-Na values, noninclusive of all important prognostic markers for ALF.

From Wiesner R, Edwards E, Freeman R, et al. Model for End-Stage Liver Disease (MELD) and allocation of donor livers. Gastroenterology 2003;124(1):p. 91–6; and Kim WR, Biggins SW, Kremers WK, et al. Hyponatremia and mortality among patients on the liver-transplant waiting list. N Engl J Med 2008;359(10):p. 1018–26; with permission.

studies have evolved based on these models to determine which indicators and modeling schemes have the most clinical fortitude. Dhiman and colleagues[50] conducted a retrospective study of a cohort of 144 patients admitted with fulminant hepatic failure secondary to acute viral hepatitis. In their statistical analysis, 6 clinical prognostic indicators of adverse outcomes related to liver failure on admission were determined: age 50 years or older, jaundice-to-encephalopathy interval greater than 7 days, grade 3 or 4 encephalopathy, presence of cerebral edema, prothrombin time 35 seconds or greater, and creatinine 1.5 mg/dL or greater. It was suggested in their study that the MELD score, in comparison with any 3 of these 6 clinical prognostic indicators, had similar sensitivity (76.1% vs 73.9%) but lower specificity (67.3% vs 86.5%), positive predictive value (80.5% vs 90.7%), negative predictive value (61.4% vs 65.2%), and diagnostic accuracy (72.9% vs 78.5%). In comparing the 6-indicator model with the King's College Criteria, it was noted that age, jaundice-to-encephalopathy interval, and prothrombin time were common in both models. However, when applying these factors to the specific cohort of patients with fulminant hepatic failure in this study, it was determined that King's College Criteria had high specificity (88.5%) and positive predictive value (87.8%), however, lower sensitivity (46.7%) and diagnostic accuracy (61.8%) in direct comparison with previously reported data of 91% and 90%, respectively, in the original King's College data.[28] There have been multiple other studies comparing the various prognostic models, each with mixed results. Just months after the Dhiman and colleagues'[50] study was published, another research article was published in the same journal suggesting the superiority of MELD to the Clichy criteria and Kings College Criteria.[51] Comparing the MELD score with the Child-Turcotte-Pugh classification, MELD has been touted and praised for clinical and statistical validity as well as being generalizable for a heterogeneous group of patients.[52–55]

OTHER CLINICAL INDICATORS OF ACUTE LIVER FAILURE

Given the multitude of clinical problems associated with the available prognostic models as well as the mixed data on their prognostic capability, the importance remains of developing the ideal model to improve sensitivity and negative predictive value for identifying appropriate candidates for orthotopic liver transplantation. Multiple serologic markers have been suggested in the literature over the past 40 years, including galactose elimination capacity,[56] serial prothrombin times,[57] arterial ketone body ratio,[58] factor V and VIII ratios,[59] plasma Gc (group-specific component) protein levels,[60] serum lactate,[61] serum phosphate,[62] and arterial sampled ammonia.[63] None of these blood markers are considered to be suitable prognostic matters.

ACUTE ON CHRONIC LIVER FAILURE

The prognostic models that were originally proposed for ALF, including Child-Turcotte-Pugh score, King's College Criteria, Clichy criteria, and the MELD score, were based on the clinical supposition that patients were without chronic liver disease before developing liver failure. Thus, investigators began trying to understand and prognosticate those patients with acute-on-chronic liver failure (ACLF), patients with established cirrhosis who developed an acute decompensation of liver disease with associated organ failure. Within the context of the European Association for the Study of the Liver–Chronic Liver Failure (EASL-CLIF), the EASL-CLIF Acute-on-Chronic Liver Failure in Cirrhosis (CANONIC) study was a prospective, observational, multicenter study of nearly 1350 patients with cirrhosis, with the aim to identify and characterize acute hepatic decompensation and determine the diagnostic criteria for ACLF.[64]

Based on the established Sequential Organ Failure Assessment (SOFA) score, which is used to diagnose organ failure in intensive care units,[65] the CLIF-SOFA score was developed for the purpose of this study based on expert opinion (**Table 4**). The CLIF-SOFA score accounts for 6 components of possible organ impairment in liver failure, including liver, kidney, brain, coagulation, circulation, and lung dysfunction. Each component has a subscore ranging from 0 to 4, with higher scores indicating severe organ dysfunction. ACLF was defined by acute hepatic decompensation (inclusion criteria, present in all of the patients in the study), organ failure based on CLIF-SOFA score, and a high 28-day mortality rate. Based on data, it was determined that those patients with ACLF were typically younger, more frequently had alcoholic cirrhosis, had a more severe grade of ACLF and associated organ failure, and higher systemic inflammatory response (increased leukocytosis and plasma C-reactive protein concentrations). In addition, ACLF was determined to be a separate entity from merely acute decompensation and considered to be a risk even if patients had no prior episodes of acute decompensation.

Stemming from the CANONIC study, another article was published by Jalan and colleagues[66] further modifying the CLIF-SOFA score into the CLIF Consortium ACLF (CLIF-C ACLF) score, attempting to improve prognostic accuracy of ACLF in direct correlation to the CLIF-SOFA score, MELD, MELD-Na, and Child Pugh scoring systems.[66] Using the population data from the CANONIC study, the study investigators first simplified the CLIF-SOFA into a score based on organ function and then further

Table 4
The Chronic Liver Failure–Sequential Organ Failure Assessment score

Organ System	Score				
	0	1	2	3	4
Liver, bilirubin (mg/dL)	<1.2	≥1.2–<2.0	≥2.0–<6.0	≥ 6.0–<12.0	≥12.0
Kidney, creatinine (mg/dL)	<1.2	≥1.2–<2.0	≥2.0–<3.5 Or use of renal-replacement therapy	≥3.5–<5.0	≥5.0
Encephalopathy grade[a]	No HE	I	II	III	IV
Coagulation, INR	<1.1	≥1.1–<2.5	≥1.25–<1.5	≥1.5–<2.5	≥2.5 or Platelets ≥20 × 10^9/L
Circulation, MAP (mm Hg)	≥70	<70	Dopamine ≤5 or dobutamine or terlipressin	Dopamine >5 or E ≤0.1 or NE ≤0.1	Dopamine >15 or E >0.1 or NE >0.1
Lungs, Pao_2/Fio_2, or SpO_2/Fio_2	>400 >512	>300–≤400 >357–≤512	>200–≤300 >214–≤357	>100–≤200 >89–≤214	≤100 ≤89

The CLIF–SOFA scale is used to assess organ failure severity using a point system based on laboratory values (bilirubin, INR, and creatinine) and clinical parameters (encephalopathy grade, pulmonary function tests [Pao_2/Fio_2 or $SpO2/Fio_2$], and MAP).

Bold format designates organ failure.

Abbreviations: E, epinephrine; Fio_2, fraction of inspired oxygen; HE, hepatic encephalopathy; MAP, mean arterial pressure; NE, norepinephrine; Pao_2, partial pressure oxygen in arterial blood; SpO_2 blood oxygen saturation level.

[a] West Haven criteria for hepatic encephalopathy.

Courtesy of European Foundation for the Study of Chronic Liver Failure EF-CLIF foundation-EASL-CLIF Consortium; with permission.

expanded it to incorporate age and leukocytosis. Furthermore, the CLIF-C ACLF was compared with the other prognostic models and deemed to have a 19% to 28% reduction in percent prediction errors observed in both the derivation and validation datasets compared with MELD, MELD-Na, and Child-Pugh scoring.

Further attempts to stratify and prognosticate subgroups of ACLF are under way. Recently, a model to assess ACLF in patients with chronic hepatitis B was developed given the high short-term mortality in this subgroup of patients.[67] In addition, acute hepatic insults in ACLF are being investigated, with one study revealing continuous alcohol use and hepatitis reactivation or superinfection as leading causes of acute hepatic insult for chronic liver failure.[68]

WEAKNESS OF CURRENT PROGNOSTIC MODELS

Physician evaluation and risk assessment of their patients with liver failure is crucial for reliable decision management about treatment options and outcome discussions with their patients. The wide variability and limited efficacy of the ALF prognostic models that are currently available is surprising given increasing clinical resources and advances in technologic capability. There are disadvantages to the current predictive models that are being used. First, despite quality-driven large-volume population studies that have been conducted over the past 50 years, significant statistical outcomes from these studies clearly do not have linear correlation with predicting patient survival with ALF. In most of the studies that have been conducted thus far, numerous variables have been identified as having a particular clinical significance in the course of liver failure, with data being collected at a specific point in time with a goal to ultimately define a specific end point (often, patient mortality). Most commonly, a linear regression analysis (ie, Cox proportional hazards ratio) has been applied for the development of the model; however, each variable has its own independent relationship with the end point that is being measured.[52,69] Most prognostic models available have been evaluated statistically by measurement of their discriminative ability, estimated by their c-statistic or AUROC. A c-statistic ranges from 0 to 1, with 0.5 indicating an outcome attributed to chance alone verses a score of 1.0 as a perfect discrimination test. Typically, a c-statistic value of greater than 0.7 indicates a useful test, with a value greater than 0.8 indicating excellent prognostication. However, c-statistic can never have a value of 1. Thus, when a prognostic model indicates AUROC of 0.8 to 0.9, this by default indicates that 10% to 20% of patients have an outcome that was not accurately predicted.[25]

Furthermore, data collection at one particular time point may be of limited utility, given the fluctuations in the clinical course of ALF. Thus, a score based on any of the available prognostic models, such as MELD-Na, is a reflection of the current state of liver failure at one time and needs to be repeatedly calculated to account for the variable clinical course. In addition, a clinical indicator of liver disease, such as serum bilirubin or INR, may be a secondary reflection of the process of ALF but may not be the true factor that allows us to understand the central process contributing to liver disease. Thus, these markers, which form the basis of many of the available scoring systems, are merely surrogates for the disease process. It is very challenging to account for the current state of liver failure as patients' clinical course and mortality risk could be determined by other factors unrelated to the liver, such as multiorgan dysfunction, infection, sepsis, and so forth. That is why the prognostic models currently available are mostly snapshots of a very dynamic process.[70]

Given the identified weakness in static binary statistical modeling and improvements with liver transplantation over the past several years, there is continued effort to modify and develop an accurate model for prognosticating ALF. Most recently in 2016, Bernal and Wang and colleagues studied a patient population of APAP-induced ALF throughout multiple intensive care units in the United Kingdom and Denmark.[71] The investigators developed prognostic models to determine mortality in patients who underwent liver transplantation for APAP toxicity. Their models were based on the AUROC and calibrated by root mean square error (RMSE). Specific admission-day variables that were evaluated included age, Glasgow coma scale, arterial pH, lactate, creatinine, INR, and cardiovascular status; a second-day model included INR and repeat lactate. Models were validated with an internal and external data set. AUROC- and RMSE-derived values from the internal and external data sets were determined for 30-day survival and applied to patients who underwent emergency liver transplantation. The median predicted 30-day survival was 51% for a transplant population (n = 116). Based on these data, it was surmised that patients with APAP-induced liver failure had improvement in rates of spontaneous recovery for ALF. Applying this type of statistical data retrospectively may be an example to help better scrutinize and ultimately identify patients who are appropriate liver transplantation candidates.

SUMMARY

Moving forward, there is a strong imperative to develop valid and accurate prognostic modeling for ALF. Despite the numerous clinical models that have been proposed thus far and the use of some such models, that is, King's College Criteria and MELD, in clinical practice to aid decision-making, there is a significant need for improvement for determining patients' clinical course, survival, and requirement for liver transplantation. Future prognostic models shall need a stronger statistical foundation and accountability for the time and variability in the clinical course of ALF and be applied for pretransplant and posttransplant outcomes.

REFERENCES

1. Trey C, Davidson C. The management of fulminant hepatic failure. In: Popper H, Schaffner F, editors. Progress in liver diseases. Volume 3. New York: Grune and Stratton; 1970. p. 282–98.
2. Lucke B, Mallory T. The fulminant form of epidemic hepatitis. Am J Pathol 1946; 22:867–943.
3. Bernuau J, Rueff B, Benhamou JP. Fulminant and subfulminant liver failure: definitions and causes. Semin Liver Dis 1986;6:97–106.
4. Tandon BN, Bernauau J, O'Grady J, et al. Recommendations of the International Association for the Study of the Liver Subcommittee on nomenclature of acute and subacute liver failure. J Gastroenterol Hepatol 1999;14:403–4.
5. Bernal W, Wendon J. Acute liver failure. N Engl J Med 2013;369(26):2525–34.
6. Ritt DJ, Whelan G, Werner DJ, et al. Acute hepatic necrosis with stupor or coma: an analysis of thirty-one patients. Medicine (Baltimore) 1969;48:151–72.
7. Ostapowicz G, Fontana RJ, Schiødt FV, et al. Results of a prospective study of acute liver failure at 17 tertiary care centers in the United States. Ann Intern Med 2002;137:947–54.
8. Reuben A, Tillman H, Fontana RJ, et al. Outcomes in Adults with acute liver failure between 1998 and 2013: an observational cohort study. Ann Intern Med 2016; 164(11):724–32.
9. Hoofnagle JH, Carithers RL Jr, Shapiro C, et al. Fulminant hepatic failure: summary of a workshop. Hepatology 1995;21(1):240–52.

10. Lee WM, Squires RH Jr, Nyberg SL, et al. Acute liver failure: summary of a workshop. Hepatology 2008;47(4):1401–15.

11. O'Grady J. Timing and benefit of liver transplantation in acute liver failure. J Hepatol 2013;60(3):663–70.

12. Germani G, Theocharidou E, Adam R, et al. Liver transplantation for acute liver failure in Europe: outcomes over 20 years from the ELTR database. J Hepatol 2012;57:288–96.

13. Freeman RB, Steffick DE, Guidinger MK, et al. Liver and intestine transplantation in the United States, 1997–2006. Am J Transplant 2008;8:958–76.

14. Rakela J, Lange SM, Ludwig J, et al. Fulminant hepatitis: Mayo Clinic experience with 34 cases. Mayo Clin Proc 1985;60:289–92.

15. Rakela J, Mosley JW, Edwards VM, et al. A double-blinded, randomized trial of hydrocortisone in acute hepatic failure. Dig Dis Sci 1991;36:1223–8.

16. Schiødt FV, Atillasoy E, Shakil AO, et al, Acute Liver Failure Study Group. Etiology and outcome for 295 patients with acute liver failure in the United States. Liver Transpl Surg 1999;5(1):29–34.

17. Williams R. Classification and clinical syndromes of acute liver failure. In: Lee WM, Williams R, editors. Acute liver failure. Cambridge: Cambridge University Press; 1997. p. 1–9.

18. Larsen FS, Kirkegaard P, Rasmussen A, et al. The Danish liver transplantation program and patients with serious acetaminophen intoxication. Transplant Proc 1995;27:3519–20.

19. Riordan SM, Williams R. Cause and prognosis in acute liver failure. Liver Transplant Surg 1999;5(1):86–9.

20. Child CG II, Turcotte JG. Surgery and portal hypertension. In: Child CG III, editor. The Liver and Portal Hypertension. Philadelphia (PA): WB Saunders; 1964. p. 50–8.

21. Conn HO. A peek at the Child-Turcotte classification. Hepatology 1981;1(6): 673–6.

22. Pugh RN, Murray-Lyon IM, Dawson JL, et al. Transection of the oesophagus for bleeding oesophageal varices. Br J Surg 1973;60(8):646–9.

23. Christensen E, Schlichting P, Fauerholdt L, et al. Prognostic value of Child-Turcotte criteria in medically treated cirrhosis. Hepatology 1984;4:430–5.

24. Christensen E. Prognostic models in chronic liver disease: validity, usefulness and future role. J Hepatol 1997;26(6):1414–24.

25. Cholongitas E, Papatheodoridis GV, Vangeli M, et al. Systematic review: the model for end-stage liver disease – should it replace Child-Pugh's classification for assessing prognosis in cirrhosis? Aliment Pharmacol Ther 2005;22(11–12): 1079–89.

26. Cooper GS, Bellamy P, Dawson NV, et al. A prognostic model for patients with end-stage liver disease. Gastroenterology 1997;113(4):1278–88.

27. Fernández-Esparrach G, Sánchez-Fueyo A, Ginès P, et al. A prognostic model for predicting survival in cirrhosis with ascites. J Hepatol 2001;34(1):46–52.

28. O'Grady JG, Alexander GJ, Hayllar KM, et al. Early indicators of prognosis in fulminant hepatic failure. Gastroenterology 1989;97(2):439–45.

29. Anand AC, Nightingale P, Neuberger JM. Early indicators of prognosis in fulminant hepatic failure: an assessment of the King's Criteria. J Hepatol 1997;26(1): 62–8.

30. Shakil AO, Kramer D, Mazariegos GV, et al. Acute liver failure: clinical features, outcome analysis, and applicability of prognostic criteria. Liver Transplant 2000;6:163–9.

31. Schmidt LE, Larsen FS. MELD score as a predictor of liver failure and death in patients with acetaminophen-induced liver injury. Hepatology 2007;45:789–96.

32. McPhail MJ, Wendon JA, Bernal W. Meta-analysis of performance of King's College Hospital Criteria in prediction of outcome in nonparacetamol-induced acute liver failure. J Hepatol 2010;53:492–9.

33. Lee WM, Larson AM, Stravitz RT. Corrections to the AASLD position paper: the management of acute liver failure: update 2011. 2011; Available at: http://www.aasld.org/practiceguidelines/Documents/AcuteLiverFailureUpdate2011.pdf. Accessed November 15, 2011.

34. Bernuau J, Goudeau A, Poynard T, et al. Multivariate analysis of prognostic factors in fulminant hepatitis B. Hepatology 1986;6(4):648–51.

35. Bernuau J, SD, Durand F, et al. Criteria for emergency liver transplantation in patients with acute viral hepatitis and factor V below 50% of normal. Hepatology 1991;14(49A).

36. Bismuth H, Samuel D, Castaing D, et al. Orthotopic liver transplantation in fulminant and subfulminant hepatitis. The Paul Brousse experience. Ann Surg 1995; 222(2):109–19.

37. Bailey B, Amre DK, Gaudreault P. Fulminant hepatic failure secondary to acetaminophen poisoning: a systematic review and meta-analysis of prognostic criteria determining the need for liver transplantation. Crit Care Med 2003;31: 299–305.

38. Bernal W, Wendon J. Liver transplantation in adults with acute liver failure. J Hepatol 2004;40(2):192–7.

39. Pauwels A, Mostefa-Kara N, Florent C, et al. Emergency liver transplantation for acute liver failure. J Hepatol 1993;17(1):124–7.

40. Huo T, Wu JC, Sheng WY, et al. Prognostic factor analysis of fulminant and subfulminant hepatic failure in an area endemic for hepatitis B. J Gastroenterol Hepatol 1996;11(6):560–5.

41. Dhiman RK, Seth AK, Jain S, et al. Prognostic evaluation of early indicators in fulminant hepatic failure by multivariate analysis. Dig Dis Sci 1998;43(6):1311–6.

42. Kamath PS, Wiesner RH, Malinchoc M, et al. A model to predict survival in patients with end-stage liver disease. Hepatology 2001;33(2):464–70.

43. Malinchoc M, Kamath PS, Gordon FD, et al. A model to predict poor survival in patients undergoing transjugular intrahepatic portosystemic shunts. Hepatology 2000;31:864–71.

44. Forman LM, Lucey MR. Predicting the prognosis of chronic liver disease: an evolution from child to MELD. Hepatology 2001;33(2):473–5.

45. Wiesner R, Edwards E, Freeman R, et al. Model for End-Stage Liver Disease (MELD) and allocation of donor livers. Gastroenterology 2003;124(1):91–6.

46. Kamath PS, Kim WR. The Model for End-Stage Liver Disease (MELD). Hepatology 2007;45(3):797–805.

47. Martin EF, O'Brien C. Update on MELD and organ allocation. Clin Liver Dis 2015; 5(4):105–7.

48. Elwir S, Lake J. Current status of liver allocation in the United States. Gastroenterol Hepatol 2016;12(3):166–70.

49. Kim WR, Biggins SW, Kremers WK, et al. Hyponatremia and mortality among patients on the liver-transplant waiting list. N Engl J Med 2008;359(10):1018–26.

50. Dhiman RK, Jain S, Maheshwari U, et al. Early indicators of prognosis in fulminant hepatic failure: an assessment of the Model for End-Stage Liver Disease (MELD) and King's College Hospital Criteria. Liver Transplant 2007;13(6): 814–21.

51. Yantorno SE, Kremers WK, Ruf AE, et al. MELD is superior to King's College and Clichy's criteria to assess prognosis in fulminant hepatic failure. Liver Transplant 2007;13(6):822–8.
52. Christensen E. Prognostic models including the Child Pugh, MELD and Mayo risk scores: where are we and where should we go? J Hepatol 2004;41(2):344–50.
53. Botta F, Giannini E, Romagnoli P, et al. MELD scoring system is useful for predicting prognosis in patients with liver cirrhosis and is correlated with residual liver function: a European study. Gut 2003;52:134–9.
54. Angermayr B, Cejna M, Karnel F, et al. Child–Pugh versus MELD score in predicting survival in patients undergoing transjugular intrahepatic portosystemic shunt. Gut 2003;52:879–85.
55. Salerno F, Merli M, Cazzaniga M, et al. MELD score is better than Child Pugh score in predicting 3-month survival of patients undergoing transjugular intrahepatic portosystemic shunt. J Hepatol 2002;36(4):494–500.
56. Ranek L, Andreasen PB, Tygstrup N. Galactose elimination capacity as a prognostic index in patients with fulminant liver failure. Gut 1976;17:959–64.
57. Harrison PM, O'Grady JG, Keays RT, et al. Serial prothrombin time as prognostic indicator in paracetamol induced fulminant hepatic failure. BMJ 1990;301(6758):964–6.
58. Saibara T, Onishi S, Sone J, et al. Arterial ketone body ratio as a possible indicator for liver transplantation in fulminant hepatic failure. Transplantation 1991;51:782–6.
59. Pereira LM, Langley PG, Hayllar KM, et al. Coagulation factor V and VIII/V ratio as predictors of outcome in paracetamol induced fulminant hepatic failure: relation to other prognostic indicators. Gut 1992;33:98–102.
60. Lee WM, Galbraith RM, Watt GH, et al. Predicting survival in fulminant hepatic failure using serum gc protein concentrations. Hepatology 1995;21(1):101–5.
61. Bernal W, Donaldson N, Wyncoll D, et al. Blood lactate as an early predictor of outcome in paracetamol-induced acute liver failure: a cohort study. Lancet 2002;359:558–63.
62. Schmidt LE, Dalhoff K. Serum phosphate is an early predictor of outcome in severe acetaminophen-induced hepatotoxicity. Hepatology 2002;36:659–65.
63. Bhatia V, Singh R, Acharya SK. Predictive value of arterial ammonia for complications and outcome in acute liver failure. Gut 2006;55:98–104.
64. Moreau R, Jalan R, Gines P, et al. Acute-on-chronic liver failure is a distinct syndrome that develops in patients with acute decompensation of cirrhosis. Gastroenterology 2013;144(7):1426–37.e9.
65. Vincent JL, Moreno R, Takala J, et al. The SOFA (Sepsis-related Organ Failure Assessment) score to describe organ dysfunction/failure. Intensive Care Med 1996;22(7):707–10.
66. Jalan R, Saliba F, Pavesi M, et al. Development and validation of a prognostic score to predict mortality in patients with acute-on-chronic liver failure. J Hepatol 2014;61(5):1038–47.
67. Li N, Huang C, Yu KK, et al. Validation of prognostic scores to predict short-term mortality in patients with HBV-related acute-on-chronic liver failure: the CLIF-C OF is superior to MELD, CLIF SOFA, and CLIF-C ACLF. Medicine 2017;96(17):e6802.
68. Shalimar KD, Kumar D, Vadiraja PK, et al. Acute on chronic liver failure because of acute hepatic insults: etiologies, course, extrahepatic organ failure and predictors of mortality. J Gastroenterol Hepatol 2016;31(4):856–64.
69. Christensen E. Multivariate survival analysis using Cox's regression model. Hepatology 1987;7:1346–58.

70. Lake JR, Sussman NL. Determining prognosis in patients with fulminant hepatic failure: when you absolutely, positively have to know the answer. Hepatology 1995;21(3):879–82.
71. Bernal W, Wang Y, Maggs J, et al. Development and validation of a dynamic outcome prediction model for paracetamol-induced acute liver failure: a cohort study. Lancet Gastroenterol Hepatol 2016;1(3):217–25.

Non–Intensive Care Unit Management of Acute Liver Failure

Andres F. Carrion, MD[a],*, Paul Martin, MD, FRCP, FRCPI[b]

KEYWORDS

- Acute liver failure • Treatment • Emergency department • Hospital ward

KEY POINTS

- Acute liver failure (ALF) is relatively uncommon with a variable and unpredictable course.
- Prompt recognition and initiation of supportive care as well as cause-specific interventions when possible may improve outcomes in ALF.
- Although many patients may benefit or require admission to an intensive care unit (ICU) (ideally one with expertise in management of ALF and at a liver transplant center), non-ICU management should focus on monitoring for progression of ALF as well as early identification and management of complications.

Acute liver failure (ALF) is a relatively uncommon clinical syndrome characterized by rapid and severe hepatic dysfunction associated with high morbidity and mortality.[1] Widespread implementation of interventions such as the use of N-acetylcysteine (NAC) for acetaminophen-induced ALF, improvements in emergency medical and critical care medicine, as well as increased availability of liver transplantation have markedly increased survival of individuals with this condition over the past few decades.[2] Management of patients with ALF typically involves multiple specialists and different levels of care, including outpatient clinics, urgent care facilities, emergency departments, general inpatient wards, intensive care units (ICU), and operating rooms if liver transplantation is performed. This review focuses on medical care of patients with ALF in non-ICU settings and will not address issues related to ICU management of ALF and its complications, liver transplantation, or liver-assist devices.

Using a standardized definition for ALF is crucial to improve communication across different levels of care within the same or across different health care systems. Results

The authors have nothing to disclose.
[a] Texas Tech University Health Sciences Center El Paso, 4800 Alberta Avenue, El Paso, TX 79905, USA; [b] Gastroenterology and Hepatology, University of Miami Miller School of Medicine, 1120 NW 14th Street, Miami, FL 33136, USA
* Corresponding author.
E-mail address: a.carrion@ttuhsc.edu

from a systematic review demonstrate significant heterogeneity in definitions used in the literature and even absence of a specific definition in many publications.[3] Current guidelines recommend defining ALF as an acute insult resulting in severe hepatic dysfunction characterized by evidence of coagulopathy (international normalized ratio [INR] $\geq$1.5) and any degree of alteration of mental status in the absence of preexisting cirrhosis and with an illness of less than 26 weeks' duration.[4] Individuals with Wilson disease, vertically transmitted hepatitis B virus (HBV) infection, or autoimmune hepatitis (AIH) may be included in this definition despite having cirrhosis if their disease has only been recognized for less than 26 weeks.[4,5] The American Association for the Study of Liver Disease guidelines discourage the use of terms such as fulminant hepatic failure or stratifying the duration of illness (ie, subacute, acute, hyperacute), because these may create confusion without adding significant prognostic value.[4] Elevation of serum aminotransferases and bilirubin commonly occurs to varying extent in ALF, but these biochemical abnormalities are not included in its definition. The term acute liver injury should be used for cases in which coagulopathy is present but there is no alteration of mental status, and acute-on-chronic liver failure should be used to describe an acute deterioration of hepatic function in individuals with underlying chronic liver disease (**Table 1**).[6]

CAUSES OF ACUTE LIVER FAILURE

It is important to review the commonest causes of ALF in order to understand some basic principles of management of this condition. There are significant differences in the epidemiology of ALF in various countries and regions of the world. For instance, drug-induced liver injury (DILI) is the commonest cause of ALF in the United States, Western Europe, and Australia. In contrast, viral infections (hepatitis A, B, and E) remain important causes in Asia, Eastern Europe, and most developing countries.[7,8] Identifying the cause of ALF provides important prognostic information and is critical for timely implementation of therapeutic interventions that may alter its natural course.[9] However, a specific cause of ALF may not be identified in a large proportion of individuals (6%–38%) despite extensive workup.[7] The commonest causes of ALF are summarized in **Table 2**.

- Acetaminophen hepatotoxicity: patients with suspect or established acetaminophen-induced hepatotoxicity usually undergo initial evaluation and management in non-ICU settings such as urgent care facilities or emergency departments. Freestanding urgent care facilities should immediately contact the nearest hospital and initiate the transfer process, because the level of care needed exceeds that available in these facilities. Data from observational studies estimate that acetaminophen overdose is responsible for up to 78,414 emergency department visits and approximately 33,520 hospitalizations annually in the United States.[10] The overwhelming majority of cases of

Table 1
Clinical characteristics of 3 different acute hepatic syndromes

Clinical Syndrome	Coagulopathy	Encephalopathy	Underlying Chronic Liver Disease
Acute liver injury	+	−	+/−
ALF	+	+	−
Acute-on-chronic liver failure	+	+	+

Table 2
Most common causes of acute liver failure

Viral	Hepatitis A, B, D, and E
	Cytomegalovirus
	Herpes simplex virus
	Hemorrhagic fever viruses
Drugs, health supplements, toxins	Acetaminophen
	Prescription drugs (ie, antibiotics, anticonvulsants, anesthetics)
	Ecstasy (MDMA)
	Herbal remedies (ie, Ma huang)
	Supplements (ie, Hydroxycut)
	Mushroom poisoning
Pregnancy-related	AFLP
	HELLP syndrome
Vascular	Budd-Chiari syndrome
	Sinusoidal obstruction syndrome
	Ischemic hepatopathy (shock liver)
Metabolic	Galactosemia
	Tyrosinemia
	Wilson disease
	Alpha 1 antitrypsin deficiency
Others	AIH
	Malignant infiltration
	Primary graft nonfunction

Abbreviation: MDMA, methylenedioxymethamphetamine.

acetaminophen overdose results in varying severity of hepatocellular injury rather than true ALF; however, acetaminophen overdose is responsible for most cases of ALF in the United States (39%) and other developed countries.[8,11] Hepatotoxicity rarely occurs when acetaminophen is used at therapeutic doses: up to 4 g per day in adults without underlying liver disease, up to 2 g per day in adults with preexisting liver disease, and up to 15 mg per kilogram of body weight in children under the age of 12 years (maximum 4 g per day). Suicidal attempts with intentional overdose are the commonest scenario for acetaminophen-induced ALF, but therapeutic misadventures (unknowingly taking multiple acetaminophen-containing formulations simultaneously) and hepatotoxicity at therapeutic doses because of induction of the cytochrome P450 system by other agents (ie, carbamazepine, phenobarbital, phenytoin, isoniazid, rifampin) also occur.[12] In contrast to other drugs causing severe DILI and ALF, widespread availability of NAC as a specific antidote for acetaminophen-induced hepatotoxicity markedly improves outcomes, particularly if administered within 8 hours following an overdose.[13] Thus, treatment with NAC should not be delayed and must be initiated upon recognition or even suspicion of acetaminophen-induced hepatotoxicity, regardless of the site of care during initial evaluation.

- DILI: similar to acetaminophen hepatotoxicity, patients with suspected or established DILI usually undergo initial evaluation and management in non-ICU settings such as urgent care facilities or emergency departments. However, because of widespread use of drugs that can potentially cause DILI in outpatient clinics as well as inpatient hospital wards, a significant proportion of patients are also initially identified in these settings.[14] Causality assignment for DILI is difficult and circumstantial in the overwhelming majority of ALF cases. DILI due to idiosyncratic drug reactions occurs less commonly than acetaminophen-induced hepatotoxicity, and agents implicated include antibiotics, nonsteroidal anti-inflammatory drugs, anticonvulsants, and health supplements, among others. Progression to ALF in individuals with non–acetaminophen DILI occurs only in approximately 10% of cases, but when it does, it is usually associated with an ominous prognosis with up to 80% of individuals dying or requiring emergency liver transplantation. There are also prognostic differences according to the subtype of DILI. For instance, purely cholestatic injury is associated with overall better prognosis compared with hepatocellular or mixed injury (spontaneous survival: 43.8% vs 26.5% vs 16.7%, respectively).[15]

- Viruses: several viruses are implicated in causing ALF, including hepatitis A, B, C, D, and E, as well as herpes simplex virus, varicella zoster virus, Epstein-Barr virus, adenovirus, cytomegalovirus, and others, including some responsible for hemorrhagic fevers. Most patients with acute viral infections receive medical care in outpatient clinics, urgent care facilities, or emergency departments, and signs of ALF must be promptly recognized in order to triage patients to an appropriate level of care. In addition to acute HBV infection, ALF may also occur as a result of HBV reactivation in chronic infected carriers receiving antineoplastic chemotherapy or immunosuppression, including biological agents for benign diseases.[16] Hepatitis C virus (HCV) and hepatitis D virus do not appear to be significant causes of ALF in the absence of coinfection with HBV. Acute hepatitis E virus (HEV) infection causes ALF in endemic areas. Individuals particularly susceptible to ALF due to acute HEV infection include the elderly, the malnourished, and pregnant women.[17,18]

- Pregnancy-related disorders: in otherwise healthy women, prenatal and postdelivery care is usually provided exclusively by obstetricians and/or midwives, who should recognize hepatic syndromes related to pregnancy. Acute fatty liver of pregnancy (AFLP) and the hemolysis, elevated liver enzymes, low platelets (HELLP) syndrome typically occur in the third trimester of pregnancy and are associated with increased fetal and/or maternal mortality, including risk of ALF.[19,20] Prompt delivery of the infant is usually followed by improvement in hepatic function, and liver transplantation is rarely necessary.[21] Severe hepatic ischemia and liver rupture associated with preeclampsia occur infrequently but may lead to ALF and should be suspected in the appropriate clinical context.[22] Importantly, ALF can present after delivery in patients with AFLP; thus, close monitoring of maternal hepatic function should continue. However, liver transplantation is rarely required.[21]

- Other causes: AIH must be considered a potential cause of ALF in middle-aged women with no other obvious cause, particularly in those with preexisting or coexisting autoimmune disorders. The presence of reactive autoantibodies, elevated globulin fraction, and specifically immunoglobulin G (IgG) levels, may suggest AIH as a cause of ALF, but histologic confirmation (demonstrating characteristic interface hepatitis with lymphoplasmacytic infiltrates) is mandatory because these may also be present in other causes of ALF.[23] Wilson disease is an uncommon cause of ALF but must be promptly identified because a fulminant presentation is typically fatal without liver transplantation.[24] Important clues to the diagnosis of acute Wilson disease include presence of acute Coombs-negative hemolytic anemia, marked elevations in the total serum bilirubin levels mainly at expense of the indirect fraction from hemolysis, very low serum uric acid and alkaline phosphatase with a bilirubin to alkaline phosphatase ratio >2, acute kidney injury from copper-induced renal tubular damage, low ceruloplasmin levels, and the presence of Kayser-Fleischer rings.[25] Hepatic hypoperfusion due to severe and sustained systemic hypotension, vasoconstrictive drugs such as cocaine, or vascular events such as Budd-Chiari syndrome and sinusoidal obstruction syndrome may rarely result in ALF. Mushroom poisoning usually by *Amanita phalloides* is rare but may progress to ALF accompanied by severe nausea, emesis, diarrhea, and acute kidney injury.[26]

DIAGNOSIS OF ACUTE LIVER FAILURE

Establishing a diagnosis of ALF can be relatively simple in individuals with an identifiable cause presenting with significant coagulopathy and obvious encephalopathy. However, it can be rather challenging when only subtle findings are present, confounding variables exist (ie, coagulopathy or changes in mental status due to other causes), or in the absence of a clear risk factor for a severe hepatic insult. A detailed history and physical examination must precede extensive workup and should emphasize risk factors for causes of liver disease.[7] Patients with biochemical evidence of acute hepatitis from any cause must be closely monitored for potential progression to ALF. Serial monitoring of coagulation and mental status is crucial. Prolongation of the prothrombin time by 4 to 6 seconds or more (or increase in the INR ≥1.5) along with any deficit in mentation is required to establish a diagnosis of ALF. Initial laboratory testing must be aimed at identifying correctable or treatable conditions that may improve outcomes and should be obtained upon suspicion or recognition of ALF (**Table 3**).

TREATMENT OF ACUTE LIVER FAILURE IN NON–INTENSIVE CARE UNIT SETTINGS

ALF is a clinical syndrome resulting from diverse hepatic insults, and its management should be guided by the following axes (**Fig. 1**): general supportive care,

Table 3 Initial testing in acute liver failure	
Routine blood work	Complete blood count, complete metabolic profile, phosphorus, magnesium, lactic acid, ABG, β-HCG
Coagulation tests	Prothrombin time, INR, activated partial thromboplastin time, fibrinogen
Blood and urine cultures	Baseline evaluation for infections
Viral tests	Anti-HAV IgM, HBsAg, anti-HBc IgM, HBV-DNA, anti-HCV antibody, HCV-RNA, anti-HEV antibody
Autoimmune markers	ANA, ASMA, IgG level
Toxicology screen	Serum and urine (as inclusive as possible), ETOH level, acetaminophen level
Abdominal imaging	Ultrasonography to evaluate hepatic parenchyma and vasculature with Doppler, or CT with intravenous contrast
Electrocardiogram	Baseline evaluation for arrhythmias and prolongation of the QT interval
Chest radiography	Baseline evaluation of cardiopulmonary status

Abbreviations: ABG, arterial blood gas; ANA, antinuclear antibody; ASMA, anti–smooth muscle antibody; CT, computed tomography; ETOH, ethanol; HAV, hepatitis A virus; HCG, human chorionic gonadotropin.

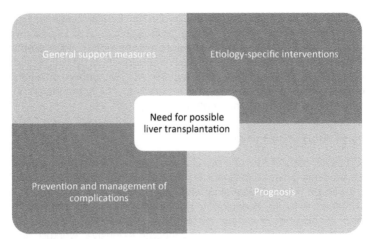

Fig. 1. Areas of focus during treatment of ALF.

cause-specific interventions, prevention and treatment of complications, and ascertaining prognosis and need for liver transplantation. For purposes of this review, the authors focus on non-ICU/nontransplant management of ALF and its complications.

General Supportive Care in Acute Liver Failure

Patients with suspected or established ALF should be closely monitored for hemodynamic derangements, electrolyte imbalances, metabolic and acid-base disturbances, changes in mental status, and infectious complications.[27] Restoration of intravascular volume is usually necessary to maintain adequate visceral perfusion because hypotension commonly occurs as result of systemic vasodilatation. The choice of intravenous fluids (crystalloid vs colloid) should be guided by clinician preference, because there are no data to provide evidence-based recommendations in ALF per se. Monitoring serum electrolytes with clinical observation to avoid fluid overload is necessary when repeated boluses and maintenance intravenous fluids are administered. Correction of coagulopathy by transfusing plasma derivatives must be avoided unless clinically evident bleeding occurs, because it may interfere with objective assessment of hepatic function through coagulation parameters.[5] Spontaneous bleeding occurs uncommonly in ALF unless a combination of profound thrombocytopenia, low fibrinogen levels, prolongation of the activated partial thromboplastin time and prothrombin time, and low factor V levels is present.[28] Recent data have disproved the common but erroneous previous belief that coagulopathy in ALF is associated with increased risk of bleeding and actually demonstrate the presence of a procoagulant imbalance in this condition.[29,30] Frequent neurologic examinations are required because encephalopathy may progress rapidly, and the need to transfer patients to an ICU must be individualized but is usually recommended for those with grade II or higher.[5] Use of sedatives is contraindicated in non-ICU settings because it interferes with neurologic examinations and may result in deeper and/or prolonged sedation because of reduced hepatic metabolism of various agents in this class. Empiric administration of broad-spectrum antibiotics has been advocated by some transplant centers, but data from observational studies have failed to support a benefit in prevention of bloodstream infections or improved survival.[31,32] Pharmacologic prophylaxis against gastrointestinal stress ulcers is recommended by guidelines, although conclusive data demonstrating improved outcomes are lacking.[33,34]

Cause-Specific Interventions in Acute Liver Failure

Rapid implementation of specific therapy, if available, may favorably alter the clinical course of ALF (**Table 4**). Acetaminophen hepatotoxicity is the best example, because timely initiation of NAC (ideally within 8 hours of ingestion) significantly improves outcomes, including transplant-free survival.[35] NAC can be administered through either enteral or intravenous routes and does not require ICU monitoring because adverse reactions are minimal (**Table 5**).[36,37] NAC has also been extensively studied in non–acetaminophen ALF with less convincing results. For instance, in the largest study to date, intravenous administration of NAC did not improve overall survival but did improve transplant-free survival in non–acetaminophen ALF compared with placebo (40% vs 27%, respectively); however, the benefits of this agent were confined to patients with less severe encephalopathy (grades I and II).[36]

In AFLP and HELLP syndrome, expedited delivery of the infant may rapidly change the course of ALF, resulting in prompt resolution.[21] However, as noted earlier, patients must be closely monitored after delivery because ALF may develop during this period.

ALF due to acute ischemic hepatic injury typically improves rapidly once hemodynamic stability and adequate hepatic perfusion are restored.

Antiviral therapy for HBV infection with a nucleos(t)ide analogue may mitigate ALF and improve outcomes, although not invariably.[38,39] Newer-generation nucleos(t)ide analogues, such as entecavir, tenofovir alafenamide, or tenofovir disoproxil fumarate, are the agents of choice.

Prompt diagnosis of Budd-Chiari syndrome resulting in ALF may permit treatment with systemic anticoagulation and angioplasty with placement of a transjugular intrahepatic portosystemic shunt, thus restoring vascular patency and improving hepatic function.[40,41]

ALF due to other causes, such as non–acetaminophen DILI, acute viral hepatitis, acute Wilson disease, AIH, and malignant infiltration of the liver, typically follows an unpredictable clinical course despite aggressive interventions.

Table 4
Cause-specific therapies that may alter the course of acute liver failure

Cause of ALF	Therapy
Acetaminophen-induced ALF	NAC
Acute HBV infection or HBV reactivation	Nucleos(t)ide analogues
AIH	High-dose corticosteroids
AFLP	Delivery of the fetus
HELLP syndrome	Delivery of the fetus
Budd-Chiari syndrome	TIPS, surgical decompression, or thrombolysis
Herpes simplex virus infection	Acyclovir
Mushroom poisoning	Activated charcoal, penicillin G, intravenous silibinin

Abbreviation: TIPS, transhepatic portosystemic shunt.

Table 5		
Protocols for N-acetylcysteine administration		
Route	Dose, mg/kg	Frequency and Intervals
Enteral route (oral or nasogastric/orogastric tube)	140 70	One dose, followed by 17 doses, every 4 h
Intravenous route	150 50 100	Infuse over 60 min, then Infuse over 4 h, then Infuse over 16 h

Management of Electrolyte, Acid-Base, and Metabolic Derangements in Acute Liver Failure

Hypokalemia is one of the commonest electrolyte abnormalities encountered in ALF and is exacerbated by diuretic therapy and increased sympathetic tone causing increased intracellular shifts. Importantly, hypokalemia increases renal tubular production of ammonia from glutamine and may result in worsening of encephalopathy; thus, efforts should focus on maintaining normokalemia.[42]

Hypophosphatemia must be recognized and treated promptly to prevent adverse cardiac events. Decreased plasma phosphate levels in ALF may indicate a favorable prognosis, particularly in acetaminophen-induced ALF, and are due to increased intracellular shifts related to metabolic demands by regenerating hepatocytes.[43]

Hyponatremia in ALF reflects enhanced release of antidiuretic hormone as well as impaired renal function due to hypoperfusion. Treatment of hyponatremia in ALF should not be overly rapid to avoid osmotic demyelination syndrome.[44]

Mixed respiratory and metabolic alkalosis is more common than acidosis during the early stages of ALF and is best managed by treating the underlying hepatic insult. Metabolic acidosis typically occurs later in ALF and is due to decreased hepatic clearance of lactate.[7]

Hypoglycemia in ALF is associated with poor prognosis and is usually multifactorial: depletion of hepatic glycogen stores, increased glycolysis, increased hepatic extraction of glucose, and impaired gluconeogenesis.[45] Close monitoring of plasma glucose concentrations is mandatory in patients with ALF, and dextrose solutions are administered intravenously to maintain levels greater than 65 mg/dL.[46] Overly aggressive glycemic corrections should be avoided because rapid boluses of concentrated glucose solutions may induce osmotic shifts in the intravascular and cerebral compartments. Hyperglycemia (>200 mg/dL) should also be avoided, because exacerbation of increased intracranial pressure has been reported.[47,48]

Hepatic Encephalopathy and Cerebral Edema

Encephalopathy is a defining feature of ALF and is primarily due to hepatic dysfunction rather than portosystemic shunting, the latter occurring in cirrhosis and end-stage liver disease. Management of hepatic encephalopathy in ALF is challenging, and routine use of lactulose is controversial, because it may not improve mentation and can lead to bowel distention resulting in technical difficulties during liver transplantation.[49] Rifaximin, which is also commonly used to manage hepatic encephalopathy in cirrhosis, has not been studied in ALF; thus, its use is not endorsed. Patients with lower grades of encephalopathy (grades I and II) may be managed in non-ICU settings with a low threshold for transfer to ICU. Patients already with more advanced grades

(III and IV) should be admitted to an ICU, because airway protection with endotracheal intubation and mechanical ventilation is recommended.[5]

Cerebral edema is uncommon in patients with grades I or II encephalopathy but is present in approximately 75% of those with grade IV encephalopathy.[50] The main concern about cerebral edema is diminished cerebral perfusion and increased intracranial pressure with risk of brainstem herniation. Cerebral edema causing increased intracranial pressure is suggested by hypertension, bradycardia, and irregular breathing (Cushing triad), as well as neurologic signs such as increased muscle tone, hyperreflexia, and altered pupillary response. Prevention of increased intracranial pressure in ALF is centered on minimizing patient agitation and neurologic stimulation, elevating the head of the bed, and maintaining optimal fluid balance with specific attention to avoiding overhydration (increases intracranial pressure) and volume depletion (decreases cerebral perfusion pressure).

Infectious Complications

Bacterial, fungal, and viral infections are a major concern in patients with ALF because severe immunologic alterations usually coexist. Furthermore, severe untreated infections may jeopardize transplant candidacy or result in postoperative complications. Recent data, however, suggest that bacteremia is not independently associated with increased mortality in patients with ALF.[51] Although empiric antibiotics are recommended for patients with ALF exhibiting signs of systemic inflammatory response syndrome, refractory hypotension, or unexplained worsening of encephalopathy, a survival benefit has not been confirmed.[32]

PROGNOSTIC MODELS IN ACUTE LIVER FAILURE

Multiple prognostic models that attempt to identify patients with ALF with a low likelihood of spontaneous recovery and who require consideration for liver transplantation have been developed. These models include the model for end-stage liver disease (MELD), King's College criteria (KCC), the sequential organ failure assessment, the Clichy criteria, the Acute Liver Failure Study Group index, among others.[52–57] Although each prognostic model has some advantages and disadvantages over others, recent guidance from the American Gastroenterology Association endorses the use of the MELD score over the KCC.[58]

The KCC were developed in the United Kingdom in the late 1980s and predict the need for liver transplantation based on the cause of ALF and several other variables listed in **Box 1**. The Clichy criteria were developed by a French group and take into consideration the presence of encephalopathy, factor V levels, and the patient's age. The predictive accuracy of the Clichy criteria is variable depending on the cause of ALF, with the highest positive and negative predictive values for viral hepatitis-induced ALF (82% and 98%, respectively). However, the predictive accuracy of the Clichy criteria was much lower than that of KCC in other populations, such as acetaminophen- and non-acetaminophen-induced ALF.[55,59] The MELD score is a well-established and validated prognostic model that predicts short-term mortality in patients with cirrhosis and is currently used for organ allocation in liver transplantation in the United States and many other countries. Results from a meta-analysis demonstrate higher overall predictive accuracy for the MELD score compared with KCC (area under the receiver operating characteristic curve values 0.78 and 0.76, respectively); however, KCC performed slightly better than the MELD score for acetaminophen-induced ALF.[60]

Box 1
King's College criteria for liver transplantation in acute liver failure

Acetaminophen-induced ALF

Arterial pH <7.3 (irrespective of the grade of encephalopathy)

OR

Grade III or IV encephalopathy *AND*

Prothrombin time >100 seconds or INR >6.5 *AND*

Serum creatinine >3.4 mg/dL

All other causes of ALF

Prothrombin time >100 seconds or INR >6.5 (irrespective of the grade of encephalopathy)

OR

Any 3 of the following (irrespective of the grade of encephalopathy):

Age <10 years or >40 years

Unfavorable cause (seronegative hepatitis or idiosyncratic drug reaction)

Duration of jaundice before the onset of encephalopathy >7 days

Prothrombin time >50 seconds or INR >3.5

Serum bilirubin greater than 18 mg/dL

SUMMARY

ALF is relatively uncommon with a variable and unpredictable course. Prompt recognition and initiation of supportive care as well as cause-specific interventions when possible may improve outcomes in ALF. Although many patients may benefit or require admission to an ICU (ideally one with expertise in management of ALF and at a liver transplant center), non-ICU management should focus on monitoring for progression of ALF as well as early identification and management of complications.

REFERENCES

1. Bower WA, Johns M, Margolis HS, et al. Population-based surveillance for acute liver failure. Am J Gastroenterol 2007;102(11):2459–63.
2. Reuben A, Tillman H, Fontana RJ, et al. Outcomes in adults with acute liver failure between 1998 and 2013: an observational cohort study. Ann Intern Med 2016; 164(11):724–32.
3. Wlodzimirow KA, Eslami S, Abu-Hanna A, et al. Systematic review: acute liver failure - one disease, more than 40 definitions. Aliment Pharmacol Ther 2012;35(11): 1245–56.
4. Polson J, Lee WM, American Association for the Study of Liver Disease. AASLD position paper: the management of acute liver failure. Hepatology 2005;41(5): 1179–97.
5. European Association for the Study of the Liver. Clinical practice guidelines panel, Wendon J, Cordoba J, Dhawan A, et al. EASL clinical practical guidelines on the management of acute (fulminant) liver failure. J Hepatol 2017;66(5): 1047–81.
6. Hernaez R, Sola E, Moreau R, et al. Acute-on-chronic liver failure: an update. Gut 2017;66(3):541–53.

7. Bernal W, Wendon J. Acute liver failure. N Engl J Med 2013;369(26):2525–34.
8. Lee WM. Etiologies of acute liver failure. Semin Liver Dis 2008;28(2):142–52.
9. Ostapowicz G, Fontana RJ, Schiodt FV, et al. Results of a prospective study of acute liver failure at 17 tertiary care centers in the United States. Ann Intern Med 2002;137(12):947–54.
10. Budnitz DS, Lovegrove MC, Crosby AE. Emergency department visits for over-doses of acetaminophen-containing products. Am J Prev Med 2011;40(6): 585–92.
11. Gill RQ, Sterling RK. Acute liver failure. J Clin Gastroenterol 2001;33(3):191–8.
12. Yoon E, Babar A, Choudhary M, et al. Acetaminophen-induced hepatotoxicity: a comprehensive update. J Clin Transl Hepatol 2016;4(2):131–42.
13. Heard K, Rumack BH, Green JL, et al. A single-arm clinical trial of a 48-hour intra-venous N-acetylcysteine protocol for treatment of acetaminophen poisoning. Clin Toxicol 2014;52(5):512–8.
14. Meier Y, Cavallaro M, Roos M, et al. Incidence of drug-induced liver injury in med-ical inpatients. Eur J Clin Pharmacol 2005;61(2):135–43.
15. Reuben A, Koch DG, Lee WM, et al. Drug-induced acute liver failure: results of a U.S. multicenter, prospective study. Hepatology 2010;52(6):2065–76.
16. Seetharam A, Perrillo R, Gish R. Immunosuppression in patients with chronic hep-atitis B. Curr Hepatol Rep 2014;13:235–44.
17. Borkakoti J, Hazam RK, Mohammad A, et al. Does high viral load of hepatitis E virus influence the severity and prognosis of acute liver failure during pregnancy? J Med Virol 2013;85(4):620–6.
18. Shalimar, Acharya SK. Hepatitis E and acute liver failure in pregnancy. J Clin Exp Hepatol 2013;3(3):213–24.
19. Hay JE. Liver disease in pregnancy. Hepatology 2008;47(3):1067–76.
20. Pereira SP, O'Donohue J, Wendon J, et al. Maternal and perinatal outcome in se-vere pregnancy-related liver disease. Hepatology 1997;26(5):1258–62.
21. Liu J, Ghaziani TT, Wolf JL. Acute fatty liver disease of pregnancy: updates in pathogenesis, diagnosis, and management. Am J Gastroenterol 2017;112(6): 838–46.
22. Frise CJ, Davis P, Barker G, et al. Hepatic capsular rupture in pregnancy. Obstet Med 2016;9(4):185–8.
23. Bernal W, Ma Y, Smith HM, et al. The significance of autoantibodies and immuno-globulins in acute liver failure: a cohort study. J Hepatol 2007;47(5):664–70.
24. Harada M. Management for acute liver failure of Wilson disease: indication for liver transplantation. Hepatol Res 2017;47(4):281–2.
25. Bandmann O, Weiss KH, Kaler SG. Wilson's disease and other neurological cop-per disorders. Lancet Neurol 2015;14(1):103–13.
26. Bonacini M, Shetler K, Yu I, et al. Features of patients with severe hepatitis due to mushroom poisoning and factors associated with outcome. Clin Gastroenterol Hepatol 2017;15(5):776–9.
27. Wang DW, Yin YM, Yao YM. Advances in the management of acute liver failure. World J Gastroenterol 2013;19(41):7069–77.
28. Habib M, Roberts LN, Patel RK, et al. Evidence of rebalanced coagulation in acute liver injury and acute liver failure as measured by thrombin generation. Liver Int 2014;34(5):672–8.
29. Hugenholtz GC, Adelmeijer J, Meijers JC, et al. An unbalance between von Wil-lebrand factor and ADAMTS13 in acute liver failure: implications for hemostasis and clinical outcome. Hepatology 2013;58(2):752–61.

30. Lisman T, Stravitz RT. Rebalanced hemostasis in patients with acute liver failure. Semin Thromb Hemost 2015;41(5):468–73.
31. Shalimar. Antibiotics in acute liver failure (ALF). J Clin Exp Hepatol 2015;5(1):95–7.
32. Karvellas CJ, Cavazos J, Battenhouse H, et al. Effects of antimicrobial prophylaxis and blood stream infections in patients with acute liver failure: a retrospective cohort study. Clin Gastroenterol Hepatol 2014;12(11):1942–9.e1.
33. Krag M, Perner A, Wetterslev J, et al. Prevalence and outcome of gastrointestinal bleeding and use of acid suppressants in acutely ill adult intensive care patients. Intensive Care Med 2015;41(5):833–45.
34. Krag M, Perner A, Wetterslev J, et al. Stress ulcer prophylaxis in the intensive care unit: an international survey of 97 units in 11 countries. Acta Anaesthesiol Scand 2015;59(5):576–85.
35. Buckley NA, Dawson AH, Juurlink DN, et al. Who gets antidotes? Choosing the chosen few. Br J Clin Pharmacol 2016;81(3):402–7.
36. Lee WM, Hynan LS, Rossaro L, et al. Intravenous N-acetylcysteine improves transplant-free survival in early stage non-acetaminophen acute liver failure. Gastroenterology 2009;137(3):856–64, 864.e1.
37. Nabi T, Nabi S, Rafiq N, et al. Role of N-acetylcysteine treatment in non-acetaminophen-induced acute liver failure: a prospective study. Saudi J Gastroenterol 2017;23(3):169–75.
38. Belongia EA, Costa J, Gareen IF, et al. NIH consensus development statement on management of hepatitis B. NIH Consens State Sci Statements 2008;25(2):1–29.
39. Miyake Y, Iwasaki Y, Takaki A, et al. Lamivudine treatment improves the prognosis of fulminant hepatitis B. Intern Med 2008;47(14):1293–9.
40. Parekh J, Matei VM, Canas-Coto A, et al. Budd-Chiari syndrome causing acute liver failure: a multicenter case series. Liver Transpl 2017;23(2):135–42.
41. Garcia-Pagan JC, Heydtmann M, Raffa S, et al. TIPS for Budd-Chiari syndrome: long-term results and prognostics factors in 124 patients. Gastroenterology 2008;135(3):808–15.
42. Tizianello A, Garibotto G, Robaudo C, et al. Renal ammoniagenesis in humans with chronic potassium depletion. Kidney Int 1991;40(4):772–8.
43. Baquerizo A, Anselmo D, Shackleton C, et al. Phosphorus ans an early predictive factor in patients with acute liver failure. Transplantation 2003;75(12):2007–14.
44. Feltracco P, Cagnin A, Carollo C, et al. Neurological disorders in liver transplant candidates: pathophysiology and clinical assessment. Transplant Rev 2017;31(3):193–206.
45. Moore JK, Love E, Craig DG, et al. Acute kidney injury in acute liver failure: a review. Expert Rev Gastroenterol Hepatol 2013;7(8):701–12.
46. Kaur S, Kumar P, Kumar V, et al. Etiology and prognostic factors of acute liver failure in children. Indian Pediatr 2013;50(7):677–9.
47. Waeschle RM, Brauer A, Hilgers R, et al. Hypoglycaemia and predisposing factors among clinical subgroups treated with intensive insulin therapy. Acta Anaesthesiol Scand 2014;58(2):223–34.
48. Kramer AH, Roberts DJ, Zygun DA. Optimal glycemic control in neurocritical care patients: a systematic review and meta-analysis. Crit Care 2012;16(5):R203.
49. Kodali S, McGuire BM. Diagnosis and management of hepatic encephalopathy in fulminant hepatic failure. Clin Liver Dis 2015;19(3):565–76.
50. Lee WM. Acute liver failure. N Engl J Med 1993;329(25):1862–72.
51. Karvellas CJ, Pink F, McPhail M, et al. Predictors of bacteraemia and mortality in patients with acute liver failure. Intensive Care Med 2009;35(8):1390–6.

52. O'Grady JG, Alexander GJ, Hayllar KM, et al. Early indicators of prognosis in fulminant hepatic failure. Gastroenterology 1989;97(2):439–45.

53. Craig DG, Zafar S, Reid TW, et al. The sequential organ failure assessment (SOFA) score is an effective triage marker following staggered paracetamol (acetaminophen) overdose. Aliment Pharmacol Ther 2012;35(12):1408–15.

54. Craig DG, Reid TW, Wright EC, et al. The sequential organ failure assessment (SOFA) score is prognostically superior to the model for end-stage liver disease (MELD) and MELD variants following paracetamol (acetaminophen) overdose. Aliment Pharmacol Ther 2012;35(6):705–13.

55. Pauwels A, Mostefa-Kara N, Florent C, et al. Emergency liver transplantation for acute liver failure. Evaluation of London and Clichy criteria. J Hepatol 1993;17(1): 124–7.

56. Bernuau J, Goudeau A, Poynard T, et al. Multivariate analysis of prognostic factors in fulminant hepatitis B. Hepatology 1986;6(4):648–51.

57. Rutherford A, King LY, Hynan LS, et al. Development of an accurate index for predicting outcomes of patients with acute liver failure. Gastroenterology 2012; 143(5):1237–43.

58. Flamm SL, Yang YX, Singh S, et al. American Gastroenterological Association Institute guidelines for the diagnosis and management of acute liver failure. Gastroenterology 2017;152(3):644–7.

59. Izumi S, Langley PG, Wendon J, et al. Coagulation factor V levels as a prognostic indicator in fulminant hepatic failure. Hepatology 1996;23(6):1507–11.

60. McPhail MJ, Farne H, Senvar N, et al. Ability of King's College criteria and model for end-stage liver disease scores to predict mortality of patients with acute liver failure: a meta-analysis. Clin Gastroenterol Hepatol 2016;14(4):516–25.e5 [quiz: e43–45].

Management of Acute Liver Failure in the Intensive Care Unit Setting

Priyanka Rajaram, MD[a], Ram Subramanian, MD[b],*

KEYWORDS

- Acute liver failure • Hepatic encephalopathy • Acute renal failure
- Intracranial hypertension • Acetaminophen toxicity

KEY POINTS

- Early recognition with serial neurologic examinations is the key to initiating appropriate management of hepatic encephalopathy and cerebral edema.
- Thrombocytopenia is not infrequently seen in acute liver failure (ALF) and is associated with increased incidence of multiorgan failure.
- The development of AKI was associated with increased mortality, with incidence being more common in patients with severe liver dysfunction.
- In patients with refractory hypotension, adrenal insufficiency should be considered.
- Patients with ALF are at high risk for bacterial and fungal infections.

INTRODUCTION

Acute liver failure (ALF) represents one of the most catastrophic conditions encountered in the intensive care unit (ICU). The severity of illness and the rapidity with which the condition progresses to multiorgan failure are alarming and prompt a high index of suspicion to arrive at a diagnosis and provide swift medical care. ALF presents a unique set of complications and management strategies with liver transplantation as the common end point in most cases. This article focuses on the management of ALF in the ICU setting.

Acute liver failure, previously known as fulminant hepatic failure, is defined as development of hepatocellular dysfunction manifesting as coagulopathy and encephalopathy in patients without pre-existing liver disease over a period of 26 weeks. There are over 2500 cases of ALF every year in the United States, with over half of them

The authors have nothing to disclose.
[a] Department of Medicine, Emory University School of Medicine, 615 Michael Street Northeast, Suite 205, Atlanta, GA 30322, USA; [b] Department of Medicine, Emory University School of Medicine, 1365 Clifton Road Northeast, B6100, Atlanta, GA 30322, USA
* Corresponding author.
E-mail address: rmsubra@emory.edu

progressing to liver transplantation.[1] Acetaminophen toxicity is by far the most common reason for liver transplantation among ALF patients, followed by other drug-related injuries, viral etiologies, and Wilson disease.[1] The major causes of mortality in ALF are intracranial hypertension (ICH) and infections; however, patients can manifest with varying degrees of hemodynamic derangements and renal dysfunction.

DIAGNOSIS OF ACUTE LIVER FAILURE

A detailed history and physical examination are key to evaluating a patient with ALF to determine the etiology of liver injury. It is important to elucidate the presence of any component of chronic liver disease to identify if this is truly ALF or a representation of acute on chronic liver failure (ACLF).[2] A thorough assessment of lack of social support, medical comorbidities, and history of malignancies should be performed, as these could preclude candidacy for liver transplantation. An initial laboratory evaluation including basic metabolic panel, liver function test, coagulation profile, arterial blood gas (ABG), serum lactate, comprehensive hepatitis panel, and toxicology screen should be obtained. All patients should undergo serial monitoring of liver function tests, coagulation profile, and mental status, given high risk for ICH and coagulopathy. Diagnostic imaging with abdominal ultrasound with Doppler to assess patency of hepatic and portal veins, presence of ascites, and liver size should be obtained. MRI of the abdomen or computed tomography (CT) of the abdomen is recommended for detailed evaluation of liver anatomy and to exclude the presence of chronic liver disease and portal hypertension.[1] Early transfer to the nearest liver transplant center is recommended given the potential for rapid deterioration. As part of the initial evaluation, a constant assessment of the patient's mental status should be performed, as changes signal the development of hepatic encephalopathy. Patients should also be evaluated for intubation, mechanical ventilation, and hemodynamic support at presentation and during the progression of ALF.

INTRACRANIAL HYPERTENSION

Intracranial hypertension (ICH) develops in 20% to 30% of patients with ALF. Hepatic encephalopathy (HE) is considered a precursor to the development of cerebral edema and ICH in these patients. In extreme cases, this can lead to transtentorial herniation, culminating in high mortality rates. The pathophysiology that leads to the development of HE is governed by the interplay between elevated levels, inflammation, and increased cerebral blood flow.[1,3] There is a strong association between elevated ammonia levels and development of ICH, particularly at levels greater than 150 to 200 micromol/L.[1] An acute rise in ammonia levels triggers osmotic shifts, which lead to astrocyte swelling and cerebral edema.

Diagnosis of Hepatic Encephalopathy

Early recognition with serial neurologic examinations is the key to initiating appropriate management of HE and cerebral edema. There are 4 grades of HE, and the grade correlates with development of cerebral edema and prognosis. Grade 1 represents a euphoric state with occasional depression or fluctuation to mild confusion. This state can be identified by an overall slowness in mentation, along with slurred speech. Grade 2 is noted to be an accentuation of grade 1 primarily dominated by drowsiness, inappropriate behavior, with an ability to maintain sphincter control. The hallmark of grade 3 is prolonged periods of sleeping with the ability to be aroused along with incoherent speech and marked confusion. Finally, grade 4 is a state where the patient is unarousable with minimal response to painful stimuli. Identification of the original stage and progression between stages is key to the management of HE and to prevent development of ICH and cerebral edema.[3]

Management of Hepatic Encephalopathy

The management of HE should begin with transfer to the ICU if the patient is on a general medical ward. The patient should undergo a noncontrast CT scan of the head[4] to rule out other causes of alteration in mental status such as intracranial hemorrhage or space-occupying lesion. The administration of sedatives should be avoided in these patients, as they might confound the signs and symptoms of progression of HE. In rare instances, short-acting antipsychotics such as haloperidol are permitted to control extreme agitation.

The treatment of grade 1 and 2 HE focuses on the administration of lactulose, particularly given the active role of ammonia in the pathogenesis of cerebral edema. Small studies have shown an improvement in survival with administration of lactulose; however, no significant change was noted in the severity of encephalopathy or overall outcome.[1] Nonabsorbable antibiotics such as rifaximin are used without any proven improvement in mortality. Of note, neomycin is rarely used in these patients given the high risk of nephrotoxicity.[1]

The progression to grade 3 HE warrants intubation for airway protection and mechanical ventilation. The mechanical ventilation strategies should target prevention of hypercapnia and possibly even aim at hyperventilation in the setting of ICH and cerebral edema. Caution should be exercised while choosing the sedative and muscle relaxant agents for intubation so as to minimize increases in intracranial pressure (ICP); propofol is a reasonable choice along with cisatracurium for neuromuscular blockade.

Monitoring Intracranial Pressures

Invasive and noninvasive neuromonitoring strategies are utilized to examine the progression of cerebral edema. The use of ICP monitoring devices has been steadily decreasing over the past few years. This is primarily related to complications such as intracranial hemorrhage, particularly in patients with grade 3 and 3 hepatic encephalopathy and infection. There is a trend toward increased use of noninvasive strategies such as serial CT head, transcranial Doppler, jugular bulb oximetry, and pupillometry.[1,4] Limitations of serial imaging include need for baseline imaging; however, this is a good modality to rule-out presence of life-threatening bleeding in the setting of worsening coagulopathy and other intracranial processes.

Strategies to Maintain Cerebral Perfusion Pressure

Cerebral perfusion pressure (CPP) is the difference between the mean arterial pressure and the ICP. The primarily goal in patients with cerebral edema is to limit ICP while maintaining adequate CPP. An ICP level greater than 40 mm Hg and CPP less than 50 mm Hg for prolonged periods of time have been associated with poor outcomes in patients with ALF. Multiple neurotherapeutic interventions are available for the management of cerebral edema and ICH.

General measures in reducing ICP involve elevation of the head of the bed to 30° along with avoidance of frequent endotracheal suctioning. Hypoxemia and hypercapnia should be avoided in these patients, as this might lead to elevation in ICP due to increased cerebral blood flow. Propofol remains the preferred sedating agent in these patients due to its rapid onset and offset of action. Opiate infusions can be used as adjunctive sedative agents with a preference for fentanyl over morphine due to fear of accumulation of metabolites in the setting of renal and hepatic dysfunction.

Mannitol

Mannitol has been proven in randomized controlled studies to reduced ICH and improve survival in patients with ALF. Mannitol through its osmotic effect reduces brain water and improves cerebral perfusion, and alkalosis induced by hyperventilation causes cerebral vasoconstriction, which leads to decreased cerebral edema and ICH.[4] No recommendations exist regarding the exact dose, but in most instances doses of 0.25 to 1 g/kg boluses are effective. Contraindications to the use of mannitol include hyperosmolality (Serum osm >320 mOsm/L) or development of acute renal failure. Limited data exist regarding the prophylactic use of mannitol in preventing cerebral edema.

Hypertonic Saline

The presence of hyponatremia can worsen cerebral edema and requires prompt treatment with hypertonic saline. This has particularly been shown to reduce the incidence of severe ICH in patients with grade 3 and 4 encephalopathy. The goal remains maintaining sodium levels between 145 and 155 mEq/L. However, no studies exist that show a survival benefit with the use of hypertonic saline. Other modalities such as barbiturate-induced coma and hypothermia,[1,3] although controversial, are available options in extreme cases.

General Management

In intubated patients, hyperventilation can be utilized to maintain the partial pressure of carbon dioxide between 25 and 30 mm Hg as this causes cerebral vasoconstriction leading to reduction in ICP in patients with cerebral edema. Of note, care should be taken to avoid marked hypocapnia to levels of no more than 25 mm Hg, as this might lead to cerebral ischemia. Maintenance of normothermia is of importance in these patients as fever exacerbates ICH.[5] Commonly used techniques include cooling blankets and fans with limited use of nonsteroidal anti-inflammatory agents and acetaminophen in the setting of renal and hepatic dysfunction.

COAGULOPATHY

Massive hepatocellular injury in ALF leads to significant reduction in procoagulation and anticoagulation factors produced by the liver. This is witnessed by the marked increases in the international normalized ratio (INR) and prothrombin time (PT), which are used to establish a diagnosis of ALF.[1] Thrombocytopenia is not infrequently seen in ALF and is associated with increased incidence of multiorgan failure. In contrast to patients with chronic liver disease, these patients have a significant decrease in factors 2, 5, 7, and 10 and an increase in factor 8, which has been attributed to acute inflammation and increased consumption.[6] Finally, because of the hypercoagulable states, there is a higher incidence of deep vein thrombosis (DVT) in the setting of elevated INR and thrombocytopenia.

Based on current guidelines, there is no role for administration of blood products such as fresh frozen plasma (FFP) to correct coagulation abnormalities in the absence of active bleeding. There has been much debate regarding the use of recombinant factor VIIa to aid in reversal of coagulopathy; however, this is limited by its increased risk of thrombosis.[6]

ACUTE KIDNEY INJURY

In the early stages, development of acute kidney injury (AKI) is attributed to direct injury caused by the agent responsible for ALF, while a later onset typically follows a pattern similar to hepatorenal syndrome (HRS) due to functional impairment. The functional impairment is caused by a complex interplay between extrarenal vasodilation and renal arteriolar vasoconstriction coupled with inadequate cardiac output.[1,7] Early initiation of renal replacement therapy (RRT) has been viewed favorably by many liver transplant centers. Studies comparing CRRT versus intermittent hemodialysis have noted greater variations in hemodynamics, with the latter along with increases in intracranial pressures, thus not recommending intermittent hemodialysis in these patients. A retrospective analysis of 1604 patients in the US Acute Liver Failure Study Group showed that 70% of patients developed AKI, with almost 30% requiring RRT. The development of AKI was associated with increased mortality, with incidence being more common in patients with severe liver dysfunction. However, while AKI affected both short- and long-term outcome it seldom led to the development of chronic kidney disease and dependence on intermittent hemodialysis.[8]

CARDIOVASCULAR AND PULMONARY COMPLICATIONS

The occurrence of hemodynamic derangements including distributive shock is common in ALF, leading to the development of multiorgan failure. With progressive disease, hypotension is encountered due to underlying arterial and peripheral vasodilation along with decreases in systemic vascular resistance (SVR). Initial steps include expanding circulating volume with administration of crystalloid solutions; however, in cases where cerebral edema and ICH are suspected, colloid administration with concentrated albumin solutions is recommended.[1] In patients with ongoing hypotension requiring vasopressor support, norepinephrine is the preferred agent of choice due to lower incidence of tachycardia compared with dopamine.

In patients with refractory hypotension, adrenal insufficiency should be considered, as this occurs in 55% to 60% of patients with ALF. Given the high incidence of adrenal insufficiency, patients benefit from administration of 200 mg/d of hydrocortisone in divided doses.[1]

The incidence of acute lung injury (ALI) has been significantly reduced in patients with ALF owing to stricter critical care and fluid management strategies.[5] In patients with advancing hepatic encephalopathy, airway compromise remains a concern. There is a strong recommendation to consider endotracheal intubation in patients who progress to grade 3 encephalopathy.[4] Given concurrent cerebral edema and ICH, rapid sequence intubation is preferred because of minimal changes in intracranial pressures. Finally, lung-protective ventilation such as low tidal volume ventilation is recommended in patients who are mechanically ventilated.[1]

INFECTIOUS COMPLICATIONS

Patients with ALF are at high risk for bacterial and fungal infections.[5] Common offenders include gram-positive cocci, enteric gram-negative bacilli, and *Candida* species. The presence of disseminated infection is a contraindication of liver transplantation. However, no survival benefit has been demonstrated with the prophylactic use of antimicrobials in patients with ALF. Based on current guidelines, broad-spectrum antibiotics should be considered in patients with grade 3/4 HE and definitely initiated in patients with positive surveillance cultures and refractory hypotension without an identified source of infection.[5] The initial antibiotic regimen should target enteric gram-negatives and anaerobes with addition of vancomycin in patients with catheter-related blood stream infections or methicillin-resistant *Staphylococcus aureus* infection.[9] There remains a low threshold for addition of antifungal coverage in patients with high suspicion for fungal etiology.[1]

GASTROINTESTINAL BLEEDING AND METABOLIC CONCERNS

All patients who are critically ill are at a high risk for gastrointestinal (GI) bleeding, particularly those with ALF. However, compared with patients with ACLF who have a high incidence of variceal bleeding, the bleeding risk in ALF is low. In patients who are mechanically ventilated or with severe hepatic dysfunction, initiation of GI prophylaxis with H2 blockers or proton pump inhibitors is recommended.[2]

Metabolic derangements are commonly seen in patients with ALF and require routine monitoring of acid-base and electrolyte status. The development of acidosis might signal the presence of acute renal failure as a potential cause. Hyperglycemia is a commonly encountered issue due to impaired hepatic gluconeogenesis in ALF. Although hyperglycemia may worsen cerebral edema, efforts should be taken to avoid hypoglycemia.[1]

SUMMARY

The care of the critically ill patient with acute liver failure involves a systematic approach to the management of hepatic and extrahepatic organ system dysfunction. The prompt recognition and management of intracranial hypertension have resulted in improved neurologic outcomes and survival. Although the major focus remains on the recognition and prevention of neurocritical illness, there should remain a high index of suspicion for the development of a systemic inflammatory response and multiorgan dysfunction.

REFERENCES

1. Kandiah P, Olson J, Subramanian RM. Emerging strategies for the treatment of patients with acute hepatic failure. Curr Opin Crit Care 2016;22:142–51.
2. Arroyo V, Moreau R, Jalan R, et al. Acute-on-chronic liver failure: a new syndrome that will re-classify cirrhosis. J Hepatol 2015;62:S131–43.
3. Karvellas CJ, Fix OK, Battenhouse H, et al. Outcomes and complications of intracranial pressure monitoring in acute liver failure: a retrospective cohort study. Crit Care Med 2014;42:1157–67.
4. Ede RJ, Gimson AE, Bihari D, et al. Controlled hyperventilation in the prevention of cerebral oedema in fulminant hepatic failure. J Hepatol 1986;2:43–51.
5. Bernal W, Wendon J. Acute liver failure. N Engl J Med 2014;370:1170–1.
6. Shami VM, Caldwell SH, Hespenheide EE, et al. Recombinant activated factor VII for coagulopathy in fulminant hepatic failure compared with conventional therapy. Liver Transpl 2003;9:138–43.
7. Larsen FS, Schmidt LE, Bernsmeier C, et al. High-volume plasma exchange in patients with acute liver failure: an open randomized controlled trial. J Hepatol 2016; 64:69–78.
8. Tujios SR, Hynan LS, Vazquez MA, et al. Risk factors and outcomes of acute kidney injury in patients with acute liver failure. Clin Gastroenterol Hepatol 2015;13: 352–9.
9. Ford RM, Sakaria SS, Subramanian RM. Critical care management of patients before liver transplantation. Transplant Rev 2010;24:190–206.

Liver Transplantation for Acute Liver Failure

Raquel Olivo, MD[a],*, James V. Guarrera, MD, FACS[b],
Nikolaos T. Pyrsopoulos, MD, PhD, MBA, FACP, AGAF, FAASLD, FRCP (Edin)[a]

KEYWORDS

- Liver transplant • Acute liver failure • Living donor liver transplant

KEY POINTS

- With the advent of liver transplant for acute liver failure (ALF), survival rate has improved drastically. Liver transplant for ALF accounts for 8% of all transplant cases.
- The 1-year survival rates are 79% in Europe and 84% in the United States, which is acceptable considering the emergent nature of the listing process and the severity of illness.
- Some patients with ALF may recover spontaneously, and approximately half will undergo liver transplant.
- It is imperative to identify patients with ALF as soon as possible to transfer them to a liver transplant center for a thorough evaluation that includes a complete socioeconomic assessment.
- Emergent liver transplant in a patient with ALF may place the patient at risk for severe complications in the postoperative period, with longer intensive care unit stays and higher retransplantation rates.

LIVER TRANSPLANTATION IN THE CONTEXT OF ACUTE LIVER FAILURE

ALF as an indication for liver transplantation (LT) was adopted in the 1980s by a consensus of the National Institutes of Health.[1] Currently, ALF accounts for approximately 8% of all liver transplants, as per data from the Scientific Registry of Transplant Recipients (SRTR) and the European Liver Transplant Registry (ELTR).[2,3] In the United Kingdom, 53% of the nonacetaminophen-related cases of ALF are transplanted, versus 40% in the United States. On the other hand, acetaminophen-related cases are transplanted only 35% of the time in the United Kingdom and 8% in the United States, respectively.[4,5] Survival of patients with ALF has significantly improved from 16% to 62% since the introduction of liver transplantation.[2] In the same series, nontransplanted

The authors have nothing to disclose.
[a] Division of Gastroenterology and Hepatology, Department of Medicine, Rutgers New Jersey Medical School, 185 South Orange Avenue, H-532, Newark, NJ 07103, USA; [b] Division of Liver Transplant and Hepatobiliary Surgery, Rutgers New Jersey Medical School, ACC Building, 140 Bergen Street. E- 1766, Newark, NJ 07103, USA
* Corresponding author.
E-mail address: rmo58@njms.rutgers.edu

patients had a survival rate improvement from 17% to 48%.[4] This improvement was most pronounced when the cause of ALF was acetaminophen toxicity, hepatitis B, and drug-induced liver injury (DILI). No significant improvement was reported in etiologies like seronegative hepatitis and in indeterminate causes of ALF.[2,4]

Approximately half of the patients admitted with ALF will receive a liver transplant, worldwide. The 1-year survival rates are 79% in Europe and 84% in the United States.[2,3] These outcomes are somewhat inferior compared with patients receiving a transplant due to chronic liver disease.[6]

ALF survival is similar to patients transplanted with a high MELD and in the intensive care unit (ICU) at the time of transplant.[3]

OPTIMIZATION OF LISTING CRITERIA

Liver transplant is a lifesaving treatment for ALF patients. The general recommendation is to transfer these patients to a facility with a liver transplant program as soon as possible.[7,8] It is imperative to thoroughly evaluate these patients and maximize medical management prior to liver transplant. Prognostic scoring systems may predict which patient will require liver transplantation versus those destined to recover (an approach favored by European Association for the Study). Alternatively, all the patients can be evaluated and listed if they fulfill the criteria for listing at the time of the presentation, an approach that is favored by the American Association for the Study of Liver Diseases, and a clinical reassessment will be performed at the time of the liver availability.[7–10] In any event, the decision to list the patient should be made expediently through a multidisciplinary approach in order to prevent further clinical deterioration that might prohibit listing.

Ethical Issues

Psychosocial assessment of the potential transplant patient is a critical aspect of the transplant evaluation process. For patients with ALF, this may prove challenging, as the patient may have already developed hepatic encephalopathy.

The extenuating circumstances may make the evaluation suboptimal compared with the full psychological assessment performed for patients undergoing nonemergent transplant evaluation. In addition, issues such as adherence, social and family support, and social environment should be discussed with the patient's family, friends, and treating physicians.[11] The etiology of ALF may present additional problems when there is an associated social stigma such as suicide attempt with acetaminophen overdose or hepatitis B transmission in the context of intravenous drug use or sexual transmission.[11,12] In addition, these cases can provide challenges in terms of bioethical principles of justice and beneficence.[12]

Additionally, in ALF cases some centers may tend to overlook traditional contraindications to LT such as alcohol abuse, drug use or suicidal attempt, a practice that is not standardized for all transplant centers. The decision to transplant or defer in this context should be done involving the multidisciplinary transplant team and a thorough documentation of the rationale is warranted.[8] Predicting compliance with posttransplant regimen can be challenging due to suboptimal evaluation,[13] but in these cases there are few alternatives to gather further information or set goals for the patient and caregivers to further assess their adherence capabilities.

Suggested Approach

Given the complex presentation and potential for rapid deterioration of patients, it is essential to have an organized and comprehensive approach in the management of

ALF. Ultimately, the goal is to provide the necessary care, in conjunction with constant reassessment of the patient for a potential liver transplant, and while targeting an optimal timing for transplantation.[14] The patient should be stabilized, and optimization of medical support should be performed.[15]

The patient should be evaluated in a liver transplant center in a multidisciplinary fashion. Evaluation for transplantation should involve a hepatologist, transplant surgeon, cardiologist, neurologist, and infectious disease specialist if warranted, as well as a social worker, transplant coordinators, financial coordinators, and any other required consultant. Financial and social support needs to be established. Candidates who meet all the listing criteria should be placed in the waiting list (**Fig. 1**). If clinical deterioration occurs or if the patient improves significantly, he or she can be delisted.

OPTIMIZING SELECTION FOR TRANSPLANT

In a matter of hours to days, the ALF patient can develop multiorgan failure, precluding transplantation and potentially leading to death. The most common contraindications for liver transplant are listed in **Box 1**.

Special attention should be placed on infectious complications in ALF patients, as they are common, occurring in up to 80% of cases. An infection may worsen the encephalopathy and can preclude transplantation. Infections account for 37% of all mortality causes in ALF patients.[16,17] At least 5% of the infections in ALF patients are fungal. If a fungal infection is confirmed, the patient should be delisted.[2,18] Thus, in patients with ALF, early and effective strategies for prevention and treatment of infections are vital.

It have been reported that approximately 50% of ALF patients may develop acute renal failure, and this has been related to poor prognosis[19] and should trigger critical care management.[14,20,21] Acute renal failure rates among ALF patients are as high as 50%, and these have a direct correlation with a poor prognosis.[22,23]

Neuro checks should be performed often, as subtler changes in mental status are an important marker of poor outcomes. Cerebral edema and herniation are contraindications for liver transplantation.[9]

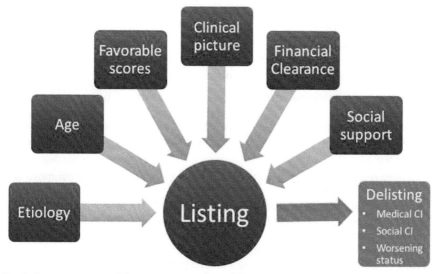

Fig. 1. Factors suggested for assessment of candidacy in ALF.

Box 1
Most common contraindications for liver transplant in acute liver failure

Evidence of brainstem herniation

Confirmed invasive fungal infection

Cardiovascular instability with increase in pressors support

Clinically unstable patient

Inadequate social support

In a series of 1457 patients from the United Network for Organ Sharing (UNOS) database who received liver transplant for ALF, it was found that a body mass index (BMI) greater than 30, serum creatinine greater than 2 mg/dL, recipient age greater than 50 years, and a history of life support were independent factors of poor post-transplant outcomes, with a survival of 47% if a patient met all the variables.[18]

An analysis of the European Liver Transplant Registry (ELTR) identify 5 major risk factors to predict mortality after liver transplant for ALF: male gender, older donor (>60 years old), older recipient (>50 years old), incompatible graft, and reduced graft size. Based on those, the group developed a model that accurately predicted mortality after liver transplant for ALF.[2]

In addition, active malignancy, dengue, and malaria, among others, are contraindications for liver transplant.

Liver Allocation

It has been reported that the mean time between listing and liver transplant is 2 days as per one large US cohort.[24] The way the allocation systems prioritize ALF patients allows most patients to be transplanted approximately 2 to 4 days after being placed on the waiting list as per other study.[6] In the United States, adult ALF is granted status 1A, placing the patient in the highest priority on the waiting list. In order to be listed as status 1A, the ALF patient must be at least 18 years old, with life expectancy of less than 7 days. Additionally, he or she must be in the intensive care unit and meet at least 1 of the following criteria:

- Ventilator dependent
- Requiring renal replacement therapy
- International normalized ratio (INR) greater than 2.0[25]

In the case of decompensated Wilson disease, the patient can be designated status 1A.[25]

In the United Kingdom, the emergency listing of an ALF patient is based on the King's College Hospital (KCH) Criteria, and the patient must be classified in one of 7 categories:

1. Acetaminophen related: pH less than 7.25 more than 24 hours after overdose and after fluid resuscitation
2. Acetaminophen related: severe coagulopathy (INR >6.5) and renal failure (anuria or serum creatinine >300 μmol/L) and grade 3 to 4 encephalopathy
3. Acetaminophen related: serum lactate greater than 3.5 on admission or greater than 3 after adequate fluid resuscitation
4. Acetaminophen related: Any 2 of the 3 criteria from category 2 combined with clinical evidence of deterioration in the absence of sepsis

5. Other etiologies: severe coagulopathy (INR >6.5) and any grade of encephalopathy
6. Other etiologies: 3 from 5 of the following: unfavorable etiology, age greater than 40 years old, jaundice greater than 7 days, serum bilirubin greater than 300 μmol/L, INR greater than 3.5, and any grade of encephalopathy.
7. Wilson disease and Budd-Chiari syndrome: any grade of encephalopathy[26]

The importance of the liver allocation is paramount. Still, of the patients with ALF listed for liver transplant in the United States, 20% succumb waiting for a liver.[27] Similar data are presented in the King's College series, where of 74 listed patients, 52 died waiting for a liver, and 15 became too ill for a transplant.[28]

Living Donor versus Deceased Donor Liver Transplantation

In Europe and United States, the graft supply is predominantly deceased donors. However, the organ availability is obviously an important issue for ALF patients in whom a rapid deterioration can occur; therefore, other alternatives solutions should be considered. In the United States, living donor transplant comprises only 4% of all transplants.[3,29] In general, ALF represents approximately 1% of all indications for living donor transplant in the United States.[30]

This is in contrast with Asia, where organ donation from deceased donors is rare, and they rely mostly on living donors. Oketani reported that 98% of liver transplants in Japan are from living donors, and in fact, only 24% of ALF patients receive a liver transplant.[31] Nevertheless, and despite some concerns in regard to results with living donor transplants, the same group reported overall comparable outcomes to deceased donor transplants, with a survival of 79% and 74% at 1 and 5 years respectively.[31] If the live donor graft is of adequate size and is from an available healthy donor, it is likely to have minimal cold ischemic time and will likely have excellent function.[9]

In regions where scarcity of donors is an issue, living donor liver transplant appears to be a viable option and is the standard of care in Asia.[32] In regions where deceased donors are relatively available, the living donor liver transplant remains somewhat controversial.[33]

There are still some ethical issues that need to be sorted out. First, living donors should only be considered in situations where the risk for the donor is justified by the possibility of recovery of the recipient. The ideal candidate should be a competent adult, willing to donate, free from coercion, medically and psychologically suitable, who has given consent and to whom all of the risks and benefits have been disclosed, including alternatives for both the recipient and the donor.[34] This is of particular importance in ALF, since it has been demonstrated that most of the living donors are close relatives who can be easily influenced by the imminent demise of their loved one.[35] Given the urgency, such decision can lead to the selection of unsuitable donor candidates. The mortality and morbidity for the living donor of a liver have been estimated to be 0.4% and 35%, respectively.[36] Therefore, it is imperative to maintain a clear communication, constantly reassessing the benefits versus the futility of the procedure, and to ensure the safety of the donor.

Special attention should be given in regard to the size of the graft. The use of the right lobe has been recommended to lessen the occurrence of small-for-size syndrome. However, the donation of the right lobe carries a higher rate of donor complications than donating the left lobe.[37,38] In a large survey from Japan involving 209 living donor liver transplants for ALF, it was reported that the right lobe was used in 50% of the cases, and the overall survival rate at 1 and 5 years was 79% and 74%, respectively.[29]

The results from the Adult-to-Adult Living Donor Liver Transplantation Cohort in the United States reported that ALF was the indication for living donor liver transplant in 1% of cases, only 14 patients; of those, 10 patients received living donor liver transplants. The recipient mortality rate was noted to be 30%, and the morbidity of the donors was 50%. The 1-year survival rate was 70%.[30]

POSTOPERATIVE CARE

The context of an emergent surgical procedure in a critically ill patient increases the risk of severe complications in the postoperative period, with longer ICU stays. Often, patients are already experiencing multiorgan failure at the time of the surgery, and marginal grafts are used frequently due to the urgency of the situation.[4] As previously discussed, infections are the most frequent cause of morbidity and mortality in the post-transplant period, which can also lead to graft dysfunction.[2,18] Retransplantation rates are approximately 10% higher in ALF patients due to primary graft nonfunction, severe graft dysfunction, and hepatic artery thrombosis.[39]

OUTCOMES

The 1-year survival rates are 79% in Europe, and 84% in the United States. The same European series reported a survival rate of 72% and 75% at 5 and 10 years, respectively.[2] Another cohort from United States reported survivals rate of 73% at 1 year and 67% at 5 years.[24] Most recently, the Acute Liver Failure Study group reported a survival of 96% at 21 years after transplant, increasing from 88% in a 16-year period.[40] Lee and colleagues[41] reported that the outcomes of liver transplant for ALF and chronic liver disease are comparable.

In general, 1-year survival of transplanted ALF patients is approximately 10% less than patients transplanted for other causes.[2,41] There is also an increase rate of postoperative complications at 3 months after transplant.[2] The most common causes of death in this period are infections (fungal in particular), neurologic complications, and multiorgan failure.[2,18,24]

Various independent risk factors have been associated with increased mortality after liver transplant (**Box 2**). One of the factors with major impact is recipient age. It was found that the mortality doubles in recipients over 50 years of age.[2,18,28,42] Etiology of ALF also plays a significant role, with the best post-transplant outcomes found in Wilson disease, and the worst outcomes are found in cases of DILI, AIH.[28,43]

As expected, patients receiving small, steatotic and ABO-incompatible grafts have inferior outcomes.[2,28] This is particularly important given that in some emergency situations, the quality of the graft can be sacrificed. That approach, however, can carry a high risk; primary nonfunction has been reported in up to 13% of patients in this setting.[24]

Box 2
Factors associated with worse outcomes after liver transplant for acute liver failure

Older patients: greater than 50 years old

Etiology: DILI, AIH

Graft factors: small, steatotic, incompatible grafts

Clinically ill patient before transplant

An important factor that should be not overlooked is the quality of life after transplant. Germani and colleagues[2] published that social issues and noncompliance with immunosuppression were related to death and graft loss as high as 10% in cases of ALF related to acetaminophen overdose.

SUMMARY

Liver transplantation can be the ultimate treatment for ALF. It has been reported that approximately 45% to 50% of ALF cases are transplanted, representing 8% of all liver transplants. Early referral and transplantation have led to an improvement of the overall survival rate to over 80%, which is comparable to a non-ALF liver transplant. It is imperative to remember that that a number of patients will recover with medical treatment. Identification of patients who will benefit from liver transplant is paramount. The context of an emergent surgical procedure in a critically ill patient places the patient at risk of severe complications in the postoperative period with longer ICU stays and with higher retransplantation rates.

REFERENCES

1. National Institutes of Health consensus development conference statement: liver transplantation–June 20-23, 1983. Hepatology 1984;4(1 Suppl):107S–10S.
2. Germani G, Theocharidou E, Adam R, et al. Liver transplantation for acute liver failure in Europe: outcomes over 20 years from the ELTR database. J Hepatol 2012;57(2):288–96.
3. Freeman RB, Steffick DE, Guidinger MK, et al. Liver and intestine transplantation in the United States, 1997-2006. Am J Transplant 2008;8(4 Pt 2):958–76.
4. Bernal W, Hyyrylainen A, Gera A, et al. Lessons from look-back in acute liver failure? A single centre experience of 3300 patients. J Hepatol 2013;59(1): 74–80.
5. Larson AM, Polson J, Fontana RJ, et al. Acetaminophen-induced acute liver failure: results of a United States multicenter, prospective study. Hepatology 2005; 42(6):1364–72.
6. O'Grady J. Timing and benefit of liver transplantation in acute liver failure. J Hepatol 2014;60:663–70.
7. Lee WM, Stravitz RT, Larson AM. Introduction to the revised American Association for the Study of Liver Diseases position paper on acute liver failure. Hepatology 2012.
8. European Association for the Study of the Liver. EASL clinical practical guidelines on the management of acute (fulminant) liver failure. J Hepatol 2017.
9. Akamatsu N, Sugawara Y, Kokudo N. Acute liver failure and liver transplantation. Intractable Rare Dis Res 2013;2(3):77–87.
10. O'Grady J, Hepatologist C. Liver transplantation for acute liver failure. Best Pract Res Clin Gastroenterol 2012;26:27–33.
11. Samuel D, Saliba F, Ichai P. Changing outcomes in acute liver failure: can we transplant only the ones who really need it? Liver Transpl 2015;21:S36–8.
12. Willey JZ, Tolchin BD. Liver transplant for intentional acetaminophen overdose and hepatic encephalopathy. Continuum (Minneap Minn) 2014;20(3 Neurology of Systemic Disease):681–5.
13. Appel J, Vaidya S. Ethical dilemmas in psychiatric evaluations in patients with fulminant liver failure. Curr Opin Organ Transplant 2014;19(2):175–80.
14. Bernal W, Wendon J. Acute liver failure. N Engl J Med 2013;26369(26):2525–34.

15. Lidofsky SD, Bass NM, Prager MC, et al. Intracranial pressure monitoring and liver transplantation for fulminant hepatic failure. Hepatology 1992; 16(1):1–7.

16. Vaquero J, Polson J, Chung C, et al. Infection and the progression of hepatic encephalopathy in acute liver failure. Gastroenterology 2003;125(3):755–64.

17. Rolando N, Philpott-Howard J, Williams R. Bacterial and fungal infection in acute liver failure. Semin Liver Dis 1996;16(4):389–402.

18. Barshes NR, Lee TC, Balkrishnan R, et al. Risk stratification of adult patients undergoing orthotopic liver transplantation for fulminant hepatic failure. Transplantation 2006;81(2):195–201.

19. O'Grady JG, Gimson AE, O'Brien CJ, et al. Controlled trials of charcoal hemoperfusion and prognostic factors in fulminant hepatic failure. Gastroenterology 1988; 94(5 Pt 1):1186–92.

20. Bagshaw SM, Uchino S, Kellum JA, et al. Association between renal replacement therapy in critically ill patients with severe acute kidney injury and mortality. J Crit Care 2013;28(6):1011–8.

21. Rutherford A, King LY, Hynan LS, et al. Development of an accurate index for predicting outcomes of patients with acute liver failure. Gastroenterology 2012; 143(5):1237–43.

22. Jain S, Pendyala P, Varma S, et al. Effect of renal dysfunction in fulminant hepatic failure. Trop Gastroenterol 2000;21(3):118–20.

23. O'Grady JG, Alexander GJ, Hayllar KM, et al. Early indicators of prognosis in fulminant hepatic failure. Gastroenterology 1989;97(2):439–45.

24. Farmer DG, Anselmo DM, Ghobrial RM, et al. Liver transplantation for fulminant hepatic failure: experience with more than 200 patients over a 17-year period. Ann Surg 2003;237(5):666–76.

25. Organ Procurement and Transplantation Network (OPTN). Policies. Available at: https://optn.transplant.hrsa.gov/media/1200/optn_policies.pdf. Accessed January 12, 2018.

26. Zalewska K. POLICY POL195/6 liver transplantation: selection criteria and recipient registration. Available at: http://www.odt.nhs.uk/pdf/non_compliance_with_selection_and_allocation_policies.pdf. Accessed January 12, 2018.

27. Organ Procurement and Transplantation Network and Scientific Registry of Transplant Recipients 2012 Data Report Available at: https://srtr.transplant.hrsa.gov/annual_reports/2012/pdf/03_liver_13.pdf. Accessed January 10, 2018.

28. Bernal W, Cross TJS, Auzinger G, et al. Outcome after wait-listing for emergency liver transplantation in acute liver failure: a single centre experience. J Hepatol 2009;50(2):306–13.

29. Yamashiki N, Sugawara Y, Tamura S, et al. Outcomes after living donor liver transplantation for acute liver failure in Japan: results of a nationwide survey. Liver Transpl 2012;18(9):1069–77.

30. Campsen J, Blei AT, Emond JC, et al. Outcomes of living donor liver transplantation for acute liver failure: the adult-to-adult living donor liver transplantation cohort study. Liver Transpl 2008;14(9):1273–80.

31. Oketani M, Ido A, Nakayama N, et al. Etiology and prognosis of fulminant hepatitis and late-onset hepatic failure in Japan: summary of the annual nationwide survey between 2004 and 2009. Hepatol Res 2013;43(2):97–105.

32. Kato T, Nery JR, Morcos JJ, et al. Successful living related liver transplantation in an adult with fulminant hepatic failure. Transplantation 1997;64(3):415–7.

33. Carlisle EM, Angelos P, Siegler M, et al. Adult living-related liver donation for acute liver failure: is it ethically appropriate? Clin Transplant 2011;25(6):813–20.

34. Wright L, Faith K, Richardson R, et al, Joint Centre for Bioethics, University of Toronto, Toronto, Ont. Ethical guidelines for the evaluation of living organ donors. Can J Surg 2004;47(6):408–13.

35. Marcos A, Ham JM, Fisher RA, et al. Emergency adult to adult living donor liver transplantation for fulminant hepatic failure. Transplantation 2000;69(10):2202–5.

36. Barr ML, Belghiti J, Villamil FG, et al. A report of the Vancouver Forum on the care of the live organ donor: lung, liver, pancreas, and intestine data and medical guidelines. Transplantation 2006;81(10):1373–85.

37. Shin M, Song S, Kim JM, et al. Donor morbidity including biliary complications in living-donor liver transplantation: single-center analysis of 827 cases. Transplantation 2012;93(9):942–8.

38. Ghobrial RM, Freise CE, Trotter JF, et al. Donor morbidity after living donation for liver transplantation. Gastroenterology 2008;135(2):468–76.

39. Marudanayagam R, Shanmugam V, Sandhu B, et al. Liver retransplantation in adults: a single-centre, 25-year experience. HPB (Oxford) 2010;12(3):217–24.

40. Fontana RJ, Ellerbe C, Durkalski VE, et al. Two-year outcomes in initial survivors with acute liver failure: results from a prospective, multicentre study. Liver Int 2015;35(2):370–80.

41. Lee WM, Squires RH, Nyberg SL, et al. Acute liver failure: summary of a workshop. Hepatology 2007;47(4):1401–15.

42. Wigg AJ, Gunson BK, Mutimer DJ. Outcomes following liver transplantation for seronegative acute liver failure: experience during a 12-year period with more than 100 patients. Liver Transpl 2005;11(1):27–34.

43. Brandsaeter B, Höckerstedt K, Friman S, et al. Fulminant hepatic failure: outcome after listing for highly urgent liver transplantation-12 years experience in the Nordic countries. Liver Transpl 2002;8(11):1055–62.

Future Approaches and Therapeutic Modalities for Acute Liver Failure

Pavan Patel, MD, Nneoma Okoronkwo, MD,
Nikolaos T. Pyrsopoulos, MD, PhD, MBA, FACP, AGAF, FAASLD, FRCP (Edin)*

KEYWORDS

- Liver assist device • Hepatocyte transplant • Stem cell transplant • ELAD
- HepatAssist • MARS • Organogenesis • Acute liver failure

KEY POINTS

- Currently available hepatic assist devices have limited studies in acute liver failure.
- Hepatocyte transplantation for acute liver failure is a promising new approach for the treatment of acute liver failure.
- The translation of mouse model stem cell transplant to humans for acute liver failure is promising but needs further research.

INTRODUCTION

Patients with acute liver failure (ALF) are usually given high priority on transplantation waiting lists. Nevertheless, because of organ shortages and the duration of the disease, many of these patients die while waiting for a transplant. Additional factors, such as psychosocial barriers and comorbid conditions, preclude these patients from transplant.

Therefore, other treatment modalities that may reduce morbidity and mortality and perhaps serve as a bridge to transplantation might be an additional option. One particular avenue that has been investigated are the hepatic assist devices. Such devices aim to temporarily assume metabolic and excretory functions of the liver and thereby allow stabilization of patients who await transplant. These devices may be categorized as biological, artificial, or bioartificial systems.[1–4]

Biological systems use whole organ perfusion (human or animal) or hepatocyte bioreactors. These devices aim to assist prominent hepatic functions. On the other hand,

Disclosure Statement: The authors have nothing to disclose.
Division of Gastroenterology and Hepatology, Rutgers New Jersey Medical School, 185 South Orange Avenue, MSB H-538, Newark, NJ 07103, USA
* Corresponding author.
E-mail address: pyrsopni@njms.rutgers.edu

artificial systems aim to detoxify via dialysis-based techniques. Bioartificial or hybrid devices combine both biological and nonbiological techniques.[2–5]

An artificial device for ALF that has been studied is the Molecular Adsorbent Recirculating System (MARS) assist device. Two bioartificial devices that use hepatocytes contained within a matrix of hollow fiber membranes include the Extracorporeal Liver Assist Device (ELAD; Vital Therapies Inc, San Diego, CA) and the HepatAssist system (Alliqua Inc, Langhorne, PA).[6]

MOLECULAR ADSORBENT RECIRCULATING SYSTEM

MARS is based on the concept of albumin dialysis and allows the removal of protein-bound as well as water-soluble toxins.[7] Albumin-bound substances can be dialyzed through a regular dialysis membrane if the dialysate contains clean albumin as a molecular acceptor. MARS was first developed in Germany in 1993 and was first commercialized and available for clinical use in 1998.[8]

Molecular Adsorbent Recirculating System Components

It comprises a modified hemodialysis with a high flux membrane permitting passage of hydrophobic, albumin-bound target substances, and an albumin-enriched dialysate. This albumin-dialysate is online regenerated by passage through a second dialyzer and 2 adsorber columns.[7] This process can be seen in **Fig. 1**.

MARS has been studied in ALF, acute on chronic liver failure, hepatic encephalopathy grade greater than II, increased intracranial pressure, acute hypoxic

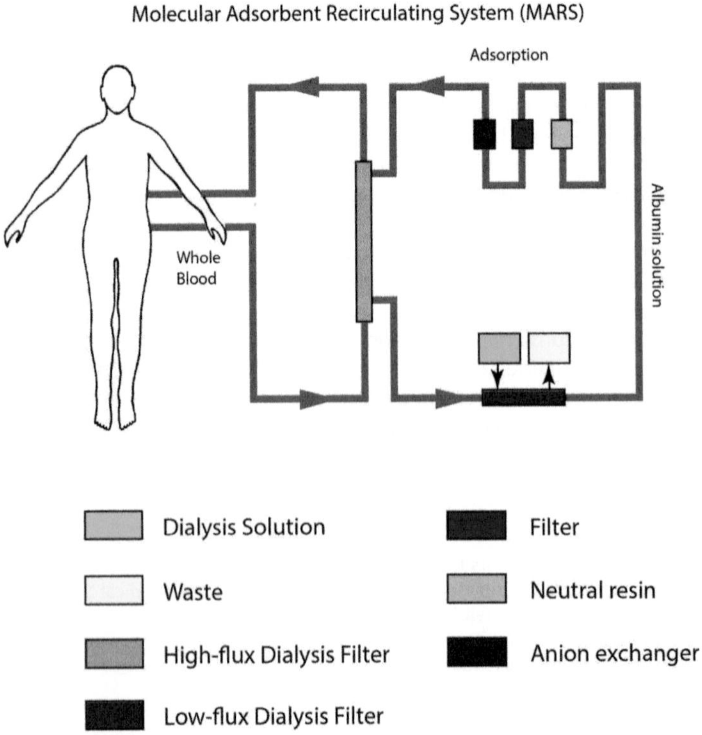
Molecular Adsorbent Recirculating System (MARS)
Adsorption
Albumin solution
Whole Blood
Dialysis Solution
Waste
High-flux Dialysis Filter
Low-flux Dialysis Filter
Filter
Neutral resin
Anion exchanger

Fig. 1. MARS diagram.

hepatitis with bilirubin greater than 8 mg/dL, hepatorenal syndrome, progressive intrahepatic cholestasis, and graft dysfunction after liver transplant.[9,10] In 2005, the Federal Drug Administration (FDA) approved MARS use for the management of drug overdose and poisoning if the drug or poison can be dialyzed (in unbound form) and bound by activated charcoal and/or anionic exchange resins.[11] In December 2012, the FDA also approved MARS for use in the treatment of hepatic encephalopathy due to decompensated of chronic liver disease.[11] MARS has not been approved by the FDA as a bridge to liver transplant, as its safety and efficacy have not been demonstrated as a bridge to transplant in controlled randomized trials. Its effectiveness in patients who are sedated could not be established in clinical studies.[11]

The risks of treatment are similar to known risks of conventional hemodialysis; but the risk of bleeding is increased, as coagulopathy disorders are common in patients with end-stage liver disease.[12] MARS has also been noted to lead to a further decrease in platelet count and fibrinogen.[13] More randomized controlled trials are needed with specific indications for treatment to gain optimal and widespread use.

EXTRACORPOREAL LIVER ASSIST DEVICE

The ELAD is a bioartificial liver assist device. Cartridges containing hollow fibers filled with human hepatoblastoma cell lines, C3A, are used in this device. These cells have hepatocyte properties, such as a functional CYP450 enzyme system and the production of liver-specific proteins. It uses whole blood for perfusion and can be continued for long periods of time.[14]

Extracorporeal Circuit

The system is connected in a closed circuit via venous access gained by placement of a double-lumen dialysis catheter in either the internal jugular or femoral vein. Four ELAD cartridges are used in this circuit to give a hepatocyte mass of 400 g. Patients' blood is ultrafiltrated to isolated plasma ultrafiltrate. This plasma is then pumped through these cartridges via a standard dialysis pump at a rate of 150 to 200 mL/min. Anticoagulation is achieved using heparin with an initial bolus and then continuous infusion to achieve an activated clotting time of 200 to 250 seconds. An oxygenator is used to ensure adequate oxygen supply to the cells. Negative pressure is applied across the membranes to achieve an ultrafiltrate before being returned to patients.[15,16] A schematic representation can be seen in **Fig. 2**.

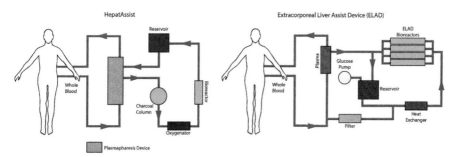

Fig. 2. Artificial Liver Assist Devices.

Studies

The pilot ELAD study enrolled 24 patients with ALF, 17 of whom had been considered to have potentially recoverable disease (group 1) and 7 who had been listed for transplant (group 2). Each of these subsets were then randomly assigned to ELAD versus control. In patients treated with ELAD, ammonia, bilirubin, and hepatic encephalopathy were improved when compared with standard medical treatment. There was no survival benefit in either group (survival rates were 78% and 75% in group 1% and 33% and 25% in group 2) for patients treated with and without ELAD, respectively.[16]

In a follow-up study in which ultrafiltrate was used instead of whole blood, Millis and colleagues[15] studied 5 patients with ALF who were bridged to transplant using ELAD. The 30-day survival rate was 75%. Other parameters that showed improvement included mean arterial pressures, cerebral perfusion pressures, and a reduction in cardiovascular and ventilator support. Additional studies investigating this population are needed.

HEPATASSIST

HepatAssist is made from porcine hepatocytes that are contained within a hollow fiber bioreactor.[17] It uses plasma that is obtained via plasmapheresis and then passed through the circuit containing porcine hepatocytes.

Extracorporeal Circuit

The system includes a perfusion pump, a charcoal column, a combined oxygenator/blood warmer, and custom tubing that connects the various components to a plasmapheresis machine.[18] During its use, plasmapheresis is performed via a double-lumen catheter. The plasma is pumped into the HepatAssist device and continuously circulates the plasma through the hollow fiber reactor. The plasma flows through the fibers that are surrounded by the porcine hepatocytes. The pore size is small enough to prevent cell debris from passing into patients.[17] This process can be seen in **Fig. 2**.

Studies

The largest, randomized, multicenter trial involving HepatAssist involved 171 patients with ALF or primary nonfunction after liver transplantation. The 30-day survival was 71% versus 62% ($P = .26$) for the HepatAssist group compared with standard medical therapy, respectively. Survival in the subgroup of patients with fulminant or subfulminant hepatic failure was significantly higher in the HepatAssist group compared with control ($P = .048$). Serum bilirubin had a statistically significant reduction in patients receiving HepatAssist; however, there were no changes in encephalopathy, hemodynamics, or other laboratory values. No zoonosis or immune reactions were reported, though this still remains a concern.[17]

PLASMA EXCHANGE

Plasma exchange involves exchanging 8 to 12 L of plasma from patients with fresh plasma per day. The benefits of exchange include removal of toxins and repletion of factors synthesized by the liver.[19]

A prospective multicenter clinical trial that randomized patients to plasma exchange plus standard medical therapy versus standard medical therapy for ALF of any cause was done. The causes of liver failure were acetaminophen (54% in treatment group vs 64% in control group) and toxic hepatitis (23% in treatment group vs 18% in control group). The overall survival was 58.7% in the treatment arm versus 47.8% in the standard medical therapy group (hazard ratio 0.56; 95% confidence interval, 0.36–0.86, P = .0083). The treatment group also had a decrease in international normalized ratio (INR), bilirubin, ammonia, and systemic inflammatory response syndrome.[20] Results should be interpreted cautiously, as plasma exchange can decrease bilirubin and INR in and of itself.[21]

LIMITATIONS

Three major systematic reviews and meta-analyses on the impact of liver support systems have been done. These reviews suggest that artificial liver support systems reduce mortality in acute-on-chronic liver failure compared with standard medical care, although these systems do not affect mortality in patients with ALF.[22,23] Detoxification of blood may be insufficient, and there is lack of cells that address more complicated metabolic pathways. Clinically, bioartificial liver support systems lack an ideal, reliable, and safe human cell source.[24] Human hepatoblastoma cells, such as the ones used in ELAD, are limited by their metabolic function; there is a theoretic risk of metastatic cell spreading by broken fibers, though this is prevented by the use of valves and membranes.[24] However, porcine hepatocytes, such as the ones used in HepatAssist, can be immunogenic and there is a risk of xenozoonoses.[25]

Furthermore, bioartificial liver support systems have a major technical limitation owing to the membranes that are used. They only allow flow rates of 100 to 200 mL/min, which is well less than those of in vivo perfusion, which is closer to 1500 mL/min. This limitation limits mass exchange and perhaps prompt overall detoxification.[26] Because of these limitations, other strategies are being evaluated that may meet more physiologic functions of the liver. These strategies include cell transplantation and bioengineering, such as organ printing and induced organogenesis.[24]

HEPATOCYTE TRANSPLANTATION

Hepatocyte transplantation is the infusion of hepatocytes that are isolated from donor organs into the porto-venous system.[27] These hepatocytes then translocate into the hepatic sinusoids and integrate into the recipient liver.[28,29] The native liver serves as a scaffolding matrix whereby infused hepatocytes can perform liver functions.[30,31]

Hepatocyte transplantation can, therefore, overcome 2 limiting problems encountered with the previously mentioned liver support systems. First, cells are part of the native liver matrix and, therefore, interact in a more physiologic manner compared with external bioreactors. Second, multiple hepatocytes can be harvested from one donor organ, which tackles the problem of donor shortages.[24]

Only small studies evaluating the efficacy of hepatocyte transplantation have been done.[31] The most promising results have been in patients with inborn metabolic liver disease, such as Crigler-Najjar syndrome type 1. In patients with this disease who have undergone hepatocyte transplantation, there has been a decrease in bilirubin of 25% to 50%, though the effect decreased over time. Whole liver transplantation was necessary in all 8 cases because of hepatocyte graft failure.[32–34]

In contrast, hepatocyte transplantation in ALF has not shown great results.[35] This finding may be partly because, in ALF, the number of hepatocytes that need to be transplanted are not sufficient for liver recompensation. There is a clinical trial underway that is currently investigating hepatocyte transplantation as a bridge to orthotopic liver transplantation during ALF.[36]

REPOPULATION OF DECELLULARIZED ORGANS

A common barrier for keeping hepatocytes metabolically active outside of their natural environment is nutrient and oxygen supply. One approach that has been studied is decellularization and recellularization of solid organs. The process of decellularization involves removal of immunogenic molecules and cells from the tissue or organ to leave an extracellular matrix. This matrix preserves the complex 3-dimensional anatomy of the organ and also includes its vascular and biliary framework.[37] The matrix is also similar across species and, therefore, less likely to be immunogenic.[38] Therefore, it can be obtained from porcine livers on a more rapid scale. The obtained matrix can be repopulated with stem cells from patients on the waiting list for transplant. After the cells mature in a bioreactor and assemble a solid organ, it can be implanted into the host without the need for lifelong immunosuppressive therapy.[39]

In vivo studies using recellularized rat livers have been done. Most have shown improvement in life span, but a limited factor is thrombogenesis.[40–42] Some studies have also looked at recellularization of ferret and porcine liver with human cells.[37,43] The limiting factor at this point seems to be reconstruction of the vascular integrity of the liver and prevention of thrombosis.[24]

STEM CELL TRANSPLANT

The use of stem cells seems to be a promising approach that will lead to donor cell–mediated rapid production of hepatocytes and improved survival rates. The use of such cells has been shown in experimental models.[44]

The main cells that have been used in clinical or experimental studies for cell transplantation are mature hepatocytes, stem/progenitor cells (embryonic stem cells, adipose-derived stem cells, umbilical stem cells, bone marrow–derived stem cells, and oval cells), and hepatocytelike cells.[44] Hepatocytes are favorable because of their high function; but limitations lie with their short survival time, large diameter leading to entrapment in hepatic sinusoids causing obstruction and portal hypertension, as well as poor engraftment rate.[45,46] Stem/progenitor type cells have high proliferative capacity but have overall weak function.[46] Clinical studies done with transplanted mature hepatocytes have shown evidence of biochemical improvement in liver injury as well as reduction in ammonia levels.[47]

However, there are still certain limitations in the use of stem cells, such as ethical concerns, long-term efficacy and safety, and the ability to obtain an adequate amount of suitable cell sources. These limitations pose challenges before stem cells can be routinely used in humans.[48]

Although most of the clinical trials in stem cell transplantation are limited because of the small sample size, there seems to be promising results; cell transplantation therapies could be one of the optimal choices for treatment of ALF or end-stage liver disease in the future.[44]

INDUCED ORGANOGENESIS

Induced organogenesis is a new frontier of implantable organs and may be a future therapy for ALF. In a study in mice, human-induced pluripotent stem cells were differentiated into endodermal cells and cultured with human mesenchymal stem cells in vitro.[49] These cells self-organized into a vascularized hepatic precursor and were implanted into immune-deficient mice. Only 48 hours after implantation the in vitro liver organoid was integrated into the vascular system of the mice. Down the line the cells matured into functional tissue and were able to rescue mice with drug-induced liver failure. This study shows encouraging results that may provide an avenue to further research and perhaps lead to new advances in liver support therapies.

SUMMARY

Although orthotopic liver transplantation is the gold standard therapy for treating ALF, there have been dramatic advances in liver support strategies to cope with the shortage in available donor organs. As outlined earlier, both biological and nonbiological liver support systems have been developed. The published results point toward the need for new trials with improvements in the system. The obvious limitations of these support systems are the membranes used for appropriate exchange and the lack of complete physiologic function.

In addition, new approaches, such as hepatocyte transplantation, repopulation of decellularized livers, organogenesis, and stem cell transplant, seem to be appealing. Further research is needed in order to increase survival of this difficult-to-manage population.

REFERENCES

1. Rahman TM, Hodgson HJ. Review article: liver support systems in acute hepatic failure. Aliment Pharmacol Ther 1999;13(10):1255–72.
2. Riordan SM, Williams R. Extracorporeal support and hepatocyte transplantation in acute liver failure and cirrhosis. J Gastroenterol Hepatol 1999;14(8):757–70.
3. Allen JW, Hassanein T, Bhatia SN. Advances in bioartificial liver devices. Hepatology 2001;34(3):447–55.
4. Keeffe EB. Liver transplantation: current status and novel approaches to liver replacement. Gastroenterology 2001;120(3):749–62.
5. Stockmann HB, Hiemstra CA, Marquet RL, et al. Extracorporeal perfusion for the treatment of acute liver failure. Ann Surg 2000;231(4):460–70. Available at: http://www.pubmedcentral.nih.gov/articlerender.fcgi?artid=1421020&tool=pmcentrez&rendertype=abstract.
6. Jauregui HO, Gann KL. Mammalian hepatocytes as a foundation for treatment in human liver failure. J Cell Biochem 1991;45(4):359–65.
7. Mitzner SR. Extracorporeal liver support-albumin dialysis with the molecular adsorbent recirculating system (MARS). Ann Hepatol 2011;10(SUPPL. 1):S21–8.
8. Kobashi-Margáin RA, Gavilanes-Espinar JG, Gutiérrez-Grobe Y, et al. Albumin dialysis with molecular adsorbent recirculating system (MARS) for the treatment of hepatic encephalopathy in liver failure. Ann Hepatol 2011;10(SUPPL. 2):S70–6.
9. Mitzner SR, Stange J, Klammt S, et al. Extracorporeal detoxification using the molecular adsorbent recirculating system for critically ill patients with liver failure. J Am Soc Nephrol 2001;12(Suppl 17):S75–82.
10. Laleman W, Wilmer A, Evenepoel P, et al. Effect of the molecular adsorbent recirculating system and Prometheus devices on systemic haemodynamics and vasoactive agents in patients with acute-on-chronic alcoholic liver failure. Crit Care 2006;10(4):R108.
11. FDA Website. FDA. 2012. Available at: https://www.accessdata.fda.gov/cdrh_docs/pdf11/K113313.pdf. Accessed December 20, 2017.
12. Saliba F. The Molecular Adsorbent Recirculating System (MARS) in the intensive care unit: a rescue therapy for patients with hepatic failure. Crit Care 2006;10(1):118.

13. Faybik P, Bacher A, Kozek-Langenecker SA, et al. Molecular adsorbent recirculating system and hemostasis in patients at high risk of bleeding: an observational study. Crit Care 2006;10(1):R24.

14. Gislason GT, Lobdell DD, Kelly JH, et al. A treatment system for implementing an extracorporeal liver assist device. Artif Organs 1994;18(5):385–9.

15. Millis JM, Cronin DC, Johnson R, et al. Initial experience with the modified extracorporeal liver-assist device for patients with fulminant hepatic failure: system modifications and clinical impact. Transplantation 2002;74(12):1735–46.

16. Ellis AJ, Hughes RD, Wendon JA, et al. Pilot-controlled trial of the extracorporeal liver assist device in acute liver failure. Hepatology 1996;24(6):1446–51.

17. Demetriou AA, Brown RS, Busuttil RW, et al. Prospective, randomized, multicenter, controlled trial of a bioartificial liver in treating acute liver failure. Ann Surg 2004;239(5):660–70.

18. Watanabe FD, Mullon CJ, Hewitt WR, et al. Clinical experience with a bioartificial liver in the treatment of severe liver failure. A phase I clinical trial. Ann Surg 1997; 225(5):484–91 [discussion: 491–4].

19. Lee W, Squires R, Nyberg S. Acute liver failure: summary of a workshop. Hepatology 2008;47(4):1401–15.

20. Larsen FS, Schmidt LE, Bernsmeier C, et al. High-volume plasma exchange in patients with acute liver failure: an open randomised controlled trial. J Hepatol 2016;64(1):69–78.

21. Karvellas CJ, Stravitz RT. High volume plasma exchange in acute liver failure: dampening the inflammatory cascade? J Hepatol 2016;64(1):10–2.

22. Liu JP, Gluud LL, Als-Nielsen B, et al. Artificial and bioartificial support systems for liver failure. Cochrane Database Syst Rev 2004;(1):CD003628.

23. Kjaergard LL, Liu J, Als-Nielsen B, et al. Artificial and bioartificial support systems for acute and acute-on-chronic liver failure a systematic review. Jama 2003; 289(2):217–22.

24. Struecker B, Raschzok N, Sauer IM. Liver support strategies: cutting-edge technologies. Nat Rev Gastroenterol Hepatol 2013;11(3):166–76.

25. Sauer IM, Kardassis D, Zeillinger K, et al. Clinical extracorporeal hybrid liver support–phase I study with primary porcine liver cells. Xenotransplantation 2003;10:460–9.

26. Iwata H, Ueda Y. Pharmacokinetic considerations in development of a bioartificial liver. Clin Pharmacokinet 2004;43(4):211–25.

27. Dhawan A, Strom SC, Sokal E, et al. Human hepatocyte transplantation. Methods Mol Biol 2010;640:525–34.

28. Gupta S, Rajvanshi P, Sokhi R, et al. Entry and integration of transplanted hepatocytes in rat liver plates occur by disruption of hepatic sinusoidal endothelium. Hepatology 1999;29(2):509–19.

29. Laconi E, Oren R, Mukhopadhyay DK, et al. Long-term, near-total liver replacement by transplantation of isolated hepatocytes in rats treated with retrorsine. Am J Pathol 1998;153(1):319–29.

30. Hughes RD, Mitry RR, Dhawan A. Current status of hepatocyte transplantation. Transplantation 2012;93(4):342–7.

31. Jorns C, Ellis EC, Nowak G, et al. Hepatocyte transplantation for inherited metabolic diseases of the liver. J Intern Med 2012;272(3):201–23.

32. Lysy PA, Najimi M, Stéphenne X, et al. Liver cell transplantation for Crigler-Najjar syndrome type I: update and perspectives. World J Gastroenterol 2008;14(22): 3464–70.

33. Fox IJ, Chowdhury JR, Kaufman SS, et al. Treatment of the Crigler–Najjar syndrome type I with hepatocyte transplantation. N Engl J Med 1998;338:1422–7.
34. Ambrosino G, Varotto S, Strom SC, et al. Isolated hepatocyte transplantation for Crigler-Najjar syndrome type 1. Cell Transpl 2005;14(2–3):151–7.
35. Dhawan A, Puppi J, Hughes RD, et al. Human hepatocyte transplantation: current experience and future challenges. Nat Rev Gastroenterol Hepatol 2010;7(5): 288–98.
36. Hepatocyte transplantation for acute decompensated liver failure - ClinicalTrials. gov. 2011. Available at: https://www.clinicaltrials.gov/ct2/show/NCT01345565. Accessed December 20, 2017.
37. Baptista PM, Siddiqui MM, Lozier G, et al. The use of whole organ decellularization for the generation of a vascularized liver organoid. Hepatology 2011;53(2): 604–17.
38. Bernard MP, Myers JC, Chu ML, et al. Structure of a cDNA for the Proα2 chain of human type I procollagen. Comparison with Chick cDNA for Proα2(I) identifies structurally conserved features of the protein and the gene. Biochemistry 1983; 22(5):1139–45.
39. Badylak SF, Weiss DJ, Caplan A, et al. Engineered whole organs and complex tissues. Lancet 2012;379(9819):943–52.
40. Bao J, Shi Y, Sun H, et al. Construction of a portal implantable functional tissue-engineered liver using perfusion-decellularized matrix and hepatocytes in rats. Cell Transpl 2011;20(5):753–66.
41. Soto-Gutierrez A, Zhang L, Medberry C, et al. A whole-organ regenerative medicine approach for liver replacement. Tissue Eng C Methods 2011;17(6):677–86.
42. Uygun BE, Soto-Gutierrez A, Yagi H, et al. Organ reengineering through development of a transplantable recellularized liver graft using decellularized liver matrix. Nat Med 2010;16(7):814–20.
43. Barakat O, Abbasi S, Rodriguez G, et al. Use of decellularized porcine liver for engineering humanized liver organ. J Surg Res 2012;173(1):e11–25.
44. Esrefoglu M. Role of stem cells in repair of liver injury: experimental and clinical benefit of transferred stem cells on liver failure. World J Gastroenterol 2013; 19(40):6757–73.
45. Weber A, Groyer-Picard MT, Franco D, et al. Hepatocyte transplantation in animal models. Liver Transpl 2009;15(1):7–14.
46. Zhang W, Tucker-Kellogg L, Narmada BC, et al. Cell-delivery therapeutics for liver regeneration. Adv Drug Deliv Rev 2010;62(7–8):814–26.
47. Strom SC, Fisher RA, Thompson MT, et al. Hepatocyte transplantation as a bridge to orthotopic liver transplantation in terminal liver failure. Transplantation 1997; 63(4):559–69.
48. Yu Y, Wang X, Nyberg S. Potential and challenges of induced pluripotent stem cells in liver diseases treatment. J Clin Med 2014;3:997–1017.
49. Takebe T, Zhang R-R, Koike H, et al. Generation of a vascularized and functional human liver from an iPSC-derived organ bud transplant. Nat Protoc 2014;9(2): 396–409.

Moving?

Make sure your subscription moves with you!

To notify us of your new address, find your **Clinics Account Number** (located on your mailing label above your name), and contact customer service at:

Email: journalscustomerservice-usa@elsevier.com

800-654-2452 (subscribers in the U.S. & Canada)
314-447-8871 (subscribers outside of the U.S. & Canada)

Fax number: 314-447-8029

Elsevier Health Sciences Division
Subscription Customer Service
3251 Riverport Lane
Maryland Heights, MO 63043

*To ensure uninterrupted delivery of your subscription, please notify us at least 4 weeks in advance of move.

Printed and bound by CPI Group (UK) Ltd, Croydon, CR0 4YY

07/10/2024

01040500-0002